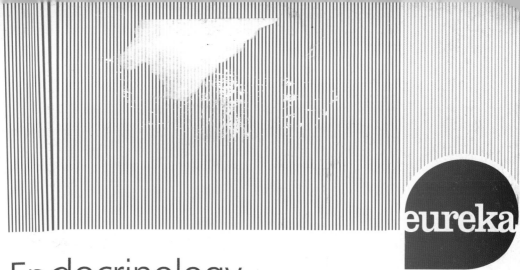

eureka

Endocrinology

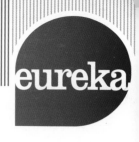

Endocrinology

Thomas Fox MBBS BSc MRCP (Endo) PGCert Med Ed
Consultant Endocrinologist
The Royal Devon and Exeter NHS Foundation Trust
Exeter, UK

Antonia Brooke MBBS MD MA MRCP
Consultant Endocrinologist
The Royal Devon and Exeter NHS Foundation Trust
Exeter, UK

Bijay Vaidya MBBS PhD FRCP (Lon & Edin)
Consultant Endocrinologist
The Royal Devon and Exeter NHS Foundation Trust
Exeter, UK

Series Editors

Janine Henderson MRCPsych MClinEd
MB BS Programme Director
Hull York Medical School
York, UK

David Oliveira PhD FRCP
Professor of Renal Medicine
St George's, University of London
London, UK

Stephen Parker BSc MS DipMedEd FRCS
Consultant Breast and General Paediatric Surgeon
St Mary's Hospital
Newport, UK

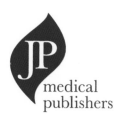

JP
medical
publishers

London • Philadelphia • New Delhi • Panama City

ISBN: 978-1-907816-71-0

British Library Cataloguing in Publication Data
A catalogue record for this book is available from the British Library

Library of Congress Cataloging in Publication Data
A catalog record for this book is available from the Library of Congress

Publisher:	Richard Furn
Development Editors:	Thomas Fletcher, Paul Mayhew, Alison Whitehouse
Editorial Assistants:	Sophie Woolven, Katie Pattullo
Copy Editor:	Kim Howell
Graphic narratives:	James Pollitt
Cover design:	Forbes Design
Page design:	Designers Collective Ltd

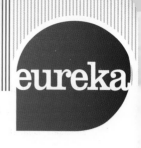

Series Editors' Foreword

Today's medical students need to know a great deal to be effective as tomorrow's doctors. This knowledge includes core science and clinical skills, from understanding biochemical pathways to communicating with patients. Modern medical school curricula integrate this teaching, thereby emphasising how learning in one area can support and reinforce another. At the same time students must acquire sound clinical reasoning skills, working with complex information to understand each individual's unique medical problems.

The *Eureka* series is designed to cover all aspects of today's medical curricula and reinforce this integrated approach. Each book can be used from first year through to qualification. Core biomedical principles are introduced but given relevant clinical context: the authors have always asked themselves, 'why does the aspiring clinician need to know this'?

Each clinical title in the series is grounded in the relevant core science, which is introduced at the start of each book. Each core science title integrates and emphasises clinical relevance throughout. Medical and surgical approaches are included to provide a complete and integrated view of the patient management options available to the clinician. Clinical insights highlight key facts and principles drawn from medical practice. Cases featuring unique graphic narratives are presented with clear explanations that show how experienced clinicians think, enabling students to develop their own clinical reasoning and decision making. Clinical SBAs help with exam revision while starter questions are a unique learning tool designed to stimulate interest in the subject.

Having biomedical principles and clinical applications together in one book will make their connections more explicit and easier to remember. Alongside repeated exposure to patients and practice of clinical and communication skills, we hope *Eureka* will equip medical students for a lifetime of successful clinical practice.

Janine Henderson, David Oliveira, Stephen Parker

About the Series Editors

Janine Henderson is the MB BS undergraduate Programme Director at Hull York Medical School (HYMS). After medical school at the University of Oxford and clinical training in psychiatry, she combined her work as a consultant with postgraduate teaching roles, moving to the new Hull York Medical School in 2004. She has a particular interest in modern educational methods, curriculum design and clinical reasoning.

David Oliveira is Professor of Renal Medicine at St George's, University of London (SGUL), where he served as the MBBS Course Director between 2007 and 2013. Having trained at Cambridge University and the Westminster Hospital he obtained a PhD in cellular immunology and worked as a renal physician before being appointed as Foundation Chair of Renal Medicine at SGUL.

Stephen Parker is a Consultant Breast and General Paediatric Surgeon at St Mary's Hospital, Isle of Wight. He trained at St George's, University of London, and after service in the Royal Navy was appointed as Consultant Surgeon at University Hospital Coventry. He has a particular interest in e-learning and the use of multimedia platforms in medical education.

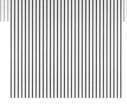

Preface

Endocrine disorders are common and becoming more prevalent, not just in the United Kingdom but worldwide. The complications of endocrine disease cause significant morbidity and mortality, so a sound understanding of their diagnosis and management is of vital importance to all clinicians. Our goal in writing *Eureka Endocrinology* is to set out this knowledge in the clearest manner possible.

The endocrine system is integral to the functioning of the human body. Chapter 1 of *Eureka Endocrinology* therefore provides the reader with a detailed overview of normal endocrine anatomy and physiology. Throughout the chapter, we have included correlating clinical information to help students understand the relevance of the anatomy, physiology and pathology to everyday practice.

In chapter 2 we explain how to take a history and examine the patient, exploring and illustrating key symptoms and clinical signs, before discussing the most important investigations and management options. In the subsequent chapters each endocrine disease is described in depth, using illustrated cases to give the student a unique insight into how patients present and how we manage their medical problems in real life.

The starter questions at the beginning of each chapter will help students consolidate and apply their learning, and the clinical SBAs at the end of the book will provide them with an invaluable revision aid.

We hope you enjoy reading and learning from *Eureka Endocrinology*.

Thomas Fox, Antonia Brooke, Bijay Vaidya
March 2015

About the Authors

Thomas Fox is lead for curriculum development in endocrinology at the University of Exeter Medical School (UEMS). He has played an active role in teaching endocrinology and clinical skills at UEMS both during specialist training and as a Consultant Endocrinologist. He delivers a special study module in metabolic medicine.

Antonia Brooke is the clinical lead for endocrinology at the Royal Devon and Exeter Hospital. She is Endocrinology Training Programme Director for the South West Peninsula, supporting registrars as they work towards becoming consultants. In her role as tutor for undergraduates and junior doctors she enjoys encouraging students into a career in endocrinology.

Bijay Vaidya is a Consultant Physician and Honorary Associate Professor of Endocrinology. As well as playing an active role in teaching endocrinology at UEMS, he has co-authored clinical reviews and learning modules on endocrine disorders for several journals, including *The BMJ* and *BMJ Learning*.

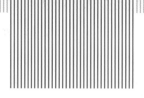

Contents

Chapter 7 Adrenal disease

Chapter 8 Calcium homeostasis and metabolic bone disease

Chapter 9 Reproductive system disorders

Chapter 10 Other endocrine disorders

Chapter 11 Endocrine emergencies

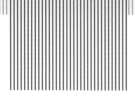

Glossary

ABPI	ankle–brachial pressure index	LDL	low-density lipoprotein
ACE	angiotensin-converting enzyme	LH	luteinising hormone
ACTH	adrenocorticotrophic hormone		
ANCA	antineutrophil cytoplasmic antibody	MEN	multiple endocrine neoplasia
		MIBG	meta-iodobenzylguanidine
BMI	body mass index	MIT	monoiodotyrosine
		MRI	magnetic resonance imaging
cAMP	cyclic adenosine monophosphate	MSH	melanocyte-stimulating hormone
CRH	corticotrophin-releasing hormone		
CT	computerised tomography	PCOS	polycystic ovary syndrome
		PET	positron emission tomography
DEXA	dual-energy X-ray absorptiometry	PKA	protein kinase A
DHEA	dehydroepiandrosterone	POMC	pro-opiomelanocortin
DIT	di-iodotyrosine	PPAR-γ	peroxisome proliferator-activated receptor-γ
ECG	electrocardiogram		
		RDA	recommended daily amount
FSH	follicle-stimulating hormone		
		SIADH	syndrome of inappropriate antidiuretic hormone
GH	growth hormone		
GHRH	growth hormone-releasing hormone	T_3	tri-iodothyronine
GnRH	gonadotrophin-releasing hormone	T_4	thyroxine
GP	general practitioner	TRH	thyrotrophin-releasing hormone
GTP	guanosine triphosphate	tRNA	transfer RNA
		TSH	thyroid-stimulating hormone
HbA1c	haemoglobin A1c		
HDL	high-density lipoprotein	UKPDS	UK Prospective Diabetes Study
HLA	human leukocyte antigen		
5-HIAA	5-hydroxyindole acetic acid	VEGF	vascular endothelial growth factor
		VIP	vasoactive intestinal polypeptide
IGF	insulin-like growth factor	VLDL	very-low-density lipoprotein

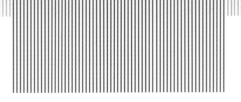

Acknowledgements

Thanks to the following medical students for their help reviewing chapters: Jessica Dunlop, Aliza Imam, Roxanne McVittie, Daniel Roberts and Joseph Suich.

Thanks to Nidhi Choudhary for her help preparing chapters.

Figure 2.35a–b is reproduced from Pachl M, et al. *Key Clinical Topics in Paediatric Surgery.* London: JP Medical, 2014.

The following figures are copyright of the Royal Devon & Exeter NHS Foundation Trust: 2.2, 2.7, 2.8a–b, 2.10, 2.11, 2.12, 2.13, 2.14, 2.15, 2.17, 2.18a, 2.19, 2.20, 2.22, 2.26, 2.29, 2.31a–b, 2.32a–b, 3.1, 3.3, 3.5, 3.6, 3.7, 3.9, 4.1a–b, 4.3, 4.5, 4.6, 4.7, 4.8, 4.9, 4.10a–b, 4.11, 4.12, 4.13, 5.2a–c, 5.3a–d, 5.4a–b, 5.5a–b, 5.7, 5.8a–b, 5.9a–b, 5.10b, 5.11, 6.3, 6.5a–b, 6.8, 7.1a–b, 7.2a–b, 7.4a–b, 8.1, 8.3a–b, 9.2, 10.1, 10.3 and 11.3a–b.

We would like to thank our families for all their support and encouragement during the process of writing *Eureka Endocrinology.*

TF, AB, BV

Chapter 1
First principles

Starter questions

Answers to the following questions are on page 63.

1. Do hormone levels change as we age?
2. Why does menstruation stop during extreme stress?
3. Do we all have the same hormone levels?

Overview of the endocrine system

The endocrine system consists of several anatomically and physiologically distinct glands. Each of these glands is a group of specialised cells that synthesise, store and secrete hormones.

Hormones are chemical messengers that travel in the bloodstream from an endocrine gland to another organ or group of organs to regulate a wide range of physiological processes. Hormones:

- stimulate or inhibit growth
- regulate metabolism by maintaining and mobilising energy stores
- promote sleep or wakefulness
- activate or suppress the immune system
- prepare the body for 'fight or flight' in response to acute stress

- produce the changes associated with puberty and reproduction
- affect mood and behaviour

Hormones also have a role in maintaining homeostasis, a state of physiological equilibrium achieved by adjusting the body's internal environment in response to changes in the external environment.

In contrast to the rapid effects of the nervous system, endocrine effects are usually slow to develop and produce a prolonged response lasting from minutes to weeks.

The human body produces many hormones for regulation of a myriad of physiological processes. New hormones continue to be discovered, and research is ongoing to explain their functions and how they interact to control the human body.

Not all hormones are essential to life.
If untreated, cortisol deficiency arising
from destruction of the adrenal cortex
by an autoimmune disease quickly leads
to severe deterioration in health and
eventually death. However, deficiency of
female sex hormones from autoimmune
destruction of the ovaries increases
morbidity but not mortality.

Endocrine glands

Endocrine glands release their products,
hormones, into the blood. They have a rich
blood supply to ensure efficient transport of
hormones around the body.

The following are the major endocrine
glands (**Figure 1.1**).

- Hypothalamus: as the main endocrine
  control centre, this tiny gland in the brain
  secretes many hormones that directly
  affect hormone production by other
  endocrine glands
- Pituitary gland: this is connected to the
  hypothalamus and produces a wide

range of hormones controlling growth,
metabolism and sexual development
- Pineal gland: this gland in the brain
  controls wakefulness
- Thyroid gland: this gland produces thyroid
  hormones, which set the body's metabolic
  rate, and calcitonin, which regulates
  calcium metabolism
- Parathyroid glands: these produce
  parathyroid hormone, which controls the
  absorption and excretion of calcium and
  phosphate
- Thymus gland: secretes thymosin, a
  hormone that stimulate the production of
  immune T cells
- Adrenal glands: these secrete many
  hormones that mediate the body's response
  to physiological and psychological stress,
  maintain fluid and electrolyte balance, and
  modulate blood pressure
- Pancreas: the endocrine cells of
  the pancreas release insulin and
  glucagon, which regulate blood glucose
  concentration
- Reproductive glands: these glands,
  the testes in males and the ovaries in
  females, produce sex hormones, which

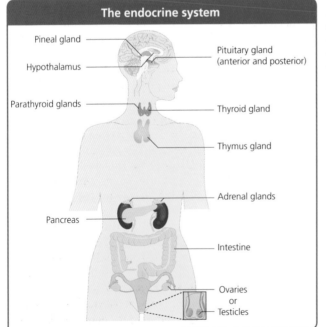

The endocrine system

Pineal gland

Hypothalamus

Pituitary gland
(anterior and posterior)

Parathyroid glands

Thyroid gland

Thymus gland

Adrenal glands

Pancreas

Intestine

Ovaries
or
Testicles

Figure 1.1 The major glands
of the endocrine system are
the hypothalamus, the pituitary
glands, the pineal gland, the
thyroid and parathyroid glands,
the thymus gland, the adrenal
glands, the pancreas and the
reproductive glands (the testes
and ovaries). The intestine also
produces and secretes hormones
as part of its function.

facilitate sexual maturation and enable reproduction

Although not major endocrine glands, the following organs produce and secrete hormones as part of their primary function.

- Intestine: several hormones are secreted from the gut to help control blood glucose concentration and growth
- Adipose tissue: hormones produced by body fat affect appetite and the feeling of fullness (satiety)

Other organs, such as the liver, kidney, heart and skin, have secondary endocrine functions unrelated to their primary function. For example, the main function of the liver is to metabolise carbohydrate, fat and protein. However, it also has secondary endocrine functions, such as producing the hormone insulin-like growth factor-1, which promotes the growth of body tissues.

An endocrine gland may produce more than one hormone, for example the thyroid gland produces thyroid hormones and calcitonin. This means that a single endocrine gland can help control multiple body functions.

Chemical classification of hormones

Hormones are grouped into three chemical classes (**Table 1.1**):

- peptides
- amines
- lipids (mainly steroids)

Peptide hormones

The hormones in this class are chains of amino acids (polypeptides). These chains range in length. They may be short and comprise only a few amino acids (e.g. antidiuretic hormone), or they may be very long molecules (e.g. follicle-stimulating hormone, FSH). Peptide hormones have a large molecular weight.

Amine hormones

Amine hormones are derived from aromatic amino acids such as tryptophan, phenylalanine and tyrosine. Aromatic amino acids have an aromatic side chain, i.e. one containing a stable, planar unsaturated ring of atoms.

Lipid hormones

Hormones in this class are derived from cholesterol and are either alcohols or ketones.

- Alcohol lipid hormones have names ending in '-ol' (e.g. oestradiol)
- Ketone lipid hormones have names ending in '-one' (e.g. aldosterone)

Hormonal signalling pathway

Hormonal signalling pathway involves hormone synthesis, storage (peptide and amine hormones only), release from endocrine cells, transport, receptor binding, release of the hormone or its breakdown products from the cells of the target organ, further transport and excretion (**Figure 1.2**).

1. Synthesis: the hormone is produced by cells in the endocrine gland
2. Storage: peptide and amine hormones are stored in preparation for rapid release when required (lipid hormones are not stored before release)
3. Release from endocrine cells: the hormone is released from the gland into the bloodstream
4. Transport: the hormone travels in the blood to the target organ either unbound, i.e. in a free state (peptide hormones and all amine hormones except thyroid hormone) or bound to transport proteins (lipid hormones and thyroid hormone)
5. Receptor binding: the hormone binds to specific receptor molecules either on the

Types of hormones		
Peptide	Amine	Lipid
Insulin	Thyroxine	Oestrogen
Parathyroid hormone	Adrenaline (epinephrine)	Testosterone
Growth hormone	Melatonin	Cortisol
Prolactin	Dopamine	

Table 1.1 Examples of different types of hormones

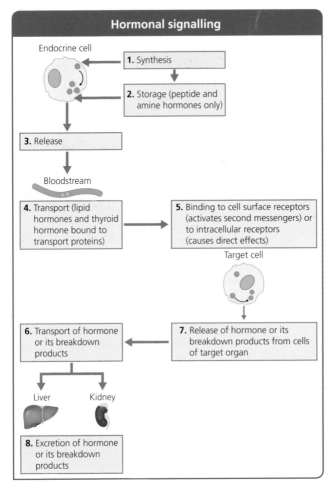

Figure 1.2 Hormonal signalling: from production to metabolism.

membrane of the cells of the target organ or inside these cells

- A hormone binding to receptor molecules on the cell membrane changes the cell's metabolism through a cascade of reactions involving various 2nd messenger chemicals
- Intracellular binding of a hormone to nuclear or cytoplasmic receptors directly affects the expression of genes in the cell

6. Release from the cells of the target organ
   - The cells secrete the hormone unchanged
   - Alternatively, the cells metabolise the hormone to an inactive form
7. Further transport: the hormone or its breakdown products travel in the bloodstream to the liver or kidneys
8. Excretion: the hormone or its breakdown are excreted by the liver (in bile) or the kidneys (in urine)

Hormone synthesis and storage

Endocrine cells synthesise peptide and amine hormones from amino acids, and lipid hormones from cholesterol.

Peptide hormones

Hormones in this class are synthesised as precursor molecules. These prohormones undergo processing in the intracellular endoplasmic reticulum and Golgi apparatus. In the Golgi apparatus, the processed peptide hormones are packaged into secretory granules. They are stored in high concentration in these granules, ready for stimulated release from the endocrine cells into the bloodstream.

Amine hormones

These hormones are synthesised from aromatic amino acids. These amino acids are chemically altered by enzymes in the cells of endocrine glands to synthesise specific hormones. For example, in cells of the adrenal medulla, adrenaline (epinephrine) is synthesised from the amino acid tyrosine. Various enzymes catalyse the steps in adrenaline production; the final step is the conversion of noradrenaline (norepinephrine) to adrenaline by the enzyme phenylethanolamine-*N*-methyltransferase. Like peptide hormones, amine hormones are stored in secretory granules.

Lipid hormones

These are synthesised from cholesterol. The cholesterol is metabolised by enzymes in the cells of an endocrine gland to produce lipid hormones that are either alcohols or ketones.

The onset of action of lipid hormones is slower than that of amine hormones. Therefore, unlike amine and peptide hormones, lipid hormones are not stored in secretory granules for rapid release. Instead, they are synthesised as required, with the rate of synthesis directly determining blood concentration.

Hormone release

When an endocrine cell is activated, secretory granules (containing peptide or amine hormones) move to the cell surface. Here, the vesicular membranes of the granules fuse with the plasma membrane of the cell surface to release their contents to the exterior of the cell. This process is called exocytosis, which literally means 'out of cell'.

Membrane transport of lipid hormones (such as testosterone) occurs in a passive manner across the cell membrane due to the non-polarised nature of the lipid-rich cell membrane. This form of hormone secretion depends upon the difference in concentration of the hormone in the intracellular space (high) to equalise with the hormone concentration in the extracellular space (low) by random motion of molecules (Brownian motion).

Hormone transport

Peptide hormones are able to travel unbound (free) in the bloodstream, because they are hydrophilic ('water loving'). Amine hormones are also hydrophilic and also able to travel unbound in the blood. The hydrophobic thyroid hormones are the exception.

Peptide and amine hormones, other than thyroid hormones, are able to pass through capillary membranes to reach their target cells.

Lipid hormones are hydrophobic ('water hating'), so they must be bound to transport proteins in plasma to enable them to travel in the bloodstream. Lipid hormones undergo continuous and spontaneous binding and unbinding from their carrier molecules. Because lipid hormones are bound to transport proteins, they have a longer half-life (the time taken for half of the hormone molecules to be excreted or metabolised) than amine hormones, which are transported unbound.

Only a small fraction of lipid hormones present in the bloodstream are in an unbound state. For example, 99% of cortisol in the blood is bound to proteins; the unbound remainder, the free cortisol, is biologically active. This is true of all lipid hormones.

Hormone receptor binding

Hormones travel through the bloodstream and thus come into contact with many cell types. However, a cellular response is initiated only in cells with the specific receptors for a hormone. These receptors may be on the cell membrane or in the cytoplasm.

Multiple types of cell may have receptors for a particular hormone. This allows a hormone, for example thyroxine (T_4), to bind to receptors in the cells of many different tissues and thus have widespread effects on metabolism throughout the body.

The effects of a hormone binding to a receptor in one type of cell will differ from those of the same hormone binding to a receptor on another type of cell due to differing downstream processes associated with each receptor. For example, when adrenaline (epinephrine) binds to β adrenergic receptors in cardiac myocytes, it causes the heart muscle to contract more forcefully; however, the same hormone causes muscle relaxation when it binds to β receptors in the bronchioles.

> **Genetic mutations of hormone receptors can lead to a failure of hormonal signalling.** For example, Laron's syndrome is caused by a mutation in the gene for the growth hormone receptor. This mutation disables the receptor and thus renders growth hormone inactive. Consequently, people with this autosomal recessive congenital disorder have a short stature.

Peptide hormone receptors

Peptide hormones are lipophobic ('lipid hating'), so they are unable to diffuse freely through the cell membrane, which consists of two layers of lipid molecules. Therefore peptide hormone receptors composed of transmembrane proteins are necessary to communicate the hormonal message from outside the cell to the target molecules inside the cell.

The peptide hormone receptor is part of a signal transduction system (**Figure 1.3**). In this system, the hormone acts as the 1st messenger by binding to its receptor on the extracellular surface of the cell. This hormone–receptor binding activates 2nd messengers such as cyclic AMP (cAMP), which relay the signal within the cell.

1. The peptide hormone binds to its specific cell surface receptor
2. Hormone binding activates a coupled G-protein (G-proteins are a class of protein present in cell membranes and that transmit signals from hormones binding extracellularly)
3. The G-protein converts guanosine diphosphate to guanosine triphosphate
4. Guanosine triphosphate binds to and thus activates the enzyme adenylate cyclase
5. Adenylate cyclase catalyses the conversion of ATP to cAMP
6. The cAMP activates protein kinase A

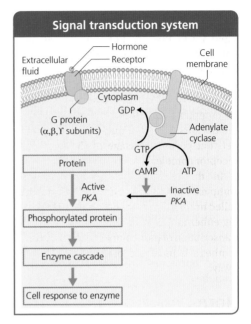

Signal transduction system

Figure 1.3 The signal transduction system activated by binding of a hormone to its receptor. cAMP, cyclic AMP; GDP, guanosine diphosphate; GTP, guanosine triphosphate; PKA, protein kinase A.

7. Now activated, protein kinase A is able to phosphorylate (add a phosphate molecule to) various cell proteins, altering their structure and function and thus producing a cellular response to hormone binding at the cell surface
8. An enzyme called phosphodiesterase breaks down cAMP, thereby inactivating it

Amine hormone receptors

Most amine hormones, for example adrenaline (epinephrine) and dopamine, are lipophobic. Therefore, like peptide hormones, they are unable to diffuse through the cell membrane and instead must bind to cell surface receptors and activate 2nd messenger systems to induce a cellular response.

Thyroxine is an exception. This amine hormone is lipophilic, so it can diffuse through the cell membrane and directly modify gene transcription in the nucleus by binding to intracellular nuclear receptors in the same way as lipid hormones.

Lipid hormone receptors

Lipid hormones are lipid-soluble, so they can diffuse freely through the cell membrane. Once in the target cell, they bind with their receptors, which are in the cytoplasm (**Figure 1.4**). The combined hormone–receptor complex then diffuses across the nuclear membrane through a nuclear pore (a channel that permits passage of the hormone–receptor complex).

In the nucleus, the hormone–receptor complex binds to specific DNA sequences called hormone response elements. This binding either amplifies or suppresses the rate of transcription of particular genes; thus, protein synthesis is increased or decreased, respectively.

Hormone degradation and clearance

The blood concentration of a hormone is affected by the speed of its production and the speed of its clearance. Circulating hormone in the blood can be cleared in several ways.

1. The hormone binds to its receptor temporarily removing it from the circulation
2. The tissues metabolise the hormone to its inactive form

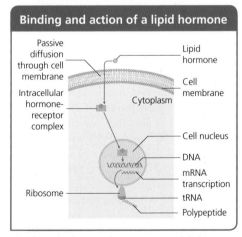

Binding and action of a lipid hormone

Passive diffusion through cell membrane
Lipid hormone
Intracellular hormone-receptor complex
Cytoplasm
Cell membrane
Cell nucleus
DNA
mRNA transcription
tRNA
Ribosome
Polypeptide

Figure 1.4 Intracellular binding and action of a lipid hormone. mRNA, messenger; RNA tRNA, transfer RNA.

3. The hormone is excreted
   ■ by the liver into the bile
   ■ by the kidneys into the urine

Hormonal regulation

All endocrine glands have precise control mechanisms to ensure appropriate hormonal secretion. Production of each hormone is altered in response to the internal and external environment; external factors include temperature, and internal factors include blood glucose concentration.

Hormones maintain a state of optimum chemical balance in which the body can function as efficiently as possible; they also enable the body to respond appropriately to illness. For example, cortisol production is increased in times of illness, to induce physiological changes that help the body to respond to the effects of the stress from the illness. However, at the same time, the production of sex hormones is decreased to reduce fertility (as reproduction is not the survival priority at that point in time).

Feedback loops

All hormone production is controlled by feedback loops. These can be negative or positive.

Negative feedback loops

Most hormonal regulation occurs through negative feedback mechanisms, through which the effects of a hormone inhibit its secretion. Thus negative feedback helps maintain homeostasis by ensuring the controlled release of hormones. Under- or overproduction of a hormone, or abnormalities in its control mechanisms, can disturb the homeostatic balance.

An example of an endocrine negative feedback loop is the hypothalamic–pituitary–adrenal axis (**Figure 1.5**). The hypothalamus secretes corticotrophin-releasing hormone (CRH), which stimulates the anterior pituitary gland to secrete adrenocorticotrophic hormone (ACTH; also known as corticotrophin). In turn, ACTH stimulates the adrenal cortex to secrete glucocorticoids, including cortisol.

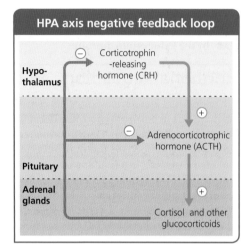

Figure 1.5 The negative feedback loop of the hypothalamic–pituitary–adrenal axis.

Glucocorticoids not only perform their respective functions throughout the body but also bind to receptors in the hypothalamus and the pituitary gland to inhibit the production of CRH and ACTH, respectively. These effects reduce the stimulus to the adrenal gland to produce cortisol and other glucocorticoids.

Positive feedback loops

In positive feedback, a hormone's effects stimulate its secretion. An example occurs in the female reproductive cycle. When luteinising hormone causes a surge in the production of oestrogen by the ovary, the released oestrogen stimulates the anterior pituitary gland to produce more luteinising hormone. This positive feedback mechanism results in the luteinising hormone surge that stimulates ovulation.

> **Without negative feedback, hormone production could become excessive and lead to endocrine disorders.** An example would be Cushing's disease, in which pituitary ACTH secretion is not inhibited by excessive cortisol.

The thyroid gland

Starter questions

The answer to the following question is on page 63.

4. Why is an adequate intake of iodine essential during pregnancy?

The thyroid gland is a bilobed (two-lobed) endocrine gland in the neck.

- The main role of the thyroid gland is secretion of thyroid hormones, which have effects on a wide variety of cells in the body; thyroid hormones help control the rate of metabolism
- The gland's secondary role is secretion of calcitonin, which plays a part in the regulation of calcium concentration in the blood

Embryology

The thyroid is the first endocrine gland to develop in utero. It originates from endoderm.

Endoderm is the innermost of the three embryological cell layers; the other two are the mesoderm (the middle layer) and the ectoderm (the outer layer).

On day 24 of gestation, the thyroid gland arises from the floor of the embryological pharynx. This site is known as the foramen caecum, and is a depression at the junction of the anterior two thirds and the posterior third of the tongue. From this depression, the thyroglossal duct invaginates (folds back into itself to form a pouch) and then descends within the neck, anterior to the pharynx (**Figure 1.6**).

If the thyroid gland fails to descend, it can remain in the base of the tongue. This results in a lingual thyroid gland, which is present

Descent of the thyroid gland

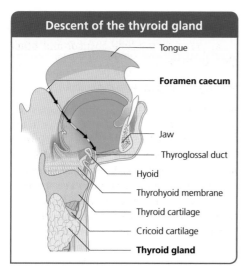

Figure 1.6 Embryological descent of the thyroid gland from its origin the foramen caecum passing down the thyroglossal duct.

Thyroid and parathyroid glands

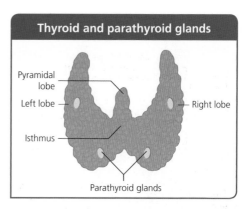

Figure 1.7 Anatomy of the thyroid and parathyroid glands (posterior view).

in 1 in 100,000 to 1 in 300,000 people. Conversely, the thyroid may descend beyond its normal anatomical position into the superior mediastinum, resulting in a retrosternal goitre.

> Thyroglossal cysts arise from remnants of the thyroglossal duct that remain at any point along its path of descent. These cysts are found in the midline of the neck, usually closely related and often attached to the hyoid bone. The results of one autopsy study showed a prevalence of 15%. However, most thyroglossal cysts are asymptomatic.

Figure 1.7 shows the structure of the thyroid gland. The distal end of the thyroglossal duct becomes bilobed to form the lateral lobes of the thyroid gland. The distal remnant of the duct may persist and become the pyramid al lobe of the thyroid gland.

> In the 1st trimester, the fetus does not have a functioning thyroid. Therefore it relies on T_4 from its mother's blood, which crosses the placenta into the fetal circulation. Untreated maternal hypothyroidism causes fetal hypothyroidism, which may result in abnormalities in fetal development.

The ultimobranchial bodies

Pharyngeal pouches are folds that appear in the anterolateral part of the foregut during early embryological development. They form cartilage, nerve, muscle and arterial tissues. Ultimobranchial bodies arise from the 4th pharyngeal pouch and become affixed to the lateral border of each thyroid lobe.

The cells of the ultimobranchial bodies originate from the neural crest, which consists of embryological cells from the ectoderm that differentiate into nerves, muscles and some endocrine glands (e.g. the adrenal medulla). Some of these cells attach to the thyroid gland and eventually become the calcitonin-secreting parafollicular C cells of the thyroid gland.

Anatomy

The thyroid is a highly vascular, butterfly-shaped gland in the anterior lower neck, in front of the trachea and larynx (**Figure 1.8**). It extends from the level of the 5th cervical vertebra down to the 1st thoracic vertebra. The thyroid gland weighs 25–30 g and is formed by two lateral lobes, each comprising a superior pole and an inferior pole. The two lobes are connected by the median isthmus, which is at the level of the 2nd to 4th tracheal ring. The gland is surrounded by a thin, two-layer sheath of fibrous tissue called the capsule.

Relation of thyroid to trachea

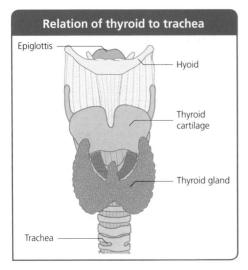

Figure 1.8 The thyroid gland in relation to the trachea (anterior view).

Posterior but separate to the thyroid are the four parathyroid glands (**Figure 1.7**) and the carotid sheath. The carotid sheath is a fibrous layer that envelops the carotid arteries, the internal jugular veins and the recurrent laryngeal nerves.

> The location of masses in the neck can provide clues to their nature. Masses in the midline are probably embryological abnormalities of thyroglossal duct, such as thyroglossal cysts. Thyroglossal cysts can be detected clinically; they elevate on protrusion of the tongue.

Vascular supply

The thyroid gland is highly vascular, with a rich arterial supply and venous drainage into the inferior jugular vein. This permits rapid transport of thyroid hormones throughout the body.

Arteries

The thyroid gland has a rich arterial supply, with four or five arteries (**Figure 1.9**).

- Two superior thyroid arteries arising from the external carotid arteries on each side supply the upper pole of each lobe
- Two inferior thyroid arteries arising from the thyrocervical trunk of the subclavian artery supply the lower pole of each lobe
- The thyroid ima artery, which is present in < 10% of people, arises inferiorly from the arch of the aorta, the brachiocephalic or inferior mammary arteries

Veins

Venous drainage is through:

- the superior thyroid vein, which drains into the internal jugular vein
- the middle thyroid vein, which drains into the internal jugular vein
- the inferior thyroid vein, which drains into the brachiocephalic vein

Lymphatics

Lymphatic vessels in the thyroid gland drain into the deep cervical nodes. These are the

Vasculature of the thyroid gland

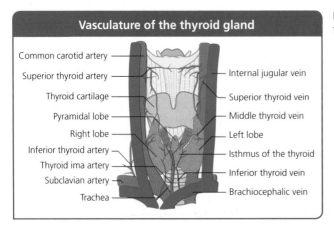

Figure 1.9 Vasculature of the thyroid gland.

periglandular, prelaryngeal, pretracheal and paratracheal lymph nodes.

> **In cases of thyroidectomy for advanced thyroid cancer,** the local lymph nodes are sometimes removed as well as the thyroid gland (depending upon the histological type and extent of the thyroid cancer). Removal of the lymph nodes reduces the risk of recurrence.

Innervation

The thyroid is supplied by autonomic nerves. Both sympathetic and parasympathetic fibres have been postulated to affect blood flow in the gland and thus have a secondary role in thyroid hormone secretion.

The autonomic nerves enter the thyroid gland alongside its blood vessels.

- Sympathetic innervation is provided by the superior, middle and inferior cervical ganglia
- Parasympathetic innervation is provided by branches of the vagus nerve

Histology

The functional unit of the thyroid gland is the thyroid follicle (**Figure 1.10**). Each follicle measures about 0.1 mm in diameter and comprises a layer of simple epithelium enclosing a cavity filled with colloid (a protein-rich fluid). The colloid contains a glycoprotein called thyroglobulin, which is a precursor of thyroid hormones. Thus the colloid serves as a reservoir for the materials needed for thyroid hormone production.

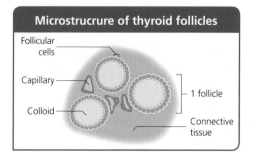

Microstrucrure of thyroid follicles

Follicular cells

Capillary

Colloid

1 follicle

Connective tissue

Figure 1.10 Microstructure of thyroid follicles.

The follicular epithelial cells:

- produce thyroglobulin
- convert thyroglobulin into the thyroid hormones (thyroxine, T_4, and tri-iodothyronine, T_3)
- secrete thyroid hormones into the surrounding capillary bed

The spaces between the thyroid follicles are filled with:

- fibroblasts (cells that produce fibrin)
- lymphocytes (immune cells)
- C cells (these produce the hormone calcitonin, which maintains calcium homeostasis)

Physiology

The primary function of the thyroid gland is to produce the hormones T_3, T_4 and calcitonin.

- T_3 and T_4 act on most cells of the body to promote carbohydrate, protein and lipid metabolism; they increase basal metabolic rate and oxygen consumption, and regulate tissue growth and development
- Calcitonin reduces serum calcium concentration by opposing the action of parathyroid hormone

Thyroglobulin

Thyroglobulin is a large glycoprotein molecule, i.e. a combination of carbohydrate and protein. It is synthesised in the follicular cells of the thyroid gland, and stored in the colloid of thyroid follicles.

Numerous tyrosine amino acids are attached to each thyroglobulin molecule. While attached, these amino acids are iodinated in the production of T_4 (**Figure 1.11**).

Thyroid hormones

The thyroid hormones (T_3 and T_4) have many actions on most cells of the body (**Table 1.2**). They affect metabolism, growth and development, and the cardiovascular, nervous and reproductive systems, and thus determine mental and physical alertness.

The two thyroid hormones differ in their effects (**Table 1.3**):

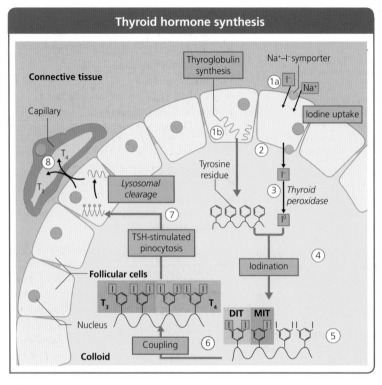

Figure 1.11 The synthesis of thyroid hormones. (1a) Iodide ion moves into the follicular cell via the iodine-sodium co-transporter. (1b) Synthesis of thyroglobulin in the follicular cells. (2) Iodide ion passes into the colloid (3) Iodide is converted to iodine by the enzyme thyroid peroxidase (4) Iodination of 3' and 5' terminals of the benzene ring of the tyrosine residues on the thyroglobulin molecule. (5) Iodination produces mono-iodotyrosine (MIT; T_1) and di-iodotyrosine (DIT; T_2). (6) Combination of MIT and DIT produces tri-iodothyronine (T_3) and combination of DIT and DIT produces thyroxine (T_4), both stored in the colloid bound to thyroglobulin. (7) Stimulation by TSH leads to cleavage of the T3 and T4 hormone from thyroglobulin and uptake into the follicular cells. (8) Release of T_3 and T_4 into systemic circulation.

Actions of thyroid hormones	
Category	Effect(s)
Metabolism	Increase basal metabolic rate and heat production
	Increase lipolysis
	Increase cellular uptake of triglycerides and cholesterol
	Increase gluconeogenesis, glycogenolysis and insulin-dependent glucose uptake
Development	Essential to fetal and neonatal brain development
Cardiovascular system	Increase heart rate, cardiac contractility and cardiac output
	Increase peripheral vasodilation
Central nervous system	Increase alertness
Reproductive system	Essential for normal reproductive function

Table 1.2 Actions of thyroid hormones

- T_3 is the active form
- T_4 is a prohormone and needs to be converted to T_3 before it can exert its effects

The synthesis of thyroid hormones relies on iodination of the amino acid tyrosine. This process, the addition of an iodide ion, is made possible by the enzyme thyroid peroxidase.

Iodine trapping

This is the process by which iodine is accumulated in the thyroid gland for the production of thyroid hormones. Iodine is a rare element, so the thyroid gland has evolved to maintain a large store of it for use in times of deficiency. Iodine, in the form of the iodide ion (I^-) present in blood, is pumped into the follicular cells by the iodide and sodium cotransporter. Thus the iodide passes into the colloid, where the enzyme thyroid peroxidase oxidises it to its active form, iodine.

Comparison of T_3 and T_4		
Property	T_3	T_4
Activity	Active hormone	Inactive pro-hormone
Relative quantity produced by the thyroid gland	1	10
Free in blood (%)	0.2	0.02
Relative potency	4	1
Half-life (days)	1	7
Speed of action	Rapid (hours)	Slow (days)

Table 1.3 Comparison of tri-iodothyronine (T_3) and thyroxine (T_4)

> The normal dietary intake of iodine is 150 µg/day, of which 125 µg is used by the thyroid gland for hormone synthesis. Seafood is a rich source of iodine, so areas of iodine deficiency are often inland or at high altitude, where the daily intake may be as low as 25 µg. About 30% of the world's population is at risk of iodine deficiency.

Iodination of thyroglobulin

As soon as it is produced by thyroid peroxidase, iodine binds to the 3' and 5' sites of the benzene ring of tyrosine residues on thyroglobulin molecules (**Figure 1.11**). Iodination with one or two iodine molecules produces the hormone precursors monoiodotyrosine and di-iodotyrosine, respectively.

Synthesis of T_3 and T_4

When monoiodotyrosine combines with di-iodotyrosine, tri-iodothyronine (T_3) is produced. When two di-iodotyrosine molecules couple, the hormone T_4 is produced. The reactions creating these combinations of iodinated tyrosine residues are catalysed by the enzyme thyroid peroxidase. The thyroid hormones are stored bound to thyroglobulin in the colloid.

> Insufficient dietary iodine can cause an increase in the size of the thyroid gland in a condition called endemic goitre. Endemic goitre results from reduced thyroid hormone synthesis and the compensatory increased secretion of thyroid-stimulating hormone (TSH), which leads to hypertrophy of thyroid cells. This enlargement of the thyroid is benign. However, it is cosmetically unappealing and may cause pain and compression of the trachea and oesophagus.

Secretion of T_3 and T_4

When stimulated to release thyroid hormones by TSH from the anterior pituitary gland, the follicular cells cleave the iodinated tyrosine residues, thus forming T_3 and T_4. Thyroid hormones are lipophilic, so they diffuse easily through the follicular cell membrane and into the blood. About 90% of hormone released from the thyroid gland is T_4; the remainder is T_3. It is T_3 that is the biologically active thyroid hormone; T_4 is readily converted to T_3 in the peripheral tissues by the deiodinase enzymes. The properties of T_3 and T_4 are compared in **Table 1.3**.

Circulation

Most T_4 produced by the thyroid gland is converted to T_3 by peripheral organs such as the liver, kidney and spleen. Both thyroid hormones are hydrophobic and therefore do not dissolve; they are transported in the circulation bound to proteins, including albumin, T_4-binding prealbumin and T_4-binding globulin. Only free hormone is physiologically active.

The lipophilic nature of thyroid hormones allows them to diffuse easily into all cells of the body.

Receptors

Tri-iodothyronine (T_3) acts by binding to thyroid receptors in cell nuclei. These receptors, which are present in nearly every cell of the body, are nuclear transcription factors that regulate gene expression. The T_3–thyroid receptor complex is able to bind to DNA in hormone response elements to stimulate gene transcription and protein synthesis. Thus the complex's binding to DNA leads to the characteristic effects of thyroid hormones (**Table 1.2**).

Calcitonin

Calcitonin is a polypeptide, a chain of 32 amino acids. This hormone is produced by parafollicular cells (cells surrounding the thyroid follicles) called C cells.

Generally, calcitonin opposes the action of parathyroid hormone on blood calcium levels; the main action of calcitonin is to decrease serum calcium concentration through its effects on various organs (**Table 1.4**). It is released in response to an increase in serum calcium.

The physiological effects of calcitonin seem minor compared with the more dominant effects of parathyroid hormone. This is apparent in patients who have undergone total thyroidectomy; the resulting calcitonin deficiency seems to have no effect on calcium homeostasis.

The calcitonin receptor is a G-protein-coupled receptor. Stimulation of the receptor by calcitonin binding activates its G-protein, which in turn activates adenylate cyclase and thus increases cAMP production in target cells. This increased cAMP production mediates the effects of calcitonin on various target tissues (**Table 1. 4**).

Hypothalamic–pituitary–thyroid axis

Thyroid hormone synthesis in the thyroid gland is controlled by hormone secretions from the pituitary gland. The pituitary gland is, in turn, regulated by the hypothalamus. This system is called the hypothalamic–pituitary–thyroid axis. Negative feedback occurs from the thyroid to the hypothalamus and the pituitary, which adds further control (see **Figure 1.18**).

Thyrotrophin-releasing hormone

Thyrotrophin-releasing hormone (TRH) is synthesised and secreted by neurosecretory cells (cells derived from the neural crest and that secrete hormones) in the hypothalamus. The hormone is cleaved from a larger precursor hormone called pro-TRH then released from the hypothalamus for transport in the blood to the anterior pituitary gland. TRH stimulates the synthesis and release of TSH from the pituitary gland. Through this action, TRH indirectly increases secretion of T_3 and T_4.

The main inhibitor of TRH secretion is negative feedback by T_3 and T_4. TRH production is also blunted by illness or starvation and by an increased amount of glucocorticoids. In these situations, a lower metabolic rate may be advantageous. In other situations, TRH secretion is increased, for example when exposure to cold activates central noradrenergic neurones; the resulting increase in T_3 and T_4 speeds up metabolism and thus generates heat.

Thyroid-stimulating hormone

The anterior pituitary gland synthesises and releases TSH, a large glycoprotein hormone. TSH increases the uptake of iodide by the thyroid gland. This effect increases thyroid peroxidase enzyme function and thus stimulates the synthesis and release of T_3 and T_4.

Thyrotrophin-releasing hormone is the main stimulus for TSH production. Therefore destruction of TRH-secreting cells leads to TSH deficiency and hypothyroidism. TSH production is suppressed when T_4 levels are high to maintain a steady amount of thyroid hormones in the circulation. The thyroid and anterior pituitary glands form a negative feedback loop.

Actions of calcitonin	
Organ	Action
Bone	Inhibits bone breakdown by osteoclasts
	Simulates bone formation by osteoblasts
Intestine	Inhibits calcium absorption
Kidney	Inhibits calcium reabsorption by the renal tubules

Table 1.4 Actions of calcitonin

The parathyroid glands

Starter questions

Answers to the following questions are on page 63.

5. Can we survive without our parathyroid glands?
6. Why do South Asian individuals in the UK have a high incidence of vitamin D deficiency?

The four parathyroid glands are in the neck, behind the thyroid. They secrete parathyroid hormone. Parathyroid hormone is the main hormone responsible for maintaining calcium and phosphate homeostasis.

Accessory or supernumerary parathyroid glands (extra glands) are common. They are present in about 10% of people. Accessory glands probably arise from fragments of tissue that detach from the parathyroid gland as it migrates during embryonic development.

Embryology

The four parathyroid glands arise from pharyngeal pouches (see page 9).

- The superior parathyroid glands develop from the 4th pharyngeal pouch
- The inferior parathyroid glands develop from the 3rd pharyngeal pouch

From their superior embryonic position, the parathyroid glands migrate inferiorly into the neck. The embryological origins explain the variable anatomical positions of the parathyroid glands.

Hyperparathyroidism occurs when one or more parathyroid glands secrete excessive parathyroid hormone. This leads to hypercalcaemia and may result in kidney stones, impaired renal function and osteoporosis.

Anatomy

The parathyroid glands usually lie on the posterior aspect of the thyroid gland (Figure 1.7). They are yellow or brown in colour about the size of a small pea, and each weighs about 30-50 mg. The superior glands have a fairly constant position, but the position of the inferior glands can be variable or aberrant. The parathyroid glands are supplied by blood from branches of the inferior thyroid arteries.

In about 5% of people, one or more parathyroid glands are absent. However, this has no detectable clinical effect provided that at least one parathyroid gland is present; the remaining gland or glands are able to secrete a sufficient amount of parathyroid hormone.

Ectopic parathyroid glands (glands in the wrong place) are present in 15–20% of patients. Common ectopic locations include the anterior mediastinum, the posterior mediastinum, and the retro-oesophageal and prevertebral regions. The parathyroid gland may become embedded in the thyroid gland, resulting in an intrathyroidal parathyroid gland.

Histology

The parathyroid glands contain two types of cell: chief cells and oxyphil cells.

- Chief cells are the predominant cell type in which parathyroid hormone is synthesised, and the hormone is stored in granules in their cytoplasm

- Oxyphil cells contain numerous mitochondria (energy producing cell organelles). These cells do not produce parathyroid hormone; their role remains unclear

Most cases of hyperparathyroidism are caused by a parathyroid adenoma (benign tumour), the common treatment for which is surgical resection. Removal of the affected gland or glands is more complicated when they are in an abnormal location, such as retrosternal.

Physiology

Parathyroid hormone is the dominant hormone controlling calcium and phosphate homeostasis (**Figure 1.12**). Vitamin D has complementary roles (i.e. facilitating increased calcium levels in the blood by increasing calcium absorption from the gut) to those of parathyroid hormone, and it depends on parathyroid hormone for activation.

Calcium

The calcium ion (Ca^{2+}) has a fundamental role in various physiological functions, including:

- bone formation
- muscle contraction
- enzymatic reactions (as a cofactor)

- stabilisation of membrane potentials in muscle cells and neurones
- blood coagulation

Mode of action of calcium

Many of the actions of calcium are brought about by the binding of Ca^{2+} to proteins, which alters their structure and function. These effects occur in calcium's role as a 2nd messenger in hormonal signalling.

1. Stimulation of G-protein–coupled extracellular hormone receptors permits opening of transmembrane Ca^{2+} channels
2. The open channels allow Ca^{2+} influx into the cell, thus increasing intracellular Ca^{2+} concentration
3. The intracellular Ca^{2+} modifies the action of extracellular signal–regulated kinases
4. The action of Ca^{2+} on these kinases changes their biological activity in the cell cytoplasm and nucleus, thus altering the intracellular environment and gene transcription, respectively

Distribution of calcium in the body

The adult human body contains about 1–2 kg of calcium, 99% of which is in teeth and bone as hydroxyapatite crystals. Of the remainder, about 1% is intracellular, and a tiny fraction, less than 0.1%, is extracellular. This small extracellular fraction determines calcium balance in the body and is regulated homeostatically by hormones.

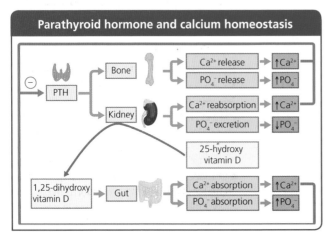

Parathyroid hormone and calcium homeostasis

Figure 1.12 Parathyroid hormone (PTH), calcium and phosphate homeostasis. .PTH acts on the bone and kidney to increase serum calcium. It causes release of phosphate by bone reabsorption and increases phosphate excretion from the kidney. Vitamin D is activated by the kidney and acts on the gut to facilitate absorption of calcium and phosphate.

Calcium in the blood

The normal range of bound calcium in the blood (serum) is narrow: 2.25–2.55 mmol/L. Only about 1 mmol/L exists as free (unbound) ionised calcium (Ca^{2+}), and that in the blood is the active calcium. About 45% of the bound calcium is bound to serum proteins (mainly albumin and, to a lesser extent, globulin), and about 10% is bound to inorganic anions such as citrate, phosphate and bicarbonate. The bound forms of calcium are in equilibrium with the free ionised calcium.

The main factor determining the amount of calcium in the blood is the concentration of albumin. In low-albumin states such as hepatic failure and nephrotic syndrome, the amount of calcium in the extracellular space is reduced.

Blood pH affects calcium protein binding:

- Acidosis reduces protein binding, thus increasing calcium concentration
- Alkalosis increases protein binding, thus reducing calcium concentration

Phosphate

Like calcium, phosphates are critical in numerous physiological processes. Such processes often require phosphorylation (addition of a phosphate ion) and dephosphorylation (removal of a phosphate ion). Examples of these processes are:

- energy transfer, in the form of conversion of stored ATP to ADP
- muscle contraction, when creatine phosphate dissociates to form creatinine and phosphate
- 2nd messenger systems, such as those including cAMP and inositol phosphates

Phosphate is also a constituent of DNA, RNA and phospholipids. These phosphate-containing compounds are termed organic phosphates, because the phosphate ion is bound to a carbon-based compound. Inorganic phosphates (negatively charged) are also present in the body and are associated with positively charged ions such as K^+ and Mg^{2+}.

Distribution of phosphate in the body

Bone contains 85% of the phosphate in the body. Just less than 5% is in the intracellular compartment, and less than 0.03% is in the serum. The total phosphate concentration in serum is normally between 0.8 and 1.5 mmol/L. About half exists in free form, and the other half is bound to serum proteins. The extracellular concentrations of phosphates are inversely related to those of Ca^{2+} and are regulated by the same hormones, i.e. parathyroid hormone and 1,25-dihydroxyvitamin D (**Figure 1.12**).

Parathyroid hormone

Parathyroid hormone is a peptide hormone produced by the parathyroid gland in response to low calcium, detected by calcium-sensing receptors on the surface of parathyroid cells. Parathyroid hormone acts on bone and the kidneys to maintain serum calcium concentration within a narrow range.

Actions

Calcium and phosphate levels depend on bone metabolism, as well as their excretion in the urine and their absorption in the gut (**Figure 1.12**).

Parathyroid hormone increase serum calcium by:

- stimulating osteoclast activity, which releases calcium from bone
- increasing renal reabsorption of calcium
- promoting renal activation of vitamin D; vitamin D facilitates calcium absorption from the intestine

The release of parathyroid hormone leads to a net decrease in serum phosphate. Parathyroid hormone–dependent bone breakdown releases phosphate. However, to prevent excessive phosphate accumulation in the serum, parathyroid hormone also acts on the kidney tubules to inhibit reabsorption of phosphate from the urine, thereby increasing renal excretion of phosphate.

Synthesis

Parathyroid hormone is produced in the cells of the parathyroid glands. Preproparathyroid hormone is cleaved to form proparathyroid hormone, which is then cleaved to form parathyroid hormone. Production of parathyroid hormone is stimulated when calcium-sensing receptors on parathyroid cells detect low calcium concentration in the blood.

Secretion and clearance

Seconds after low calcium is detected, the cells of the parathyroid gland release their stored parathyroid hormone. This process occurs by exocytosis.

An increase in Ca^{2+} binding to the calcium-sensing receptor reduces the release of parathyroid hormone. Consequently, parathyroid hormone secretion is inversely proportional to serum calcium concentration and is thus controlled by negative feedback.

Parathyroid hormone is transported unbound in the serum, has a short half-life of a few minutes and is cleared by the kidney and liver. The rapid release and breakdown of parathyroid hormone mean that this hormone system is very quick to respond to changes in blood calcium and thus maintain the serum calcium concentration within its narrow range.

Receptors

Parathyroid hormone receptors are G-protein–coupled receptors. They are present predominantly in bone and the kidneys, the main sites of action of parathyroid hormone.

Vitamin D

Vitamin D is a lipid hormone derived from cholesterol. In contrast to other vitamins, its active form is not available in the diet. Instead, vitamin D requires activation through a series of metabolic steps. This means that activated vitamin D deficiency can develop in people on a normal diet, for example in cases of renal failure.

Vitamin D exists in several forms:

- Vitamin D2 (ergocalciferol) is absorbed from the gut from plants and fungi; it is also used in some vitamin supplements

- Vitamin D3 (cholecalciferol) is synthesised from 7-dehydrocholesterol in the skin on exposure to sunlight; vitamin D3 can also be absorbed from the gut from foods such as oily fish, milk and eggs, but because it is very difficult to obtain enough vitamin D3 from the diet, synthesis on exposure to sunlight is the main source (**Table 1.5**)
- 25-Hydroxyvitamin D (calcifediol) is synthesised in the liver from hydroxylation of vitamin D3 and vitamin D2
- 1,25-Dihydroxyvitamin D (calcitriol) is the biologically active form of vitamin D; it is produced when 25-hydroxyvitamin D is hydroxylated in the kidneys

> **Vitamin D deficiency can result in demineralisation of bones, causing rickets in children and osteomalacia in adults.** Risk factors include malnutrition, inadequate exposure to sunlight, dark skin pigmentation and obesity.

Actions

In calcium and phosphate homeostasis, active vitamin D facilitates calcium and phosphate absorption from the gut.

Sources of vitamin D	
Source	Amount of vitamin D
Exposure to ultraviolet light in sunlight (10–30 min)*	90% of RDA
Cod liver oil (one capsule)	25–100% of RDA
Fortified breakfast cereal (one serving)	10–20% of RDA
Oily fish such as trout, salmon and mackerel (100 g)	10% of RDA
Egg yolk	2.5% of RDA
Margarine and infant formula milk containing vitamin D†	<5% RDA

RDA, recommended daily amount.

*The time required to synthesise vitamin D depends on the time of year (e.g. summer or winter), the degree of skin pigmentation and the amount of skin exposed.

†Vitamin D is supplemented to these foods in the UK and other countries.

Table 1.5 Sources of vitamin D

In the bone, active vitamin D stimulates activation of osteoclasts to enhance bone resorption. In the kidneys, it increases the effect of PTH in the renal tubular reabsorption of calcium.

Vitamin D receptors are expressed in many cell types throughout the body, including immune cells, neurones and skin cells. The wide expression of these receptors suggests that vitamin D has functions in addition to those in calcium and phosphate physiology and bone formation. For example, vitamin D appears to have a role in immunity, because vitamin D deficiency is linked to increased rates of infectious illness.

Synthesis

Steps in the synthesis of active 1,25-dihydroxyvitamin D are shown in **Figure 1.13**.

Receptors

The vitamin D receptor is a nuclear receptor. It is activated by the binding of 1,25-dihydroxyvitamin D. The activated receptor then forms a transcription factor that facilitates gene transcription.

The role of the vitamin D receptor is best understood in the following:

- In the bone, binding of 1,25-dihydroxyvitamin D to the receptor causes activation of osteoclasts (specialised cells involved in reabsorption of bone)
- In the gut, activation of the vitamin D receptor facilitates absorption of calcium and phosphate

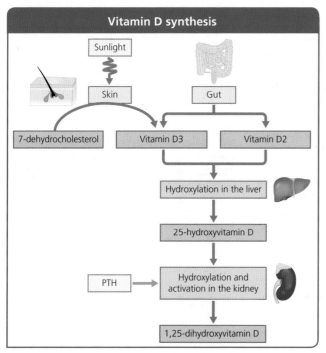

Figure 1.13 Vitamin D synthesis pathway. Vitamin D3 (cholecalciferol) is either synthesised in the skin or absorbed from the gut, along with vitamin D2 (ergocalciferol). Vitamin D2 and D3 undergo hydroxylation in the liver to produce 25-hydroxyvitamin D. The final hydroxylation and activation occurs in the kidney (catalysed by PTH) resulting in the formation of 1,25-hydroxyvitamin D.

The hypothalamus

Starter questions

Answers to the following questions are on page 63.

7. How does the body control its temperature if the hypothalamus is damaged?
8. Can hormones be replaced if the hypothalamus is damaged?

The hypothalamus is an almond-sized symmetrical structure in the brain. It is below and anterior to the thalamus, superior to the pituitary gland and either side of the 3rd ventricle.

As an endocrine gland, the hypothalamus is responsible for control of the pituitary gland. It also has major effects on other, non-endocrine physiological processes, such as regulation of body temperature.

Embryology

The hypothalamus develops from the neural tube at about 5 weeks' gestation. The neural tube is a group of cells that develops into the brain, spinal cord and autonomic ganglia. The neural origin of the hypothalamus underlies its role as a neuroendocrine gland and allows neural connections with many other parts of the central nervous system, such as the thalamus and the midbrain, which determine the hypothalamus's wide-ranging effects on the body.

Anatomy

The hypothalamus is surrounded by the thalamus laterally and superiorly. The medial border is the wall of the 3rd ventricle, and the inferior border includes the pituitary stalk, a structure connecting the hypothalamus and posterior pituitary (also known as the neurohypophysis) and the continuation of the floor of the 3rd ventricle.

There are three main anatomical areas of the hypothalamus (medial, paraventricular

and lateral), some of which share neuroendocrine functions (**Figure 1.14**).

The medial hypothalamus has projections to the paraventricular hypothalamus as well as the anterior and posterior pituitary glands; it regulates higher functions such as body temperature, appetite, thirst, the sleep–wake cycle and sexual behaviour.

The paraventricular hypothalamus, which borders the 3rd ventricle, has neurones that project to the anterior and posterior pituitary glands.

The lateral hypothalamus is a 'relay centre' containing the medial forebrain bundles, which have neuronal connections to the amygdala, the hippocampus and olfactory system, and the medial hippocampus.

Two different types of neuroendocrine cell in the hypothalamus separately regulate the anterior and posterior pituitary glands:

- The neuroendocrine cells that make up the tuberoinfundibular tract project into the capillary bed, where they form synapses (the end terminal of a nerve cell that

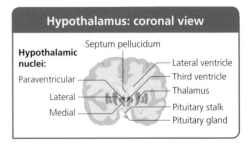

Figure 1.14 The hypothalamus and its relations (coronal view).

transmits the cells electrical or chemical signal to another cell) and release hormones that stimulate or inhibit the anterior pituitary

- The neuroendocrine cells that make up the magnocellular–neurohypophysial tract synapse directly in the posterior pituitary gland and release the hormones antidiuretic hormone and oxytocin.

Arterial supply

Arterial blood is supplied to the hypothalamus from terminal branches of the circle of Willis. These branches are, in turn, fed by the two major arteries supplying the brain: the internal carotid and basilar arteries.

Venous drainage

Hormones from the hypothalamus are transported in blood to the anterior pituitary gland through the median eminence. This midline structure comprises the hormone-secreting terminals of the hypothalamic neuroendocrine cells, as well as a capillary bed that transports hormones to the anterior pituitary gland (termed the hypothalamic-pituitary portal system).

The capillaries drain directly into the anterior pituitary gland, where the hypothalamic hormones act on pituitary cells. The remaining venous drainage from the hypothalamus occurs through the anterior cerebral and basilar veins.

Histology

The hypothalamus consists of neurones (nerve cells) and neuroendocrine cells (cells that receive neuronal input and release hormones into the blood).

The neuroendocrine cells synthesise two sets of hormone (**Table 1.6**):

- The first set are hormones (i.e. antidiuretic hormone and oxytocin) are synthesised in the hypothalamus and transported down axons for storage and release from the posterior pituitary gland
- The second set are hormones (e.g. growth hormone–releasing hormone, GHRH; somatostatin; corticotrophin-releasing hormone, CRH; thyrotropin releasing hormone, TRH; gonadotrophin-releasing hormone, GnRH; and dopamine) are synthesised in the hypothalamus and reach the anterior pituitary gland through the hypothalamic–pituitary portal system (a network of arteries and capillaries carrying blood from the hypothalamus to the anterior pituitary) to stimulate or inhibit secretion of anterior pituitary hormones

Hypothalamic hormones: sites of release and effects		
Hypothalamic hormone	**Site of release**	**Effect**
Antidiuretic hormone	Posterior pituitary gland	Promotes renal reabsorption of water
Oxytocin		Stimulates uterine contraction
Growth hormone–releasing hormone	Anterior pituitary gland	Induces secretion of growth hormone
Somatostatin		Inhibits secretion of growth hormone
Corticotrophin-releasing hormone		Induces secretion of adrenocorticotrophic hormone
Thyrotrophin-releasing hormone		Induces secretion of thyroid-stimulating hormone
Gonadotrophin-releasing hormone		Stimulates secretion of luteinising hormone and follicle-stimulating hormone
Dopamine		Inhibits secretion of prolactin

Table 1.6 Hypothalamic hormones: their sites of release and effects

Physiology

The hypothalamus is considered the body's 'master control centre' for hormone secretion. In this role, it controls and receives feedback signals from other endocrine glands. End organs controlled by the hypothalamus through hormones released by the anterior pituitary include:

- thyroid gland
- adrenal glands
- gonads

Body temperature is controlled by the hypothalamus, which also has effects on appetite and thirst, the sleep–wake cycle and sexual behaviour. Emotion is influenced through connections to the limbic system. The hypothalamus affects the autonomic nervous system (which regulates involuntary body systems such as the heart and the smooth muscle of the vascular system and gastrointestinal tract) through projections to spinal and brain stem nuclei.

Hypothalamic hormones (**Table 1.6**) are secreted either directly into the systemic circulation through the posterior pituitary or into the hypothalamic–pituitary portal system to reach the cells of the anterior pituitary. Here, they stimulate or inhibit the release of anterior pituitary gland hormones.

Antidiuretic hormone

Antidiuretic hormone (also known as vasopressin) is a polypeptide hormone. It is synthesised by hypothalamic neuroendocrine cells that project into the posterior pituitary gland, from which the hormone is secreted. Antidiuretic hormone is stored in granules at the terminal ends of magnocellular neuroendocrine cells in the posterior pituitary gland.

Actions

The overall action of antidiuretic hormone is to increase the water content of the body. This is primarily achieved through its effect on the collecting ducts of the kidney, where antidiuretic hormone causes aquaporin 2 channel proteins to migrate to the luminal membrane. Aquaporin 2 channels permit water absorption from the urine into the kidney. Thus water transport across the impermeable membrane is increased, and more water is reabsorbed from the collecting duct.

> **Insensitivity of antidiuretic hormone receptors leads to their under-activation by the hormone.** For example, in nephrogenic diabetes insipidus, the target cells in the kidney are insensitive to antidiuretic hormone resulting in excessive free water excretion in the urine.

Antidiuretic hormone also binds to receptors on the vascular smooth muscle in blood vessel walls; it causes vasoconstriction and thus increases blood pressure.

Secretion

Antidiuretic hormone secretion is stimulated by increased serum osmolarity (the concentration of solute in the blood), which reflects water deficiency (**Figure 1.15**). Changes in osmolarity are sensed by specialist cells called osmoreceptors in the hypothalamus and other areas of the brain (**Figure 1.14**).

The release of antidiuretic hormone is also stimulated by low blood pressure, which is sensed by baroreceptors (blood pressure detectors) in the large blood vessels and heart. This mechanism is influenced by the autonomic nervous system being up-regulated by sympathetic drive (which is synergistic in increasing blood pressure).

Antidiuretic hormone is transported unbound in the plasma.

> **Antidiuretic hormone receptors are present in many types of body tissue.** They exert a wide range of effects, including conserving water and increasing blood pressure. Therefore polyuria and the inability to conserve water appropriately are features of antidiuretic hormone deficiency (cranial diabetes insipidus).

Receptors

The three major antidiuretic hormone receptors have various functions (**Table 1.7**).

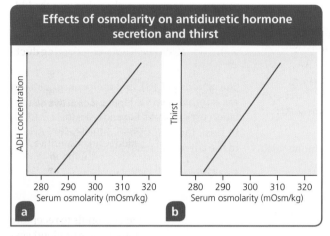

Figure 1.15 (a) Secretion of antidiuretic hormone (ADH) increases with increasing serum osmolarity, and there is no secretion below osmolarity of about 285 mOsm/kg. (b) Thirst also increases as serum osmolarity increases.

Type of receptor	Location	Effect
ADH 1a	Vascular smooth muscle	Increases blood pressure
ADH 1b	Corticotrophs (cells in the anterior pituitary gland that produce ACTH)	Increases ACTH secretion
ADH 2	Collecting duct of kidney	Increases water reabsorption

Antidiuretic hormone receptors: locations and effects

ACTH, adrenocorticotrophic hormone; ADH, antidiuretic hormone.

Table 1.7 The locations of different antidiuretic hormone receptors and the physiological effects when activated

The receptors are G-protein–coupled receptors (see page 6).

Oxytocin

This peptide hormone is synthesised in magnocellular cells of the hypothalamus and secreted from their terminal ends in the posterior pituitary.

Actions

The main roles of oxytocin are to stimulate:

- uterine contraction during labour
- milk let-down to facilitate lactation

Oxytocin also has roles in the menstrual cycle in women and in erectile function in men but these are poorly understood.

Secretion

Oxytocin is released from projections of the magnocellular neurones of the hypothalamus into the posterior pituitary gland. Like most peptide hormones, oxytocin is transported unbound in the serum.

Receptor

The oxytocin receptor is a G-protein–coupled receptor present in the uterus and breasts. It is also in the central nervous system, which suggests that oxytocin also has roles outside childbirth, such as the establishment of complex bonding behaviours with the baby.

Labour can be induced by using synthetic oxytocin to stimulate uterine contraction. The procedure is used, for example, for women with life-threatening diabetes or pre-eclampsia, or if the baby is overdue and labour has not occurred spontaneously.

Growth hormone–releasing hormone and somatostatin

Growth hormone–releasing hormone and somatostatin are peptide hormones produced in the tuberoinfundibular tract of the hypothalamus that bind to G-protein–coupled receptors in somatotrophs (cells in the anterior pituitary gland that produce growth hormone).

Actions

Growth hormone–releasing hormone and somatostatin have antagonistic actions on the somatotrophs (**Figure 1.16**):

- GHRH stimulates the production and release of growth hormone
- Somatostatin inhibits growth hormone production

Growth hormone–releasing hormone also promotes somatotroph replication.

As well as reducing the production of growth hormone in the pituitary, somatostatin inhibits the production of GHRH in the hypothalamus. Somatostatin also has other endocrine effects; for example, it is produced in the pancreas and inhibits insulin secretion.

Secretion

The control of GHRH and somatostatin release is shown in **Figure 1.16**. The release of GHRH is inhibited by negative feedback from circulating growth hormone and insulin-like growth factor-1. GHRH release is also inhibited by somatostatin-secreting neurones in the hypothalamus.

Both GHRH and somatostatin are released into the blood of the hypothalamic-pituitary portal system and transported to the anterior pituitary gland. These hormones are transported unbound in the blood.

Corticotrophin-releasing hormone

Corticotrophin-releasing hormone is a peptide hormone produced in the hypothalamus.

It binds to a G-protein–coupled receptor on corticotrophs (ACTH-producing cells in the anterior pituitary gland).

Actions

The actions of CRH, and their consequences, are summarised in **Figure 1.5**. CRH stimulates corticotrophs to produce ACTH. ACTH, in turn, increases the production of cortisol in the adrenal glands (see page 31).

Secretion

Figure 1.5 shows the feedback loops for CRH. Release of CRH is stimulated by the neurotransmitters noradrenaline (norepinephrine) and acetylcholine, histamine, thus 'stress' neurotransmitters influence the cortisol-secreting system. CRH therefore acts a final common pathway messenger of physiological stress that results in the up-regulation of cortisol production. Conversely, CRH release is inhibited by negative feedback to the hypothalamus from ACTH and cortisol.

Corticotrophin-releasing hormone is released from hypothalamic neurones into the blood of the hypothalamic-pituitary portal system, where it is transported in an unbound state to the anterior pituitary gland.

Thyrotrophin-releasing hormone

Thyrotrophin-releasing hormone is a peptide hormone produced in the paraventricular nucleus of the hypothalamus. It binds to G-protein–coupled receptors on thyrotrophs

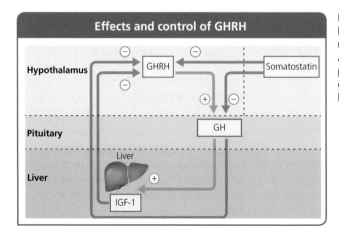

Effects and control of GHRH

Figure 1.16 Secretion of growth hormone–releasing hormone (GHRH) from the hypothalamus, and its effects on the anterior pituitary gland. IGF1, insulin-like growth factor 1; GH, growth hormone.

(cells in the anterior pituitary gland that produce TSH) to stimulate the production and release of TSH (**Figure 1.17**).

Secretion

The release of TSH is controlled by negative feedback from the thyroid hormones, T_3 and T_4 (**Figure 1.17**). In the physiological states of fasting and illness, TRH production is downregulated by inhibitory neuronal input of multiple cells of the peripheral and central nervous system. This effect conserves energy by producing a state of low thyroid hormone levels and a reduced metabolic rate.

Transport

Thyrotrophin-releasing hormone is transported unbound in the blood. Once secreted into the median eminence from granules at the distal end of the hypothalamic neurons it travels to the anterior pituitary gland in the blood via the hypothalamic-pituitary portal system the hypothalamic-pituitary portal system.

Gonadotrophin-releasing hormone

Gonadotrophin-releasing hormone is a peptide hormone produced by cells widely distributed throughout the medial hypothalamus. GnRH binds to a G-protein–coupled receptor on cells of the anterior pituitary gland.

This hormone promotes sexual development, sex hormone production and reproduction by stimulating production of the gonadotrophins (hormones that stimulate gonadal function, e.g. luteinising hormone and FSH).

Actions

Gonadotrophin-releasing hormone stimulates gonadotrophin production by gonadotrophs (cells in the anterior pituitary that produce gonadotrophins) (**Figure 1.18**). GnRH activity is low in childhood but is activated around puberty when genetic triggers are activated by hypothalamic hormones called Kisspeptins.

Secretion

Gonadotrophin-releasing hormone is released in pulses. The pulsatile nature of GnRH is reflected in its effects on the gonadotrophs. For example, changes in the frequency of GnRH pulses determine the frequency of pulses of gonadotrophins from the pituitary.

- In women and girls, such changes enable progression through the phases of the menstrual cycle, as when a surge of luteinising hormone precipitates ovulation (see page 34)
- In men, the pulsatility of GnRH and thus gonadotrophins is less variable

The pulsatile nature of GnRH release is vital during puberty. There is an increase in the

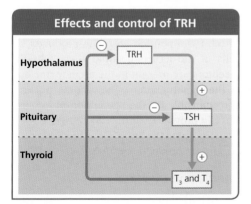

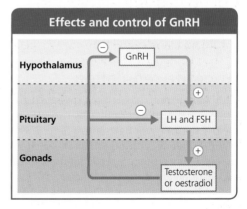

Figure 1.17 Secretion of thyrotrophin-releasing hormone (TRH) from the hypothalamus, and its effects on the anterior pituitary gland. T_3, tri-iodothyronine; T_4, thyroxine; TSH, thyroid-stimulating hormone.

Figure 1.18 Secretion of gonadotrophin-releasing hormone (GnRH) from the hypothalamus, and its effects on the anterior pituitary gland. FSH, follicle-stimulating hormone; LH, luteinising hormone.

frequency and amplitude of GnRH pulses that 'wakes up' the entire reproductive system that has previously laid dormant.

Gonadotrophin-releasing hormone pulsatility is controlled by kisspeptin hormones, which are produced in cells of the hypothalamus. These peptide hormones are vital triggers for sexual development and reproduction.

The frequency and amplitude of GnRH release provide chemical signals to the gonadotrophs to commence production of gonadotrophins. Production of luteinising hormone and FSH is stimulated or inhibited accordingly.

Oestradiol and testosterone have a negative feedback effect on the hypothalamus that down-regulates GnRH release (**Figure 1.18**).

Transport

From the median eminence, where it is secreted, gonadotrophin-releasing hormone is transported unbound in the blood through the hypothalamic-pituitary portal system to the anterior pituitary gland.

> Women undergoing in vitro fertilisation have daily injections of a GnRH analogue to obliterate luteinising hormone-FSH pulsatility. Once the normal menstrual cycle is switched off this way, subcutaneous injections of a combination of luteinising hormone and FSH are used to artificially stimulate egg development and ovulation. The resulting ova are then harvested and fertilised.

Appetite regulation

The hypothalamus has a role in appetite regulation. Appetite is determined by two contradictory impulses: hunger and satiety. These impulses, along with other factors, such as the availability of food, social impulses, smell and taste, determine energy intake.

The hypothalamus controls eating behaviour by:

- responding to afferent nervous and endocrine stimuli
- acting through efferent nervous pathways to control eating behaviour

Signals to the hypothalamus

Appetite is affected by nervous impulses and hormonal signals (transported from endocrine cells through the blood) to the hypothalamus.

Satiety signals

Food entering the gut stretches the intestinal wall and thus stimulates the vagus nerve. This effect signals 'fullness' to the hypothalamus.

In addition, gut hormones such as glucagon-like peptide-1, cholecystokinin and peptide YY are released from the gut in response to ingestion of food. These hormones provide hormonal feedback to the hypothalamus to increase the feeling of satiety.

Leptin is produced by adipose (fat) cells to help regulate the amount of fat stored in adipose tissue. Leptin provides an endocrine signal to the hypothalamus to decrease appetite and thus reduce food intake if fat stores are sufficient.

> In the rare cases of congenital leptin deficiency, administration of leptin suppresses appetite and promotes weight loss. However, leptin therapy does not reverse excessive body weight in the vast majority of cases of obesity, in which the causes are dietary and lifestyle factors.

Hunger signals

Ghrelin is a peptide hormone produced by cells of the gastrointestinal tract. Ghrelin receptors are present in the arcuate nucleus of the hypothalamus. The arcuate nucleus is responsible for the perception of hunger. Ghrelin provides a hormonal 'hunger signal' from the gut to the brain. Once food is ingested, ghrelin production wanes.

Integration of signals

The hypothalamus integrates the endocrine and neural impulses that it receives, and communicates them through neural projections to the cerebral cortex. These hypothalamic signals are reincorporated with other higher impulses, such as the hedonic (pleasure) signals associated with food intake. The cerebral cortex then acts on these signals to determine food-seeking behaviour and food intake.

Temperature regulation

The preoptic region of the hypothalamus is responsible for regulation of body temperature (thermoregulation). The temperature is maintained at 36–37.5°C to maximise metabolic efficiency; enzymes function optimally in this range.

The hypothalamus assesses temperature:

- peripherally through nerves in the skin that sense external temperature
- centrally through temperature-sensing nerves that detect the temperature of blood around the hypothalamus

These nervous signals feed back to the hypothalamus, which then activates appropriate cooling or warming actions (**Figure 1.19**).

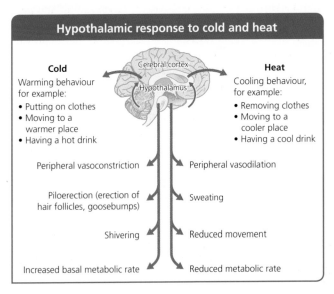

Figure 1.19 The response of the hypothalamus to cold and heat.

The pituitary gland

Starter questions

Answers to the following questions are on page 63–64.

9. Does prolactin play a role in men?
10. Why does the anterior pituitary gland have little direct blood supply?
11. Why is the pulsatility of pituitary hormone secretion so important?

The pituitary gland lies in the pituitary fossa at the base of the skull. Although small (about 0.5 cm in diameter), the gland controls many of the body's endocrine systems.

The gland is anatomically and functionally separated into two parts:

- the anterior pituitary gland (also known as the adenohypophysis)

- the posterior pituitary gland (also known as the neurohypophysis)

A wide variety of hormones are secreted from multiple cell types in the anterior pituitary gland (**Table 1.8**). Hormones of the posterior pituitary gland (antidiuretic hormone and oxytocin) are released in the posterior pituitary having been synthesised in the hypothalamus.

Embryology

The anterior and posterior pituitary glands have different embryological origins (**Figure 1.20**).

- The anterior pituitary is an upgrowth from the oral ectoderm of the stomodeum (primitive oral cavity) called the Rathke's pouch
- The posterior pituitary derives from nervous tissue (the diencephalon) and forms from an out-pouching of the neural ectoderm or diencephalon that forms the floor of the 3rd ventricle

Therefore the anterior pituitary has a rich vascular supply but no neural tissue, whereas the posterior pituitary comprises mainly neurones originating in the hypothalamus.

Development of the pituitary gland starts at 4 weeks' gestation. By 6 weeks of gestation, the anterior pituitary gland has been formed by cleavage of Rathke's pouch. The border between the anterior pituitary and the posterior pituitary remains and is termed the pars intermedia.

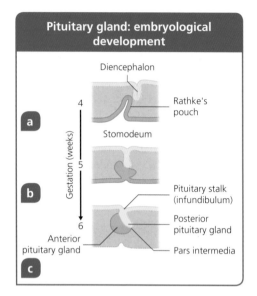

Pituitary gland: embryological development

Figure 1.20 Embryological development of the pituitary gland. (a) Development starts at 4 weeks of gestation by upgrowth of the stomodeum to form Rathke's pouch and downgrowth of the diencephalon to form the posterior pituitary; (b), the two structures meet; (c) the anterior pituitary gland has been formed by cleavage of Rathke's pouch and is attached to the posterior pituitary gland.

Anterior pituitary gland hormones			
Hormone	Pituitary cell type	Target	Hormone effect(s)
Growth hormone	Somatotrophic	Hepatocytes and adipose cells	Promotes growth and regulates metabolism. Stimulates IGF-1 production in the liver
Adrenocorticotrophic hormone	Corticotrophic	Adrenal cortex	Increases secretion of corticosteroids
Thyroid-stimulating hormone	Thyrotrophic	Thyroid gland	Stimulates secretion of thyroxine and tri-iodothyronine
Luteinising hormone	Gonadotrophic	Testes (in males) or ovaries (in females)	Increases sex hormone secretion
Follicle-stimulating hormone	Gonadotrophic	Testes	Stimulates spermatogenesjs
		Ovaries	Stimulates follicle production
Prolactin	Lactotrophic	Mammary glands	Promotes lactation

Table 1.8 Hormones secreted by the anterior pituitary gland, their cell type, hormone target and effects

A Rathke's cleft cyst is thought to arise as an overgrowth of the remnant from the Rathke's pouch. This fluid-filled, benign structure is usually small and discovered incidentally on radiographic imaging. However, the cyst can enlarge, even in adulthood, to compress the optic chiasm causing a visual field defect.

the pituitary stalk and into the anterior pituitary gland (**Figure 1.21**).

If the pituitary fossa enlarges, for example as a result of pituitary adenoma, it compresses local structures, including the infundibulum, the optic chiasm and the pituitary gland itself (**Figure 1.22**). The result may be pituitary hormone dysfunction or loss of field of vision (bitemporal heminaopia).

Anatomy

The pituitary gland is in the pituitary fossa and weighs about 0.5 g. The posterior pituitary is connected to the median eminence of the hypothalamus through the pituitary stalk, also known as the infundibulum. The anterior pituitary makes up 80% of the pituitary gland and lies in contact with the posterior pituitary.

The pituitary gland is surrounded by a thick covering (dura mater). The pituitary gland lies in the pituitary fossa, in the sella turcica of the sphenoid bone.

Magnocellular neurosecretory cells, which originate in the hypothalamus and terminate in the posterior pituitary, produce antidiuretic hormone and oxytocin.

The tuberoinfundibular pathway is a collection of dopamine-transmitting neurones that emanate from the hypothalamus and feed into the pituitary stalk (infundibulum). These terminate in a rich capillary bed of the hypothalamic-pituitary portal system (in which dopamine can circulate), passing down

Structures lying close to the pituitary gland in the pituitary fossa include:

- optic chiasm superiorly (where the tracts of the optic nerves carrying signals from the temporal field of vision in each side cross)
- cavernous sinus laterally
- internal carotid arteries laterally
- sphenoid bone inferiorly
- 3rd ventricle posteriorly

Arterial supply

The two parts of the pituitary gland receive blood from different sources.

- The posterior pituitary receives most of its blood supply from the inferior hypophyseal artery
- The anterior pituitary receives blood directly from the superior hypophyseal artery and indirectly from the same artery through the hypothalamic-pituitary portal system from the median eminence

Figure 1.21 Anatomy of the pituitary gland.

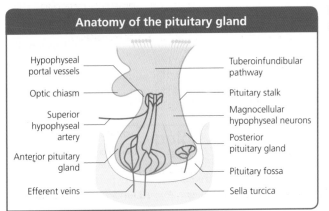

Anatomy of the pituitary gland

Hypophyseal portal vessels

Optic chiasm

Superior hypophyseal artery

Anterior pituitary gland

Efferent veins

Tuberoinfundibular pathway

Pituitary stalk

Magnocellular hypophyseal neurons

Posterior pituitary gland

Pituitary fossa

Sella turcica

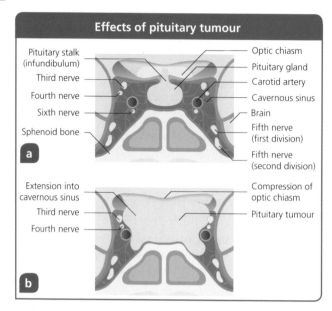

Figure 1.22 Coronal sections through the pituitary gland. (a) The normal pituitary gland. (b) A large pituitary tumour occupies the pituitary fossa, extending into the cavernous sinus and compressing the optic chiasm.

The blood in the portal system is rich in hypothalamic stimulating and inhibitory hormones, such as CRH, TRH, GHRH, somatostatin, GnRH and dopamine. These hormones are conveyed to the anterior pituitary gland to control the synthesis and release of anterior pituitary hormones.

The hypophyseal arteries are terminal branches from the internal carotid artery.

Venous drainage

The pituitary gland is drained by the hypophyseal veins. This blood now contains hormones from the anterior and posterior pituitary glands. These veins drain into the petrosal sinuses and then the jugular vein, from which the hormones are disseminated systemically to their target tissues.

Innervation

The posterior pituitary is directly innervated by nerves from the magnocellular pathway from the hypothalamus. At the termination of these neurones, oxytocin and antidiuretic hormone are released. Oxytocin is released during labour and breastfeeding and causes uterine contraction and help lactation. Antidiuretic hormone is released in response to increased blood osmolarity, decreased blood volume and stress.

There is no direct innervation of the anterior pituitary gland. Information from the brain is translated into hormones from the hypothalamic cells. These hormones are released into the blood supply of the pituitary to stimulate hormonal release. The connection between the hypothalamus and the anterior pituitary gland is therefore purely vascular.

Histology

The secretory area of the anterior pituitary gland is the pars distalis (anterior lobe). The pars distalis contains various types of epithelial cell. These are divided into two groups:

- chromophils (cells that stain with dye)
- chromophobes (cells that do not stain)

The chromophilic epithelial cells are further subdivided into acidophilic and basophilic cells (**Table 1.9**).

The posterior pituitary consists of a vascular bed and the terminal ends of myelinated axons projecting from the hypothalamus.

Physiology

Hormone release from the anterior pituitary gland is controlled by hypothalamic hormones (see page 20). Anterior pituitary hormone production is also affected by negative feedback from the target endocrine gland, such

Histology of anterior pituitary cells			
Type of epithelial cell	Secretory protein	Class	Hormone secreted
Acidophilic	Polypeptide	Somatotrophic	Growth hormone
		Lactotrophic	Prolactin
Basophilic	Glycoprotein	Corticotrophic	Adrenocorticotrophic hormone
		Gonadotrophic	Luteinising hormone and follicle-stimulating hormone
		Thyrotrophic	Thyroid-stimulating hormone
Chromotrophic	No hormones	-	-

Table 1.9 Histology of the anterior pituitary cells

as T_4 acting directly on the pituitary to inhibit TSH release but also to inhibit TRH release from the hypothalamus.

Adrenocorticotrophic hormone

This peptide hormone is derived from a large precursor molecule called pro-opiomelanocortin. Cleavage of this polypeptide produces several peptides, including ACTH. ACTH is synthesised by the corticotrophs of the anterior pituitary gland. These cells make up about a quarter of the anterior pituitary gland.

Actions

Adrenocorticotrophic hormone binds to ACTH receptors, which are transmembrane receptors in the zona fasciculata and zona reticularis of the adrenal cortex. Binding of ACTH to its receptor stimulates the production of cortisol (see page 41).

In addition, ACTH binds to cells in the zona glomerulosa and zona reticularis to stimulate synthesis of aldosterone and adrenal androgens. However, these hormones have other, more potent stimuli for secretion. For example, aldosterone secretion is primarily stimulated by angiotensin II.

Aside from its role in hormone production, ACTH also stimulates proliferation of adrenal cortex cells to maintain the adrenal cortex at a size sufficient to produce adequate amounts of cortisol.

Secretion

The secretion of ACTH is stimulated by CRH from the hypothalamus. The hormone is transported unbound in the systemic circulation.

There are many other physiological stimuli for ACTH secretion. These include antidiuretic hormone, catecholamines and growth hormone (i.e. other hormones that control the stress response and affect metabolism). ACTH secretion has physiological characteristics that directly influence the reactive production of cortisol:

■ ACTH secretion is pulsatile
■ ACTH secretion has a circadian rhythm
■ ACTH release is stimulated by stress

The circadian rhythm is a pattern of secretion that follows a 24-h cycle set by a hypothalamic pacemaker. ACTH is not unique in having such a rhythm; other hormones, such as testosterone and growth hormone, also follow a circadian pattern.

The frequency of ACTH pulses remains constant, but circadian rhythm occurs by changes in the quantity of ACTH released with each pulse. The highest peaks are early in the morning, and the lowest troughs are in the middle of the night.

Stress leads to cytokine, hormone and neurotransmitter release, which stimulates the release of CRH. CRH, in turn, increases overall ACTH secretion and cortisol production. For example, ACTH release can be caused by hypotension, pain, emotional strain and metabolic stressors such as hypoglycaemia.

ACTH stimulates the release of cortisol, which reduces the immune response and stimulates cytokine production; it also has other effects, such as increasing blood pressure.

Pituitary function is tested by using intravenous insulin to deliberately induce hypoglycaemia; this is the insulin stress test. Hypoglycaemic stress normally causes cortisol to peak. Failure to do so confirms pituitary or adrenal failure.

Receptors

Adrenocorticotrophic hormone receptors are G-protein–coupled transmembrane receptors. Once bound with ACTH, they transmit their signal by activating the adenylate cyclase pathway (see page 6). ACTH receptors are present in the zona reticularis and the zona fasciculata of the adrenal cortex.

Growth hormone

Growth hormone is a polypeptide hormone released from somatotrophs in the anterior pituitary gland. It is the most abundant anterior pituitary hormone.

In childhood, growth hormone has a key role in promoting growth. It also has a role in adulthood in increasing muscle growth and increasing blood glucose, even after the body has reached its final height.

Actions

The biological effects of growth hormone are varied and complex, but almost all its actions are through its effector hormone, insulin-like growth factor-1. Growth hormone stimulates the production of insulin-like growth factor-1 (a peptide hormone with a similar chemical structure to insulin) in the liver via activation of growth hormone receptors.

Insulin-like growth factor-1 has effects on multiple tissues, including promotion of cellular proliferation and stimulation of metabolism (Table 1.10). However, the key target organ of IGF-1 in childhood is the epiphyseal growth plates in long bones; therefore ICF-1 stimulates long bone growth children.

Physiological effects of growth hormone and IGF-1

Cells (tissue)	Active hormone(s)	Effect(s)
Chondrocytes (cartilage)	Growth hormone and IGF-1	Promote proliferation and growth
Myoblasts (muscle)	IGF-1	Promotes proliferation
		Increases amino acid uptake
Adipocytes (adipose tissue)	IGF-1	Stimulates adipose metabolism to release fatty acids
Hepatocytes (liver)	IGF-1	Increases gluconeogenesis
Peripheral tissues	IGF-1	Impairs glucose uptake
		Increases amino acid uptake and protein synthesis

Table 1.10 The physiological effects of growth hormone and insulin-like growth hormone (IGF)-1

Growth hormone also affects tissues directly to cause growth by cellular proliferation. The precise mechanism for this is unclear.

Secretion

The transcription and release of growth hormone are stimulated by GHRH. Growth hormone secretion is also stimulated by ghrelin produced by the stomach, because ghrelin augments GHRH and inhibits somatostatin (an inhibitor of growth hormone release).

The release of growth hormone is pulsatile. Pulses occur less than a dozen times per day. During the intervening times, growth hormone levels are low. Growth hormone secretion has a circadian pattern; pulses occur in greater frequency and amplitude during sleep, when peak growth occurs in children (Figure 1.23).

Growth hormone is present from birth. However, the onset of puberty causes a marked increase in the amplitude of growth hormone pulses as a result of genetic stimuli. In adulthood, growth hormone secretion declines with age but the pulse frequency remains constant.

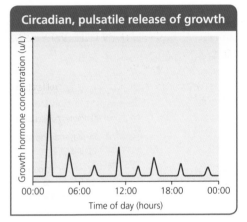

Circadian, pulsatile release of growth

Growth hormone concentration (u/L)

Time of day (hours)

00:00   06:00   12:00   18:00   00:00

Figure 1.23 The normal circadian, pulsatile release of growth hormone.

Growth hormone is not the only hormone to promote growth. Growth velocity decreases during periods of illness in childhood, and multiple factors produce the 'catch-up growth' that occurs after a period of prolonged illness; this type of growth is the result of a complex interaction of hormones and physical state (e.g. nutritional status).

Growth hormone is transported bound to proteins in the blood.

> The oral administration of glucose tests the ability of the pituitary gland to suppress growth hormone production. Therefore the oral glucose tolerance test is used to detect uncontrolled, excessive growth hormone production in suspected cases of acromegaly.

Receptor

The growth hormone receptor is a transmembrane receptor expressed widely in the body, including in the skeletal muscle, heart, brain and liver.

The binding of growth hormone to its receptor leads to activation by receptor dimerisation (two receptor subunits combining to form one active hormone-receptor complex). Dimerisation results from protein kinase activation and consequent phosphorylation cascade of proteins within the cytoplasm.

The main result of growth hormone activation is production of insulin-like growth factor-1. Insulin-like growth factor-1, in turn, promotes growth by binding to insulin-like growth factor-1 receptors in body tissues.

Thyroid-stimulating hormone

Thyroid-stimulating hormone is a glycoprotein synthesised in the anterior pituitary. Through its actions on TSH receptors in the thyroid, it is a major stimulus for thyroid cell growth, differentiation and function.

TSH has two subunits.

- The α subunit is nearly identical to that of human chorionic gonadotrophin, luteinising hormone and FSH
- The β subunit is unique to TSH and is responsible for binding to the TSH receptor

Actions

Thyroid-stimulating hormone promotes production of the thyroid hormones, T_3 and T_4, by the follicular cells of the thyroid gland. TSH also stimulates thyroid cell growth and differentiation.

Secretion

Thyroid-stimulating hormone secretion is pulsatile and circadian, peaking in the evening. Secretion from the anterior pituitary gland is stimulated by TRH from the hypothalamus.

Factors affecting TSH production	
Clinical situation	Effect on TSH production
Fasting state	↓
Illness	↓
Depression	↓
Use of certain medications (e.g. corticosteroids and opiates)	↓
Cortisol deficiency	↑

Table 1.11 Factors affecting production of thyroid-stimulating hormone (TSH)

The production and secretion of TSH by the anterior pituitary gland are directly inhibited by negative feedback from T_3 and T_4. Other factors that modulate TSH secretion are shown in **Table 1.11**.

The hormone is transported unbound in the serum.

Receptor

The TSH receptor is a G-protein–coupled transmembrane receptor. It is predominantly present in the thyroid gland but is also in muscle, bone and adipose tissue.

Receptor activation leads to gene activation and nuclear transcription.

Luteinising hormone and follicle-stimulating hormone

Luteinising hormone and FSH are called gonadotrophins, because they stimulate the gonads (the testes in males and the ovaries in females). They are glycoproteins produced by the gonadotrophs of the pituitary gland.

Similar to TSH and human chorionic gonadotrophin, they comprise homologous α chains and unique β chains. The β chains bind to activate the receptors.

The gonadotrophins are not essential to life (as individuals with genetic disorders of gonadotrophin deficiency, e.g. Kallman's syndrome, have only partially reduced life-expectancy). However, they are essential for pubertal development and fertility.

Actions

Luteinising hormone and FSH stimulate sex hormone (see pages 51 and 56) and gamete production in both males and females (**Table 1.12**). FSH is responsible for stimulating:

- development of the ovarian follicles in women
- spermatogenesis (sperm-production) in the Sertoli cells in men

Luteinising hormone stimulates production of the sex steroids. In response to luteinising hormone, testosterone is secreted from the Leydig cells in men and from theca cells in women. In women, the testosterone is then

Actions of luteinising hormone and FSH

Hormone	Sex	Action(s)
Luteinising hormone	Female	Stimulates ovulation
		Maintains the corpus luteum (the remnant of the developing ovum the remains in the ovary secreting hormones after ovulation)
		Stimulates the corpus luteum to produce oestradiol and progesterone
	Male	Stimulates the Leydig cells of the testes to produce testosterone
FSH	Female	Promotes development of the ovarian follicle
		Stimulates the follicle to produce oestradiol
	Male	Stimulates differentiation of the Sertoli cells and spermatogenesis

Table 1.12 Actions of luteinising hormone and follicle-stimulating hormone (FSH) in females and males

converted into oestrogen in ovarian granulosa cells, adjacent to the theca cells, during the follicular phase of the menstrual cycle (in which the developing follicle produces oestrogen in response to stimulation by LH and FSH).

Secretion

Luteinising hormone and FSH are produced in response to pulses of GnRH from the hypothalamus. The increased frequency and amplitude of these pulses are detected by activation of the GnRH receptors on the gonadotrophs and increase the amount of luteinising hormone and FSH produced.

In women, there is a surge in gonadotrophins, predominantly luteinising hormone, just before ovulation. The luteinising hormone helps turn the remaining follicle into the corpus luteum. The corpus luteum secretes progesterone, which helps prepare the endometrium for possible implantation. The cyclicity of gonadotrophin secretion in women is not present in men as semen production and fertility are continuous rather than cyclical as in the female.

The hormones that inhibit luteinising hormone and FSH production are shown in

Hormones that inhibit luteinising hormone and FSH production	
Hormone	Organ of origin
Inhibin	Ovaries (females)
	Testes (males)
Oestradiol	Ovaries (females)
Testosterone	Testes (males)
Prolactin	Anterior pituitary gland

Table 1.13 Hormones that inhibit gonadotrophin (luteinising hormone and follicle-stimulating hormone, FSH) production

Actions of prolactin	
Tissue	Action(s)
Mammary gland	Promotes growth and development
	Stimulates synthesis of milk
	Maintains lactation
Central nervous system	Stimulates sexualised behaviour
Ovaries	Promotes persistence of corpus luteum

Table 1.14 Actions of prolactin

Table 1.13. Both luteinising hormone and FSH are transported unbound in the serum.

> Androgens such as testosterone are common drugs of abuse in professional and amateur sports, especially body building. The prolonged use of androgens may cause temporary or permanent hypothalamic dysfunction (luteinising hormone and FSH deficiency).

Receptors

The luteinising hormone receptor is present in Leydig cells in the testes, and theca and granulosa cells in the ovaries. The FSH receptor is on Sertoli cells in the testes and granulosa cells in the ovaries. These receptors are G-protein–coupled receptors.

The luteinising hormone receptor also binds human chorionic gonadotrophin, because of the similarity in the two hormones' structures. If a pregnancy occurs:

- luteinising hormone concentration decreases
- human chorionic gonadotrophin concentration increases

The binding of human chorionic gonadotrophin to the luteinising hormone receptor helps support progesterone secretion and implantation of the embryo.

Prolactin

Prolactin is a single-chain polypeptide hormone produced by lactotrophs (prolactin-synthesising cells in the anterior pituitary gland). Prolactin was originally so named because it promotes lactation (milk production). However, this is only one of prolactin's various effects, which primarily relate to reproduction and lactation (**Table 1.14**).

Secretion

Prolactin is primarily secreted from lactotrophs in the anterior pituitary gland. However, it is also produced in the hypothalamus, placenta, uterus and mammary glands, and binds to local receptors to affect behaviours such as maternal behaviour and mating instincts.

Secretion of prolactin from the anterior pituitary gland is determined by tonic inhibition. In this type of inhibition, small amounts of dopamine are released independently of neural stimulation, which leads to inhibition of prolactin release.

Physiological triggers also stimulate prolactin release by direct neural or hormonal signals to the hypothalamic dopaminergic neurons. These include:

- breastfeeding
- stress
- oestradiol and progesterone

Prolactin is transported unbound in the serum.

> Dopamine receptor agonists such as cabergoline are used clinically to inhibit prolactin production by increasing the tonic flow of dopamine. These drugs are the mainstay of treatment for prolactin excess associated with prolactin-secreting pituitary tumours and usually obviate the need for surgery.

Receptor

The prolactin receptor is a single-protein transmembrane receptor. The receptor is part of the cytokine receptor superfamily. It is expressed in the breast, where its activation leads to proliferation of breast tissue and stimulation of the mammary glands to produce milk. It is also widely expressed in other tissues such as the brain, uterus and ovary.

The adrenal glands

Starter questions

Answers to the following questions are on page 64.

12. Why do people with absent or non-functioning adrenal glands crave salt?
13. Why is adrenaline not replaced when the adrenal glands are removed?

An adrenal gland lies above each kidney. The adrenal glands have two distinct layers: the cortex and the medulla (**Figure 1.24**). The outer cortex comprises three functionally different layers that secrete different hormones:

- the zona glomerulosa
- the zona fasciculata
- the zona reticularis

The adrenal medulla is at the centre of the gland and forms part of the sympathetic nervous system, which activates the fight or flight response and produces the catecholamines adrenaline (epinephrine) and noradrenaline (norepinephrine).

Adrenal gland in cross-section

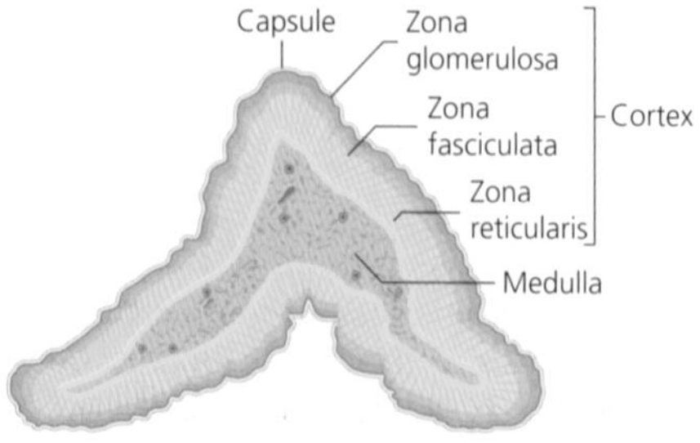

Figure 1.24 Cross-section of the adrenal gland.

Embryology

The two layers of the adrenal gland have different embryological origins.

- The adrenal medulla develops from cells of the neural crest
- The adrenal cortex develops from the mesoderm (the middle germinal layer between the ectoderm and the endoderm and formed in early embryonic life)

Failure of the cortex, and occasionally the medulla, to develop is called adrenal agenesis. If the condition is bilateral, it can lead to life-threatening cortisol deficiency at birth. It can also be associated with ipsilateral renal agenesis.

Anatomy

Each gland weighs about 5 g and is 5 cm long, 3 cm wide and 1 cm thick. The adrenal glands look yellow because of their high cholesterol content; cholesterol is the substrate for lipid hormone production. Each adrenal gland is surrounded by a protective lipid-rich capsule.

Arterial supply

The adrenal glands are highly vascular organs; they require a good blood supply

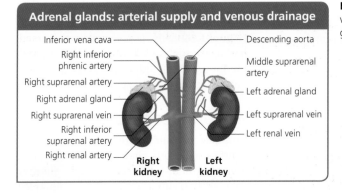

Adrenal glands: arterial supply and venous drainage

Inferior vena cava
Right inferior phrenic artery
Right suprarenal artery
Right adrenal gland
Right suprarenal vein
Right inferior suprarenal artery
Right renal artery

Descending aorta
Middle suprarenal artery
Left adrenal gland
Left suprarenal vein
Left renal vein

Right kidney   **Left kidney**

Figure 1.25 Arterial supply and venous drainage of the adrenal glands (anterior view).

because of their high metabolic rate. The glands receive blood from three suprarenal arteries (**Figure 1.25**):

- the superior suprarenal artery (from a branch of the inferior phrenic artery)
- the middle suprarenal artery (arising from the abdominal aorta)
- the inferior suprarenal artery (arising from the renal artery)

Venous drainage

Venous drainage arises from the adrenal medulla and continues through the adrenal vein. The suprarenal vein drains into the inferior vena cava on the right and into the renal vein on the left (see **Figure 1.26**).

> During adrenal venous sampling to detect ipsilateral aldosterone excess, an intravenous catheter is passed from the femoral vein up the inferior vena cava. The acute angle of the right suprarenal vein means that it can be technically challenging to pass the catheter into the right suprarenal vein.

Innervation

Innervation of the adrenal glands arises mainly from the coeliac plexus and splanchnic nerves. Innervation of the adrenal medulla is by preganglionic sympathetic autonomic fibres that synapse directly with the chromaffin cells (catecholamine-secreting cells) rather than synapsing in the coeliac ganglion. This feature permits very rapid conversion of autonomic signals to a systemic catecholamine response (often termed the 'fight or flight' response).

Acetylcholine is the neurotransmitter released from the autonomic fibres. On stimulation of the sympathetic nerves, catecholamines are released directly into the systemic circulation through the medullary vein.

Innervation of the adrenal cortex comes from postganglionic sympathetic adrenergic nerves.

Histology

The boundaries of the three layers of the adrenal cortex are not easily distinguishable, and some function is shared within each layer.

- The zona glomerulosa columnar cells secrete mineralocorticoids and tend to be arranged in irregular rows
- The polyhedral cells of the zona fasciculata have pale-staining cytoplasm because of their high lipid content and secrete mainly glucocorticoids (cholesterol is required for glucocorticoid hormone synthesis)
- In the zona reticularis, there are fewer lipid droplets, and the cells mainly produce androgens

The histologically distinct adrenal medulla consists of many columnar-shaped chromaffin cells oriented around medullary veins, into which they secrete catecholamines. The cytoplasm of these cells is granular; the granules contain stored peptide hormone.

Unlike the adrenal cortex, the adrenal medulla contains little lipid.

There is extensive sympathetic nervous innervation.

Physiology

The three layers of the adrenal cortex and the adrenal medulla control a wide range of physiological processes through the production of steroid and amine hormones, respectively.

■ Mineralocorticoids (e.g. aldosterone) from the zona glomerulosa reduce the excretion of sodium and in favour of potassium from the kidney and increase blood pressure
■ Glucocorticoids (e.g. cortisol) from the zona fasciculata control the metabolism of carbohydrate, fats and protein
■ Adrenal androgens from the zona reticularis are less influential than sex hormone production from the adult gonads but help promote the development of secondary sexual characteristics such as hair growth and adrenarche (the early stage of development before puberty)

Catecholamines such as adrenaline (epinephrine) and noradrenaline (norepinephrine) from the adrenal medulla rapidly bind to adrenergic receptors in several systems, including the heart, lungs, blood vessels, skeletal muscle and liver. They prepare these systems for 'fight or flight' by increasing heart rate and contractility, blood flow to muscles and glucose production by the liver.

Cholesterol is the lipid precursor of all hormones produced by the adrenal cortex. Cholesterol undergoes multiple stages of enzymatic metabolism (alterations in chemical structure) to produce many functionally distinct hormones. Thus from a small number of chemical precursors a huge variety of hormones are produced, from cortisol to sex hormones to aldosterone (**Figure 1.26a**).

Inherited enzymatic deficiencies can block production of some hormones in the pathway for steroid hormone synthesis and thus cause their precursors to accumulate. For example, 21-hydroxylase deficiency results in a build-up of progesterone, the precursor for the production of adrenal androgens. This leads to excessive testosterone, which causes the symptoms of congenital adrenal hyperplasia (**Figure 1.26b**). The prenatal accumulation of androgens such as testosterone can result in the formation of ambiguous genitalia apparent in affected females at birth.

Mineralocorticoids

Mineralocorticoids are lipid hormones synthesised from cholesterol in the zona glomerulosa of the adrenal cortex. Aldosterone is the primary endogenous mineralocorticoid and regulates blood pressure. Other hormones that are not classified as mineralocorticoids, such as cortisol, can have weak mineralocorticoid activity and have a role in salt and water balance (the blood contains a much higher concentration of cortisol than of aldosterone).

Actions

Aldosterone causes extracellular volume expansion and increases blood pressure by enhancing active sodium reabsorption in the distal renal tubules, thus increasing sodium concentration outside the tubules and promoting passive water reabsorption.

Secretion

The mineralocorticoid aldosterone is regulated by a feedback mechanism called the renin–angiotensin–aldosterone system (**Figure 1.27**). Renin is produced by specialised juxtaglomerular cells in the kidney in response to low renal perfusion and low circulating blood volume. Renin stimulates the conversion of angiotensinogen to angiotensin I. In the lungs and other tissues, angiotensin I is then converted by angiotensin-converting enzyme to angiotensin II.

Angiotensin I is biologically inactive and therefore an intermediate chemical in this pathway. In contrast, angiotensin II has strong vasopressor actions; it increases blood pressure through vasoconstriction, by increasing sympathetic activity and augmenting the secretion of ADH from the posterior pituitary gland. Angiotensin II also stimulates the zona glomerulosa of the adrenal gland to produce aldosterone.

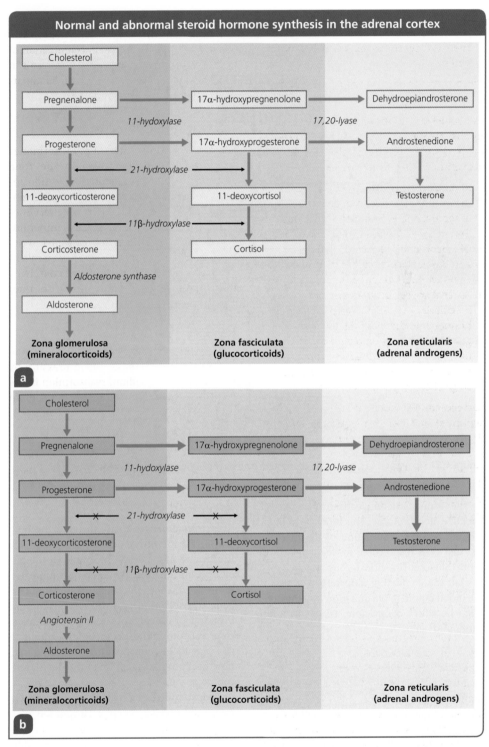

Figure 1.26 Steroid hormone synthesis in the adrenal cortex. (a) Normal steroid hormone synthesis.
Enzyme names are italicised. (b) Steroid hormone synthesis in cases of 21-hydroxlase deficiency, which
results in reduced aldosterone and cortisol synthesis (red) and increased adrenal androgen synthesis (green).
These effects underlie the symptoms of congenital adrenal hyperplasia.

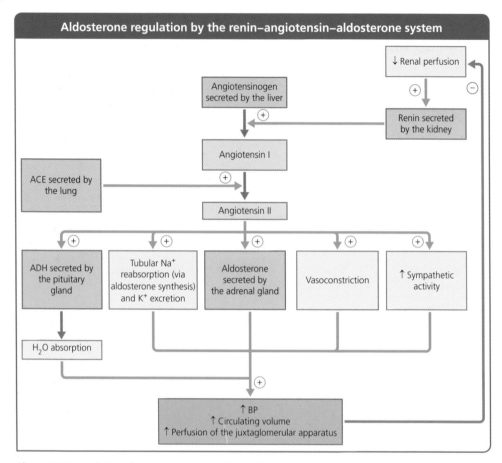

Figure 1.27 Regulation of aldosterone production by the renin–angiotensin–aldosterone system.

The vasoconstriction leads to an increase in effective blood volume. This increase in blood volume reduces stimulation of the juxtaglomerular cells responsible for feedback in the renin–angiotensin–aldosterone system.

Half the circulating aldosterone travels in the blood bound to plasma proteins. The other half, the active component, travels in a free (unbound) state.

> **Drugs that inhibit the renin–angiotensin–aldosterone system are used to reduce blood pressure in patients with hypertension.** Antihypertensive agents include angiotensin-converting enzyme inhibitors, angiotensin II receptor blockers and aldosterone antagonists.

Receptor

Aldosterone passes easily through the lipophilic cell membrane to act intracellularly. Binding to aldosterone receptors in the cell cytoplasm enables the receptor-bound hormone to pass into the cell nucleus, the site of gene transcription and protein production. Proteins produced in response to aldosterone receptor binding include subunits of the Na^+-K^+-H^+ cotransporter, which facilitates sodium reabsorption in the distal renal tubule.

Aldosterone has a high affinity (attraction) for the aldosterone receptor. However, cortisol also binds to the aldosterone receptor with high affinity. Therefore to prevent overstimulation of the aldosterone receptor by the more abundant cortisol, the enzyme 11b-hydroxysteroid dehydrogenase coverts cortisol to inactive cortisone in the tissues. Cortisone does not bind at the aldosterone receptor.

Glucocorticoids

Glucocorticoids are lipid hormones produced in the zona fasciculata of the adrenal cortex. Like other adrenal hormones, glucocorticoids are synthesised from cholesterol.

The glucocorticoids have a key role in carbohydrate, protein and lipid metabolism. Although the body produces other glucocorticoids and their metabolites (such as corticosterone), cortisol is the most biologically active and therefore the most important in terms of function.

Actions

Cortisol has the following physiological effects, which occur continuously with its secretion:

- It facilitates hepatic gluconeogenesis (glucose production) by mobilising amino acid and lipid stores, which are used in the liver to synthesise glucose; other biological stimuli, such as the release of adrenaline (epinephrine) and glucagon in response to hypoglycaemia, trigger gluconeogenesis
- Cortisol inhibits glucose uptake in extrahepatic tissues such as muscle
- Cortisol inhibits protein synthesis
- It reduces inflammatory processes

Cortisol secretion is increased at times of physiological and psychological stress. By ensuring a ready supply of glucose and down-regulating unnecessary body processes (such as inflammation), cortisol maximises energy supplies to deal with the stressor.

Synthetic glucocorticoids ('steroids') are one of the most commonly prescribed groups of drugs, and are used for their anti-inflammatory and immunosuppressive properties. Different glucocorticoids suppress the immune system to different extents; methylprednisolone is the most powerful suppressor and hydrocortisone is the weakest.

Secretion

The secretion of cortisol is related to the release of ACTH from the anterior pituitary gland (**Figure 1.28**). ACTH production is stimulated by CRH from the hypothalamus, and the released ACTH stimulates cortisol secretion. Therefore ACTH release, which is pulsatile, results in pulsatile cortisol secretion (**Figure 1.29**).

There is a circadian rhythm to the release of ACTH and cortisol; they are highest in the early morning and lowest at about midnight (**Figure 1.29**).

Physical and emotional stress increase CRH and ACTH production, so cortisol levels increase in consequence. A negative feedback loop means that ACTH production decreases when cortisol increases.

Cortisol is mainly metabolised in the liver, where the hormone undergoes hydroxylation

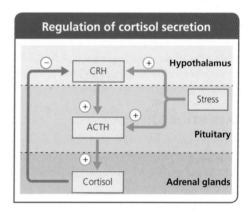

Figure 1.28 Regulation of cortisol secretion. ACTH, adrenocorticotrophic hormone; CRH, corticotrophin-releasing hormone.

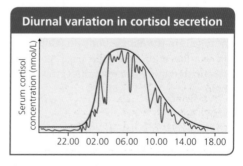

Figure 1.29 Pulsatile cortisol secretion with diurnal variation.

(addition of a hydroxyl group, –OH). Hydroxylation produces its inactive metabolite, cortisone, which is then excreted by the kidneys.

Transport

About 90% of the body's cortisol is bound in the blood to corticosteroid-binding globulin and albumin. The remaining 10% is in the blood in a free state, in which the hormone can pass into cells and is therefore biologically active. Bound cortisol functions as a reservoir of the hormone and balances the clearance of cortisol by preventing enzymatic metabolism to less active or inactive metabolites.

Receptor

Like aldosterone, lipophilic cortisol is able to pass freely through the lipid-rich cell membrane. Once in the cell, the hormone binds to a cytoplasmic glucocorticoid receptor. The cortisol–glucocorticoid receptor complex then enters the cell nucleus by passive diffusion. In the nucleus, the complex binds to specific glucocorticoid response elements on DNA to promote gene expression and protein transcription. These effects on DNA underlie the biological effects of cortisol.

Adrenal androgens

Adrenal androgens are a group of related steroid hormones synthesised in the zona reticularis of the adrenal cortex. The main adrenal androgens are:

- dehydroepiandrosterone (DHEA)
- DHEA sulphate
- androstenedione

The exact role of and control mechanisms for adrenal androgens are unclear. However, they promote sexual maturation, and as the major androgens in the female body (in addition to the ovarian androgens; see page 59), their presence is required for pubic hair growth and libido.

Actions

The zona reticularis, where adrenal androgens are synthesised, enlarges during childhood as part of sexual maturation. Adrenal androgens are produced in increasing quantities from the age of 7 years until puberty. These hormones are responsible for adrenarche, a stage of development that includes the growth of pubic and armpit hair and skin changes such as oily skin (and consequently acne). Adrenarche precedes the release of sex hormones from the gonads that occur at puberty.

In women, the adrenal gland is a major source of androgens. Less androstenedione is secreted than DHEA and DHEA sulphate, but it is more readily converted to testosterone and dihydrotestosterone. These converted adrenal androgens have clearer physiological roles; they bind to the testosterone receptor to exert their effects on pubic hair growth and libido.

In men, the physiological role of adrenal androgens is unknown, because it seems unnecessary for adrenal androgens to be produced given the large quantities of androgens produced by the male testes.

Secretion

Adrenal androgens are produced in response to stimulation by ACTH. Therefore production of adrenal androgens, like that of cortisol, has a circadian rhythm.

In the liver, metabolism of adrenal androgens results in their biological inactivation, and the breakdown products are rendered more water-soluble to permit urinary excretion from the kidneys.

Most adrenal androgen in the body is transported bound to albumin; only a small amount is bound to the sex hormone–binding globulin. The remainder is free in the plasma.

Receptors

Adrenal androgens are biologically inactive. To become active, they must be converted to testosterone and dihydrotestosterone; these reactions occur in peripheral tissues such as the skin.

Testosterone and dihydrotestosterone are lipophilic, so they passively enter the cell through the cell membrane. In the cytoplasm, testosterone binds to the androgen receptor. Subsequently, the hormone–androgen receptor complex enters the nucleus passively, by diffusion, where it results in gene transcription and protein synthesis.

Catecholamines

The amine hormones adrenaline (epinephrine) and noradrenaline (norepinephrine) are the main catecholamines produced in the adrenal medulla. The adrenal medulla responds directly to sympathetic nervous impulses to release preformed adrenaline (80%) and noradrenaline (20%), as well as a small amount of dopamine.

Adrenaline and noradrenaline are monoamine hormones synthesised from the amino acids phenylalanine and tyrosine. They act as both neurotransmitters and endocrine hormones.

Adrenaline and noradrenaline are released rapidly to increase available glucose, as well as cardiac output, blood pressure and blood supply to the muscles, in readiness for 'fight or flight' response.

Actions

Adrenaline and noradrenaline have a multitude of effects throughout the body. They stimulate the adrenergic receptors of the autonomic nervous system. These receptors are usually stimulated by noradrenaline as a neurotransmitter released at the synapses between neurones. However, they are also stimulated by adrenaline and noradrenaline circulating as hormones in the blood.

The physiological effects of adrenaline and noradrenaline are:

- increased heart rate and contractility
- vasoconstriction, leading to increased blood pressure
- increased circulating glucose (through promotion of glycogenolysis and gluconeogenesis in the liver)
- bronchodilation, which increases airflow into the lungs

All these effects prime the body to mobilise blood, glucose and oxygen to the muscles and thus prepare to move immediately and as quickly as possible. This system has evolved to allow humans to escape predators and pursue prey as efficiently as possible.

Secretion

Catecholamine release is entirely managed by the autonomic nervous system; this makes the adrenal medulla a truly neuroendocrine gland. Direct nervous stimulation by the preganglionic sympathetic nerve fibres causes the exocytotic release of preformed adrenaline and noradrenaline (stored in granules in the chromaffin cells of the adrenal medulla) directly into the systemic circulation. This system permits the most rapid response possible, with almost instantaneous effects on the body's physiology.

There is no hormonal feedback to the adrenal glands. Instead, the amount of circulating adrenaline and noradrenaline is limited by their rapid metabolism and inactivation by the enzymes monoamine oxidase and catechol-O-methyltransferase. Once the adrenaline and noradrenaline have enacted their physiological effects, their production is reduced by decreased stimulation of the autonomic nervous system.

Adrenaline and noradrenaline are peptide hormones. Therefore they travel unbound in the systemic circulation.

Receptors

There are four major types of adrenergic receptor (**Table 1.15**). Each receptor has a

Adrenergic receptors: types, locations and actions		
Type	Location	Action
α_1	Venous and arterial smooth muscle	Causes smooth muscle contraction and vasoconstriction
α_2	Presynaptic vascular smooth muscle	Inhibits synaptic release of acetylcholine, thus counteracting the effect of α_1 receptors
β_1	Heart	Increases heart rate, contractility, conduction velocity and relaxation rate
	Kidneys	Increases renin release
β_2	Venous and arterial smooth muscle	Caues vasodilation
	Bronchial smooth muscle in the lungs	Causes bronchodilation
	Liver	Increases glycogenolysis

Table 1.15 Types, locations and actions of adrenergic receptors

different function depending on the tissue in which it is present.

The α adrenergic receptors are G-protein–coupled receptors. The binding of noradrenaline to these receptors causes an inositol triphosphate (second messenger) intracellular chemical cascade leading to vascular smooth muscle contraction.

The β adrenergic receptors are also G-protein–coupled receptors. The binding of noradrenaline to these receptors causes adenylate cyclase to convert ATP into cAMP. The cAMP then triggers various signalling cascades, depending on the tissue type. For example, cAMP

increases Ca^{2+} influx into cardiac myocytes to promote depolarisation and contraction.

Many drugs bind to adrenergic receptors to either agonise or antagonise them. These drugs have a wide range of therapeutic applications and are used to treat many common clinical conditions **(Table 1.16)**. β_2 agonists such as salbutamol are used as bronchodilators, and α_1 antagonists such as doxazosin are used as fit on one line agents.

Adrenergic drugs and their actions

Adrenergic receptor targeted	Action	Clinical use(s)	Example
α_1	Antagonist	Antihypertensive agents	Doxazosin
α_1	Agonist	Pressor agents (produce systemic vasoconstriction)	Phenylephrine
α_2	Agonist	Centrally acting vasodilators or antihypertensive agents	Clonidine
β_1	Antagonist	Antihypertensive agents or negative chronotropes (decrease heart rate)	Bisoprolol
β_1 and β_2	Antagonist	Antihypertensive agents or negative chronotropes	Propranolol
β_2	Agonist	Bronchodilator agents	Salbutamol

Table 1.16 Drugs acting on adrenergic receptors and their actions

The pancreas

Starter questions

Answers to the following questions are on page 64.

14. Why is glucose so important?
15. What is the body's physiological response to low blood glucose?

The pancreas lies towards the back of the abdomen, behind the stomach. It has both endocrine and exocrine functions.

The predominant endocrine roles of the pancreas are the control of blood glucose and the regulation of gut hormones. Pancreatic hormones are produced by the islets of Langerhans. These clusters of hormone-secreting

beta and alpha cells produce two hormones that affect glucose homeostasis:

■ Insulin is secreted from the beta cells in response to increased blood glucose; this hormone stimulates cellular uptake of glucose and amino acids, inhibits gluconeogenesis and promotes protein and fat synthesis

- Glucagon is secreted from the alpha cells in response to hypoglycaemia; it stimulates the conversion of glycogen stored in the liver to glucose

The pancreas secretes exocrine enzymes, which are released into the gut. These enzymes include:

- amylase, which breaks down starch into smaller carbohydrates
- lipase, which breaks down fat
- proteases (trypsin and chymotrypsin), which breakdown proteins

Embryology

The pancreas develops from the endodermal layer. Two buds develop either side of the foregut (the ventral and dorsal side). The ventral bud forms the uncinate process of the pancreas, and the dorsal bud forms the head, body and tail. The two buds fuse at about 7 weeks' gestation, with the two developing ducts combining to form the pancreatic duct.

Developmental abnormalities of the pancreas are rare. They include pancreatic agenesis, abnormal pancreatic fusion, ectopic pancreas and annular pancreas (in which the pancreas forms a ring around the duodenum).

Anatomy

The pancreas is retroperitoneal (behind the fibrous peritoneal cavity). It is posterior to the stomach and anterior to the spine, aorta and inferior vena cava.

The pancreas is 12–15 cm long and has four main regions: the head, the uncinate process, the body and the tail (**Figure 1.30**). The head lies in the curve of the duodenum, and the body crosses over the midline at the level of the L1 vertebra. The tail extends towards the spleen.

The pancreatic duct collects exocrine secretions from the pancreatic acini (secretory sacs formed by clusters of cells). It joins the common bile duct to drain into the duodenum through the sphincter of Oddi.

Because the pancreas is formed by the fusion of two embryological buds, distinct areas of the pancreas are supplied by distinct groups of arteries and veins: those to the head and those to the tail.

Arterial supply

Blood is supplied to different regions of the pancreas by different arteries (see **Figure 1.30**).

The head and uncinate process are supplied by:

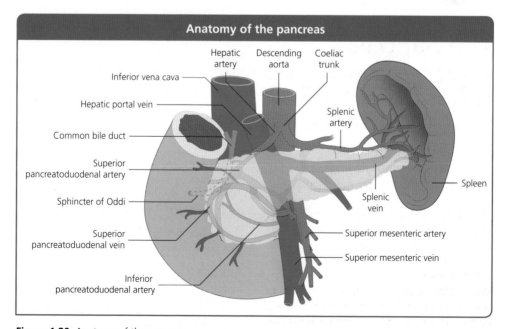

Anatomy of the pancreas

Hepatic artery
Descending aorta
Coeliac trunk
Inferior vena cava
Hepatic portal vein
Common bile duct
Superior pancreatoduodenal artery
Sphincter of Oddi
Superior pancreatoduodenal vein
Inferior pancreatoduodenal artery
Splenic artery
Splenic vein
Spleen
Superior mesenteric artery
Superior mesenteric vein

Figure 1.30 Anatomy of the pancreas.

- the superior pancreatoduodenal artery, a branch of the common hepatic artery from the coeliac trunk
- the inferior pancreatoduodenal artery, a branch of the superior mesenteric artery

The body and tail of the pancreas are supplied by multiple branches of the splenic artery. The inferior border of the pancreas is supplied by the pancreatic artery.

Venous drainage

The superior and inferior pancreatoduodenal veins drain similar areas to their paired arteries: the hepatic portal vein and the superior mesenteric vein, respectively. The remainder of the venous drainage of the pancreas is through numerous branches that drain into the splenic vein.

Innervation

Parasympathetic nervous supply is provided through the coeliac branch of the vagus nerve. Sympathetic innervation arises from the T6–T10 splanchnic and coeliac plexus.

Histology

The endocrine and exocrine cells of the pancreas form different arrangements.

Endocrine cells

The endocrine cells of the pancreas are arranged in irregular collections called islets of Langerhans. The islets are highly vascular; their rich fenestrated capillary bed facilitates the secretion of pancreatic hormones into the systemic circulation.

Two cell types predominate:

- beta cells, which produce insulin
- alpha cells, which produce glucagon

The islets of Langerhans also contain PP cells, which secrete pancreatic polypeptides, and D cells, which secrete somatostatin.

Exocrine cells

Most of the pancreas consists of groups of columnar exocrine cells arranged in acini. Each exocrine cell contains many secretory granules. When the contents of these granules are released, they collect in the acinar lumen (the cavity within each acinus).

The secretions of multiple acini then drain into a series of ducts. The ducts coalesce to form interlobular ducts and ultimately the pancreatic duct.

Physiology

The primary role of insulin and glucagon is to maintain blood glucose concentration within a narrow range. Tight blood glucose homeostasis is vital, because the brain is very sensitive to low blood glucose, which can produce confusion and seizures. The pancreas produces two counter-regulatory hormones with essentially opposite actions.

- Insulin promotes the cellular uptake of glucose and the synthesis of protein and fat
- Glucagon stimulates glucose release from glycogen stores in the liver and promotes the breakdown of protein and lipids to produce glucose

Insulin

Insulin is a peptide hormone comprising 35 amino acids arranged in an A chain and a B chain linked by a disulphide bridge.

Preproinsulin is produced in the rough endoplasmic reticulum of pancreatic beta cells. This molecule is cleaved rapidly by proteolytic enzymes into proinsulin. The insulin molecule is then created by cleavage of the C chain from the larger proinsulin molecule. This process produces equal amounts of insulin and C-peptide (**Figure 1.31**).

> C-peptide is measured in the blood and urine of patients to assess the production of endogenous insulin. C-peptide is a useful clinical marker, because insulin itself is difficult to measure; most insulin is metabolised as it passes through the liver.

Actions

Insulin is an anabolic (growth-promoting) hormone with various effects on different tissues (e.g. muscles and adipose tissues). Insulin

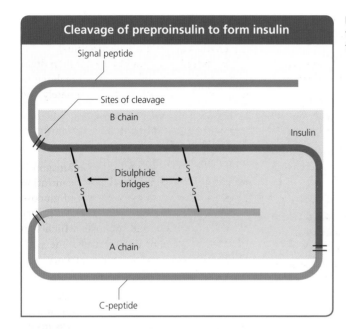

Cleavage of preproinsulin to form insulin

Signal peptide

Sites of cleavage

B chain

Insulin

S S

Disulphide bridges

S S

A chain

C-peptide

Figure 1.31 Sites of cleavage on the preproinsulin molecule to form the insulin molecule.

Physiological effects of insulin over time

Timing of effect(s)	Effect(s)	Location(s)
Immediate	Transports glucose and amino acids to the intracellular space	Liver, muscle and adipose tissue
Intermediate	Promotes glycogen synthesis and inhibits gluconeogenesis	Liver
	Increases lipogenesis and protein synthesis	Liver, muscle and adipose tissue
Long term	Stimulates cell growth and division	Liver, muscle and adipose tissue

Table 1.17 The physiological effects of insulin over time

reduces blood glucose after a meal and promotes its storage in tissues; it also increases synthesis of both protein and fat (**Table 1.17**).

Secretion

Glucose is the major stimulus for insulin secretion from the endocrine pancreas. Other factors that regulate insulin secretion are listed in **Table 1.18**.

Control of insulin secretion occurs through the following steps:

1. Glucose in the blood enters the pancreatic beta cell through the glucose transporter 2 protein
2. Once inside the beta cell, glucose is oxidised by the glucokinase protein, which acts as a glucose sensor

Factors affecting insulin release

Stimulatory	Inhibitory
Glucose and fructose	Hypoglycaemia
Amino acids	Hormones, such as adrenaline (epinephrine), noradrenaline (norepinephrine) and somatostatin
Fatty acids	
Hormones, such as growth hormone, glucagon and glucagon-like peptide-1	
Drugs, such as sulfonylureas	Drugs, such as diazoxide

Table 1.18 Factors affecting insulin release

3. If serum glucose concentration is >5 mmol/L, insulin is released from the beta cell

Insulin secretion from the pancreas occurs in two phases:

- Phase 1 insulin secretion is rapid: preformed insulin stored in Golgi granules is released within seconds
- Phase 2 insulin secretion occurs in response to cAMP activation in the minutes after stimulation

High blood glucose stimulates insulin release from the pancreas; low or decreasing blood glucose inhibits it.

> Genetic abnormalities of glucokinase enzyme, the 'glucose sensor', lead to an increased glucose set point. The condition causes mild hyperglycaemia and is characterised by increased fasting glucose concentration with a small increase in postprandial glucose. Glucokinase diabetes may be mistaken for other types of diabetes, such as gestational diabetes and type 2 diabetes.

Receptors

Insulin receptors are present in many body tissues, including hepatic, muscle and adipose tissue. Each of these transmembrane receptors consists of an α subunit and a β subunit.

Insulin has high affinity for its receptor. Binding of insulin activates tyrosine kinase in the β subunit of the receptor, an effect that triggers a cascade of intracellular phosphorylation in the target cell. As a result, the glucose transporter 4 protein is transferred from the cytoplasm to the cell membrane. Once inserted into the cell membrane, the glucose transporter 4 protein is activated, i.e. able to carry extracellular glucose into the cell.

As the cells absorb glucose through the glucose transporter 4-mediated movement of glucose from the blood into the cells, blood glucose concentration decreases.

Transport

Insulin is transported away from the pancreas in the portal system. It first arrives at the liver before being carried more widely in the systemic circulation to induce its more distal effects. Insulin travels freely in the circulation in an unbound form.

Clearance

About 70% of endogenous insulin is metabolised in the liver during first pass (hepatic metabolism resulting in reduced concentration before reaching systemic circulation). Endogenous insulin is that made in the body, as opposed to exogenous insulin, which is injected as a therapy for diabetes mellitus.

A high glucose concentration reduces insulin metabolism in the liver. This effect allows greater insulin activity in the systemic circulation.

The remaining insulin in the systemic circulation is removed from the body by hepatic clearance as well as renal excretion into the urine.

Glucagon

Glucagon is a peptide hormone comprising a single chain of 29 amino acids. It is the counter-regulatory hormone to insulin; insulin decreases blood glucose whereas glucagon increases it. The equilibrium between insulin and glucagon maintains euglycaemia (normal blood glucose concentration).

The release of glucagon from the alpha cells of the islets of Langerhans is stimulated by hypoglycaemia and high amino acid concentration.

Actions

Glucagon acts predominantly in the liver to stimulate glycogenolysis (production of glucose from glycogen stores). Glucagon also induces hepatic gluconeogenesis from non-carbohydrate stores such as amino acids. Its non-hepatic actions include stimulating the breakdown of lipids to provide an alternative energy source through ketogenesis (production of ketone bodies).

> Glucagon is used to treat severe hypoglycaemia, because it causes the rapid release of glucose from hepatic glycogen stores. Glucagon is used to treat hypoglycaemia in patients unable to take oral glucose, for example those with a reduced level of consciousness.

Secretion

Glucagon is produced in pancreatic alpha cells from proglucagon. Proglucagon is also expressed in the intestine. This precursor molecule is cleaved to form other peptide hormones in addition to glucagon: these are the glucagon-like peptides-1 and -2.

In contrast to the biphasic release of insulin, glucagon is released gradually in the blood stream after a meal. Glucagon release is inhibited by high blood glucose concentration and insulin. Glucagon travels freely in the circulation in an unbound form.

Receptor

The glucagon receptor is a G-protein–coupled receptor. It is expressed throughout the body, but its predominant role is in the liver and pancreas.

Somatostatin

Somatostatin is a peptide hormone produced by the D cells of the pancreas. However, the factors that stimulate its release are poorly understood.

The hormone inhibits release of both insulin and glucagon. Other effects include reducing gastrin production, gastric emptying and splanchnic blood flow to the intestine.

Pancreatic polypeptide

This peptide hormone is produced by the PP cells of the pancreas in response to the ingestion of food. The actions of pancreatic polypeptide reduce pancreatic exocrine activity, gastric motility and gall bladder activity. It may also suppress appetite.

The gut

Starter questions

The answer to the following question is on page 64.

16. Why does oral glucose cause more insulin secretion than intravenous glucose?

The human intestinal walls contain many endocrine cells, which secrete a wide range of hormones. Many help regulate digestion and glucose homeostasis. Endocrine cells in the walls of the small intestine secrete incretin hormones in response to food. These decrease gut motility and appetite, and increase insulin secretion.

Apart from incretin hormones, the following hormones are also secreted from the gut:

- Gastrin: a peptide hormone that causes gastric acid secretion and aids gastric motility
- Vasoactive intestinal peptide: this hormone stimulates the secretion of water and electrolytes from the intestinal mucosa and into the bowel
- Ghrelin: this is secreted by the intestinal wall in response to fasting, and communicates a hunger signal to the hypothalamus

Incretin hormones

The incretins are polypeptide hormones. The two identified incretin hormones are:

- Glucagon-like peptide-1: this hormone is derived from glucagon precursors; it is released in response to food ingestion and augments insulin release, slows gastric emptying and provides a satiety signal to the hypothalamus
- Glucose-dependent insulinotrophic polypeptide (also known as gastric

inhibitory polypeptide): this hormone also augments insulin secretion from the pancreas

Actions

Incretin hormones increase insulin secretion in response to high blood glucose. Thus they reduce glucose concentration after a meal. Other effects of glucagon-like peptide-1 are shown in **Table 1.19**.

Secretion

The incretins are secreted by different cells:

Effects of glucagon-like peptide-1	
Organ	Effect
Pancreas	Increases insulin secretion
	Increases beta-cell proliferation
	Reduces beta-cell apoptosis
Gastrointestinal tract	Reduces gastric emptying
Brain	Increases satiety
Liver	Reduces glucose production
Muscle	Increases insulin sensitivity

Table 1.19 Physiological effects of glucagon-like peptide-1

- Glucagon-like peptide-1 is secreted by the L cells (specialised endocrine cells) of the small and large intestine
- Glucose-dependent insulinotrophic polypeptide is secreted from the K cells (specialised endocrine cells) of the small intestine

Production of the incretin hormones is glucose-dependent; more incretin is released as blood glucose increases.

The 'incretin effect' is the increased release of insulin when glucose is administered enterally (for ingestion in the gut) rather than intravenously (thereby bypassing the stomach) (**Figure 1.32a**). This phenomenon is caused by the effects of glucagon-like peptide-1 and glucose-dependent insulinotrophic polypeptide, neither of which is released when glucose is administered intravenously.

> The incretin effect is much less apparent in people with type 2 diabetes mellitus (**Figure 1.32b**). The reduced incretin effect contributes to increased blood glucose concentration. New therapies have been developed to increase incretin levels in this patient group (see page 65).

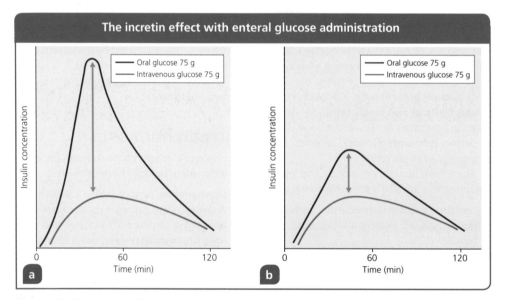

Figure 1.32 The 'incretin effect'. (a) In people with normal glucose metabolism, insulin release is increased when glucose is administered orally as opposed to intravenously. (b) This incretin effect is much reduced in people with type 2 diabetes mellitus.

Transport and clearance

The incretins are transported in the blood in their unbound form, because they are water-soluble. Both glucagon-like peptide-1 and glucose-dependent insulinotrophic polypeptide are rapidly metabolised by the enzyme dipeptidyl peptidase-4. This process produces inactive metabolites of glucagon-like peptide-1 and glucose-dependent insulinotrophic polypeptide.

Receptors

Both glucagon-like peptide-1 and glucose-dependent insulinotrophic polypeptide bind to G-protein–coupled receptors that are expressed in the pancreas (where they increase insulin secretion) and other non-endocrine tissues (where they decrease gut motility or appetite).

Gastrin

Gastrin is a peptide hormone synthesised from preprogastrin in the wall of the stomach, near the pylorus. It is stored in secretory granules in G cells (gastrin-secreting cells).

Secretion of gastrin is stimulated by dilation of the intestinal wall by food, as well as by vagal nerve impulses. The hormone stimulates secretion of gastric acid by the stomach's parietal cells.

Vasoactive intestinal peptide

Vasoactive intestinal peptide is widely produced in the digestive tract, pancreas and central nervous system. This peptide hormone has several neuroendocrine effects:

- It causes vasodilation, thus slowing blood flow in the intestine
- It causes contraction of smooth muscle in the gut
- It increases secretion of water and electrolytes from the gut epithelial cells

Ghrelin levels are markedly increased by an unknown mechanism in people with Prader–Willi syndrome. This syndrome is characterised by obesity and excessive appetite, as well as learning difficulties.

Ghrelin

Ghrelin is a peptide hormone produced in the stomach and intestinal wall. Its levels increase in the fasting state, thus communicating a hormonal hunger signal to the brain. Ghrelin acts on receptors that are widely expressed in the hypothalamus, anterior pituitary gland and other areas of the brain.

The male reproductive system

Starter questions

Answers to the following questions are on page 64.

17. Is there a male menopause?
18. Why do the testes sit outside the abdomen?

Hormones released by the male reproductive endocrine system promote sexual maturation, determine sexual behaviour and facilitate the production of gametes.

The system comprises:

- the hypothalamic–pituitary–gonadal axis
- the testicles
- the adrenal glands

The testes are the major site for androgen (testosterone) production in the male endocrine reproductive system. By the time of birth, the anatomical reproductive system organs are complete. The reproductive organs undergo growth and maturation during puberty.

The roles of the testis are to:

- secrete testosterone to maintain male secondary sexual characteristics and libido
- produce gametes, in the form of spermatozoa

Spermatozoa are transmitted through the penis to the uterus. In the uterus, a single spermatozoon fertilises an ovum to create a zygote in the process of sexual reproduction.

Embryology

The male reproductive system develops throughout the embryonic and fetal stages, infancy and childhood before sexual maturity is reached at puberty.

0-6 weeks

Embryological development of the reproductive system is initially the same in males and females (**Figure 1.33**); the so-called indeterminate phase of development persists for the first 6 weeks of life. Were it not for the effect of SRY (sex-determining region Y), a gene on the short arm of the Y chromosome that determines testis formation and male phenotype, all embryos would develop into females by default.

The reproductive system begins as a layer of mesoderm. The mesoderm develops into long nephrogenic cords (precursors of the urogenital tract) that give rise to the reproductive organs as well as the urinary tract and kidneys, whose development is closely associated with that of the reproductive system.

7–13 weeks

At 7 weeks, the SRY gene produces the SRY protein, which differentiates the two sexes by facilitating development of the male testes and inhibiting development of the ovaries and female external genitalia.

Differentiation of cells in the developing testes leads to formation of different tissue types.

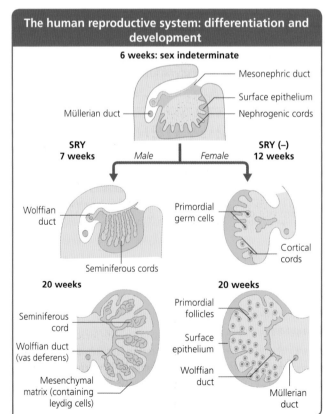

Figure 1.33 Differentiation and development of the human reproductive system

The human reproductive system: differentiation and development

6 weeks: sex indeterminate

Mesonephric duct
Surface epithelium
Müllerian duct
Nephrogenic cords

SRY 7 weeks — Male — Female — SRY (–) 12 weeks

Wolffian duct
Primordial germ cells
Seminiferous cords
Cortical cords

20 weeks

Seminiferous cord
Wolffian duct (vas deferens)
Mesenchymal matrix (containing leydig cells)

20 weeks

Primordial follicles
Surface epithelium
Wolffian duct
Müllerian duct

- Sertoli cells produce antimüllerian hormone, which inhibits development of the müllerian duct (the embryological precursor of the female uterus)
- Leydig cells also produce hormones, the androgens testosterone and androstenedione

Thus this combination of antimüllerian, testosterone and androstenedione hormones determines male sex.

14 weeks to term

The testes form in the abdominal cavity. Their descent through the abdomen occurs between 14 and 23 weeks of gestation. At 24 weeks, the testes enter the inguinal canal and descend to the scrotum. The testes are fully descended by 35 weeks.

Anatomy

The male reproductive organs comprise the two testes and the penis (**Table 1.20** and **Figure 1.34**).

- The testes synthesise androgens and produce spermatozoa
- The penis introduces spermatozoa into the vagina during sexual intercourse; this may lead to fertilisation of the ovum

Anatomy of the male reproductive system	
Organ	Function(s)
Testes	Spermatogenesis (spermatozoa production) and androgen production
Epididymis	Through contraction of the epidydimal wall, transmission of spermatozoa into the vas deferens on ejaculation
Pampiniform plexus	A network of veins surrounding the testes and epididymis, which in addition to venous return from the testes, also helps temperature regulation of the testes
Vas deferens	Transports spermatozoa from the testes to the penis
Prostate	Secretes prostate fluid which is a component of seminal fluid
Seminal vesicles	Secretes and stores lubricating fluid to accompany the spermatozoa in semen
Prostate	Secretes an alkaline fluid into semen to neutralise the acidity of the female reproductive tract and prolong spermatozoa survival
Urethra	Transmits spermatozoa through the penis on ejaculation
	Transports urine from the bladder during excretion
Penis	Contains an expandable, highly vascular bed of arterioles (the corpus cavernosum) that cause the penis to become erect on stimulation

Table 1.20 Parts of the male reproductive systems and their roles

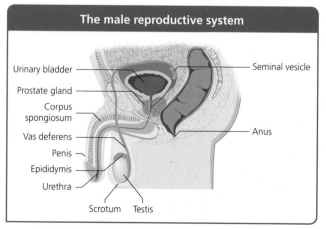

The male reproductive system

Urinary bladder
Prostate gland
Corpus spongiosum
Vas deferens
Penis
Epididymis
Urethra
Scrotum   Testis
Seminal vesicle
Anus

Figure 1.34 The male reproductive system.

Arterial supply

Blood supply to the penis is determined by the embryological origin of the testes before they descend. Therefore blood supplied to the penis is superior in origin.

The testicular arteries arise directly from the abdominal aorta inferior to the renal arteries. They pass in the retroperitoneal space, then through the inguinal canal to the testes.

The deep structures of the penis are supplied by the internal pudendal artery, a branch of the femoral artery.

Venous drainage

The testicular veins drain blood from the pampiniform plexus.

■ The right testicular vein drains into the inferior vena cava
■ The left testicular vein drains into the left renal vein

Blood from the penis drains through the superficial, intermediate and deep venous systems. The deep system drains into the internal pudendal veins.

Innervation

Nervous supply to the penis is both autonomic and somatic (sensory and motor nerves). The testes receive autonomic innervation.

Autonomic nervous supply to the penis

The autonomic fibres determine whether the penis is flaccid or erect.

■ Nitric oxide is the major mediator of penile erection; it relaxes smooth muscle in the arteriole wall, and the resulting arteriolar dilation allows more blood to flow into the penis, making it tumescent and erect
■ Sympathetic nervous stimulation of the vascular smooth muscle causes vasoconstriction, thus reducing blood flow to the penis, which then becomes flaccid

There are two sources of nitric oxide. The synapses of parasympathetic nerves innervating the smooth muscle release nitric oxide as a neurotransmitter to elicit its effects directly.

Nitric oxide is also synthesised in the smooth muscle walls of the arterioles in response to stimulation by acetylcholine secreted from parasympathetic nerves.

Somatic nervous supply to the penis

Somatic fibres provide the penis with sensation. They also stimulate its non-vascular muscles to contract.

Autonomic nervous supply to the testes

The testes are supplied by autonomic nerves (both sympathetic and parasympathetic). The parasympathetic stimulation results in vasodilation and erection, while the sympathetic stimulation causes vasoconstriction and ejaculation.

Histology

The testes comprise multiple lobes containing seminiferous tubules, which produce spermatozoa. The tubules are folded into convolutions (coils) to increase their internal surface area.

The seminiferous tubules contain several cell types (**Figure 1.35**):

■ germ cells at various stages of maturation as they develop from spermatogonia (primitive male germ cells) into mature spermatozoa
■ Sertoli cells, which provide nutritional and mechanical support to these cells as they mature to form spermatozoa

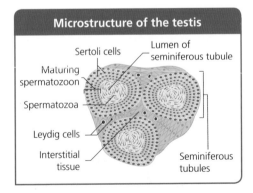

Microstructure of the testis

Sertoli cells

Lumen of seminiferous tubule

Maturing spermatozoon

Spermatozoa

Leydig cells

Interstitial tissue

Seminiferous tubules

Figure 1.35 Microstructure of the testis; there 400–600 seminiferous tubules in each testis.

Outside the tubules is the elastic interstitium. The interstitium contains Leydig cells, which secrete testosterone.

Multiple seminiferous tubules merge to form efferent ducts, which then undergo further merging to form the duct known as vas deferens. It is joined by the duct from the seminal vesicle to form the ejaculatory duct. The ducts transport spermatozoa from the seminiferous tubules to the epididymis and then to the ejaculatory duct.

The ducts are lined with stereocilia, microvilli-like projections that absorb fluid. This absorption creates the fluid current needed to propel the spermatozoa along the ducts.

Physiology

Male sex hormones are called androgens. Testosterone is the main androgen; others include dehydroepiandrosterone, androstenedione and dihydrotestosterone (metabolite of testosterone).

Testosterone

The androgen testosterone is derived from cholesterol. Its major source is the Leydig cells of the testes.

Testosterone has multiple effects in boys and men. For example, it:

- stimulates pubertal development
- underlies development of secondary sexual characteristics
- increases muscle strength
- enhances libido

Furthermore, sufficient quantities of testosterone are necessary for penile erection.

Testosterone is also converted by 5α-reductase to its active metabolite, dihydrotestosterone, in tissues such as the prostate, skin and testes. The conversion of testosterone to dihydrotestosterone is essential in the normal embryonic development of the male reproductive organs.

Deficiency of 5α-reductase results in deficiency of dihydrotestosterone in the embryo causing insufficient development of the reproductive organs. Babies affected by 5α-reductase are genetically male but have ambiguous genitalia.

Secretion

Low-density lipoprotein cholesterol is absorbed by the Leydig cells as the precursor to testosterone production. Testosterone is synthesised as part of the steroid synthesis pathway.

The secretion of testosterone is controlled by a negative feedback system. Pulsatile release of GnRH from the hypothalamus stimulates production of gonadotrophins in the pituitary gland. Gonadotrophin production is inhibited by negative feedback from testosterone, which reduces the release of both GnRH and gonadotrophins.

During embryonic development and infancy, a small amount of testosterone is required for growth and development in the male. Adrenarche is the early stage of sexual maturation in childhood. It is stimulated by production of androgens of adrenal origin (DHEA and DHEA sulphate) rather than those of testicular origin. In males, adrenarche is responsible for the development of adult body odour, early pubic hair growth and greasiness of the skin.

At the initiation of puberty (at an average age of 12–13 years), gonadotrophin-dependent maturation of the testes occurs, and there is a corresponding surge in testosterone production. This results in testicular growth and growth of the penis. The male voice deepens as the vocal cords slacken. There is a surge in height.

Men with a inactivating mutation in the androgen receptor develop with phenotypically female external genitalia and small, undescended testes (pseudohermaphroditism). They appear phenotypically female. Chromosomal analysis confirms the XY karyotype.

Transport

Most testosterone travels in the blood in a bound state, because it is a poorly soluble lipid hormone. Testosterone is bound either to:

- sex hormone–binding globulin (a carrier plasma protein)
- albumin

Testosterone is active only when unbound (in its free state).

Receptor

The androgen receptor has a fivefold higher affinity for dihydrotestosterone than for testosterone. The androgen receptor is a member of the nuclear receptor superfamily, whose members are in the nucleus of target cells. Testosterone and dihydrotestosterone pass through the cell membrane to activate the androgen receptor and thus induce gene transcription.

Actions

The actions of testosterone are outlined in **Table 1.21**. Testosterone is vital in males for sexual differentiation, pubertal development and virilisation. The voice deepens, body fat is reduced, muscle bulk is increased, and fusion of the epiphyses (bone growth plates) is stimulated in response to testosterone.

Actions of testosterone	
Target organ	Action(s)
Testes	Initiates production of spermatozoa
	Promotes maturation of spermatozoa
External genitalia	Stimulates growth and development in the embryo and at puberty
Multiple organs (such as, facial and body hair, larynx, muscles)	Initiate and promote development of secondary sexual characteristics at puberty
Bone	Promote mineralisation
Muscle	Stimulate muscle growth

Table 1.21 Actions of testosterone

The female reproductive system

Starter questions

The answer to the following question is on page 65.

19. Do menstrual cycles synchronise when women live in close proximity?

Hormones produced by the female reproductive system:

- promote sexual maturation
- influence sexual behaviour
- facilitate the production of gametes
- create the ideal conditions for fertilisation of the ova, development of the embryo, and delivery of the baby

The female reproductive system starts to develop during the embryonic stage before progressing through the fetal stage, infancy and childhood until sexual maturity is reached at puberty. In women, the period of fertility is finite, and its end is marked by the menopause.

The female reproductive endocrine system consists of:

- the hypothalamic–pituitary–gonadal axis
- the ovaries and uterus
- the adrenal glands

The female sex hormones, oestrogen and progesterone, are secreted by the ovaries. Their release is regulated by the gonadotrophins (luteinising hormone and FSH), which are produced by anterior pituitary, and GnRH, which is produced by the hypothalamus.

The sex hormones are responsible for sexual maturation in girls. Furthermore, changes in oestrogen and progesterone release produce the cyclical changes in the uterus that make it suitable for implantation of an embryo in the event of fertilisation and the subsequent growth and nourishment of the developing fetus during gestation.

Embryology

The embryological development of female reproductive organs is contingent on the absence of androgens (testosterone and androstenedione) rather than any hormonal action.

The ovarian structures do not begin developing until the 10th week of gestation. They start as primordial follicles, each of which contains an oogonium surrounded by a layer of follicular cells. Each oogonium is derived from a primordial germ cell. The oogonium has the potential to develop into an ovum.

Two million oogonia are formed, but many degrade before adulthood. No further potential ova are produced after the embryological stage.

Anatomy

The following are the key components of the female reproductive system (**Figure 1.36**).

- ovaries
- fallopian tubes
- uterus
- vagina

The roles of these components are shown in **Table 1.22**. Ovaries contain developing ovarian follicles and secrete female sex hormones. The uterus has a rich vascular internal lining (called endometrium) that permits the implantations of a fertilised embryo.

Function of the female reproductive system	
Organ	Function(s)
Ovaries	Contain developing follicles and secrete female sex hormones
Uterus	Hosts the fertilised ovum during gestation
Fallopian tubes (oviducts)	Transport the mature ovum towards the uterus to allow fertilisation by spermatozoa
Vagina	Receives the penis during sexual intercourse, so that spermatozoa can reach the uterus to fertilise the ovum
	Provides a passage for menstrual blood loss
	Acts as a birth canal
Breasts	Secrete milk to nourish the infant

Table 1.22 Parts of the female reproductive systems and their roles

Arterial supply

The female reproductive system has a rich vascular supply. The arterial supply to female reproductive organs are:

- Ovaries: ovarian arteries branch directly off the descending aorta at the level of L2
- Uterus and fallopian tubes: uterine arteries which are braches of the internal iliac arteries and ovarian arteries
- Vagina: vaginal arteries which are branches of the anterior iliac artery

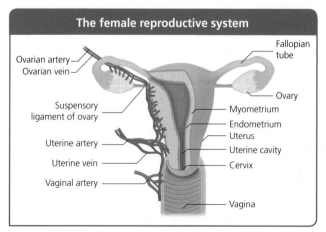

The female reproductive system

Ovarian artery
Ovarian vein
Suspensory ligament of ovary
Uterine artery
Uterine vein
Vaginal artery

Fallopian tube
Ovary
Myometrium
Endometrium
Uterus
Uterine cavity
Cervix
Vagina

Figure 1.36 The female reproductive system

Venous drainage

Venous drainage is provided by the following.

- Ovarian veins: the left ovarian vein drains into the left renal vein, whereas the right ovarian vein drains directly into the inferior vena cava
- Uterine vein: this drains the uterine venous plexus into the internal iliac vein
- Vaginal veins: these veins drain the vaginal venous plexus into the hypogastric veins

Innervation

The ovary, uterus and vagina have complex autonomic innervation with both sympathetic and parasympathetic nerves. Nerve supply to the ovaries runs alongside the vascular supply in the suspensory ligaments.

Histology

The uterus has three layers (**Figure 1.37**).

1. The perimetrium is the outer single layer of mesothelial cells (cells derived from embryonic mesothelium)
2. The myometrium is the middle smooth muscle layer. It is further divided into three layers:

   - outer longitudinal layer, called stratum supra-vascularae
   - the middle vascular layer called stratum vasculare
   - inner longitudinal layer

3. The endometrium is the inner mucous membrane layer, which undergoes cyclical changes in the menstrual cycle
   - The luminal part of the endometrium (the striatum functionalis, further subdivided into the stratum compactum and the stratum spongiosum) is sloughed off during menstruation
   - The deepest layer (the stratum basalis) is retained and serves as the regenerative layer after menstruation

Ovaries have two histological layers: the outer cortex and the inner medulla (**Figure 1.38**). The ovarian cortex contains developing ovarian follicles, whereas the medulla contains a rich vascular bed.

> **A minority of ovarian tumours (5–10%) are associated with hormone production.** Testosterone-secreting tumours may present with hirsutism and male pattern balding. Oestrogen-secreting tumours may present with precocious puberty, abnormal menstrual bleeding or postmenopausal bleeding, depending on the age of the patient.

Physiology

Oestrogen and progesterone are the main female sex hormones. Both of these hormones are secreted by ovaries and play key roles in female reproduction.

Ovarian hormones

The two main hormones secreted by the ovary are oestrogen and progesterone. Ovaries also secrete small amounts of androgens.

The principle hormones secreted by the ovary and their actions are summarised in **Table 1.23**.

Secretion

Oestrogen and progesterone secretion are stimulated by the anterior pituitary hormones

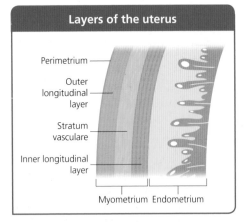

Layers of the uterus

Perimetrium
Outer longitudinal layer
Stratum vasculare
Inner longitudinal layer
Myometrium   Endometrium

Figure 1.37 Layers of the uterus (cross-section). The uterus is divided into three layers: the perimetrium, myometrium and endometrium.

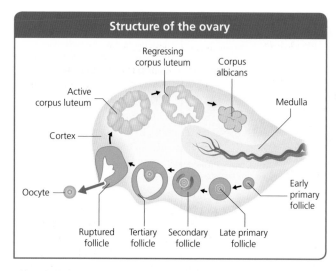

Structure of the ovary

Regressing corpus luteum

Corpus albicans

Active corpus luteum

Medulla

Cortex

Oocyte

Early primary follicle

Ruptured follicle   Tertiary follicle   Secondary follicle   Late primary follicle

Figure 1.38 Structure of the ovaries. Each ovary contains an outer cortex and an inner medulla.

Ovarian hormones

Hormone	Site of production	Action(s)
Oestrogen	Developing follicles and corpus luteum	Inhibits excessive follicle development
		Promotes development of female sex organs at puberty
		Promotes female pattern of fat distribution
Progesterone	Corpus luteum	Helps maintain the endometrium
		Thickens vaginal secretions
		Prepares the breasts for lactation
Androgens	Follicles	Promotes bone mineralisation

Table 1.23 Ovarian hormones and their actions

luteinising hormone and FSH. The release of luteinising hormone and FSH are, in turn, stimulated by the hypothalamic hormone GnRH. Oestrogen has a negative feedback effect on the secretion of luteinising hormone, FSH and GnRH.

Transport

Most oestrogen circulating in the blood is bound to either sex hormone–binding globulin or serum albumin. Only a small proportion of oestrogen (about 1%) circulates as free (unbound) hormone. The unbound oestrogen is the biologically active form of the hormone.

Receptors

As with other steroid hormones, the receptors for both oestrogen and progesterone are predominantly intracellular nuclear receptors. Activation of these receptors by their respective hormones results in gene transcription and protein synthesis, and the consequent hormonal effects.

The menstrual cycle

The menstrual cycle is the series of cyclical changes that the ovaries and uterus undergo to prepare for possible pregnancy (**Figure 1.39**). The onset of menstrual cycles (called menarche) usually occurs at about the age of 12 years.

Menses

Menstrual bleeding marks the start of the menstrual cycle (day 1). When the corpus luteum degenerates at the start of a new monthly cycle (day 1), no oestrogen or progesterone is secreted for a few days. This lack of stimulatory hormones results in contraction of the arterioles supplying the endometrium. Arteriolar

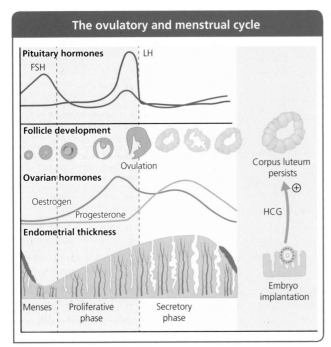

The ovulatory and menstrual cycle

Pituitary hormones — LH, FSH

Follicle development — Ovulation — Corpus luteum persists — HCG

Ovarian hormones — Oestrogen, Progesterone

Endometrial thickness — Embryo implantation

Menses | Proliferative phase | Secretory phase

Figure 1.39 The ovulatory and menstrual cycle. Follicular phase (blue); luteal phase (yellow); fertilisation (orange). FSH, follicular stimulating hormone; HCG, human chorionic gonadotrophin; LH, luteinising hormone.

contraction causes the very rapid necrosis of the superficial two thirds of endometrium, resulting in menstruation. The blood loss lasts about 4 days.

The follicular phase

After menstruation, new ovarian follicles start to develop. FSH stimulates the initial growth of the ovarian follicle. On the subsequent days of the follicular phase, both FSH and luteinising hormone stimulate oestrogen secretion.

Specialised cells (the granulosa and theca cells) surrounding a small number of ova in the ovaries proliferate and secrete oestrogen and fluid-forming follicles. The ova mature in the follicles.

Ovulation

On about day 14 of the cycle, a large amount of luteinising hormone is released from the anterior pituitary; this luteinising hormone surge triggers ovulation.

One of the developing follicles breaks open and releases a mature ovum, ready for fertilisation, into the abdominal cavity. The remaining follicles degenerate rapidly.

The luteal phase

Soon after release of the ovum, the granulosa and theca cells of the follicle enlarge with vascularisation and lipid accumulation (a process known as luteinisation) to become a corpus luteum.

Luteinising hormone stimulates the corpus luteum to produce progesterone and oestrogen. The oestrogen and progesterone secreted by the ovaries thicken the endometrium in preparation for implantation of a fertilised ovum.

The combined oral contraceptive pill contains oestrogen and progesterone, which inhibit the production of GnRH and the gonadotrophins (luteinising hormone and FSH). By inhibiting the cycle of FSH and luteinising hormone, follicular development is blocked. A break of 5 days in the cycle allows a withdrawal bleed, which diminishes the risk of developing endometrial cancer.

- If the ovum is not fertilised, the corpus luteum degenerates after about 14 days. This leads to a rapid drop in oestrogen and progesterone leading to menstrual bleeding
- If fertilisation occurs and the embryo implants into the endometrium, β-human chorionic growth hormone produced by the developing placenta stimulates the corpus luteum to continue to secrete progesterone and oestrogen to support pregnancy

The menopause

The period in which a woman can reproduce is limited. At the age of about 50 years, all ova in the ovaries have either been used or have degenerated in the ovaries, resulting in menopause.

Menopause is the end of reproductive function in the female. The period is associated with cessation of ovulation and the menstrual cycle. The lack of follicles and development of corpus luteum results in a failure of the ovaries to secrete oestrogen and progesterone.

> **Post-menopausal women have high serum concentrations of the gonadotrophins luteinising hormone and FSH.** FSH can be purified from the urine of post-menopausal women and used therapeutically to stimulate follicle development in women with infertility.

The deficiency of oestrogen during menopause often manifests with menopausal symptoms, such as hot flushes, sweating and irritability. The decrease in oestrogen during menopause also results in unopposed increased pituitary secretion of the gonadotrophins (luteinising hormone and FSH).

The pineal gland

Starter questions

The answer to the following question is on page 65.

20. Why does the pineal gland contain light-sensitive cells?

The pineal gland is a small neuroendocrine gland shaped like a pine cone, hence the name ('pineal'). It is inferior to the diencephalon in the brain.

The main role of the pineal gland is nocturnal secretion of the hormone melatonin. Melatonin is the major determinant of the sleep–wake cycle and the internal 'body clock'.

Histology

The pineal gland is about the size of a pine nut. It consists of two cell types: pinocytes and astrocytes.

- Pinocytes (principal cells of the pineal gland) are specialised neuronal cells histologically similar to the rods and cones (light-sensing cells) of the retina
- Astrocytes are star-shaped neuronal cells with long spindle processes that contact pinocytes

The pinocytes receive sympathetic nervous innervation from the retina. Therefore they are able to transfer information on light and dark into a hormonal response in the form of melatonin production.

The astrocytic processes form the infrastructure to which pinocytes are tethered. Astrocytes also form part of the blood–brain barrier.

Physiology

Sympathetic nervous input from the retina controls the main functions of pinocytes: the synthesis and secretion of melatonin into the circulation. Melatonin is synthesised and released during the dark phase of the day–night cycle. Exposure of the eye to light halts melatonin secretion.

The pineal gland, through its production of melatonin, therefore seems necessary for maintenance of the sleep–wake cycle and circadian rhythm. The circadian rhythm is a physiological, psychological and behavioural cycle (lasting 24–25 h) that causes changes in hormone secretion and wakefulness. These actions ensure that:

- physiological processes suited to sleep time, such as growth, occur at night
- those necessary for daytime, such as alertness and easy availability of glucose, occur during the day

> Melatonin is used to treat conditions thought to be caused by disruption of normal circadian rhythm, such as jet lag, primary sleep disturbances and sleep disturbances related to blindness.

Melatonin

Melatonin is an amine hormone. Its production is cyclical across the day–night (light–dark) cycle, being greater at night (**Figure 1.40**).

The normal pattern of melatonin production is disturbed by exposure to bright artificial light during the night. It is also affected by crossing time zones rapidly; for example, long-distance air travel results in jet lag.

Receptors

Melatonin receptors are G-protein–coupled transmembrane receptors. The activated receptors exert their intracellular effects through the second messenger cAMP.

Melatonin is lipophilic. Therefore it passes readily through the cell membrane and probably has biological effects resulting from binding to cytoplasmic or nuclear receptors as well as those on the cell surface.

Both benign and malignant tumours may develop in the pineal gland. The most common of these are germinomas; these develop from embryonic cells that have migrated through midline structures such as the pineal gland.

Disorders of melatonin production occur when the usual sleep–wake cycle is disturbed. This leads to the following conditions:

- jet lag
- shift work disorder
- insomnia in people with poor vision (caused by a failure of light detection)

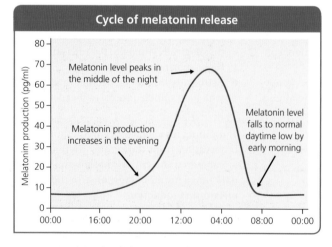

Cycle of melatonin release

Melatonin level peaks in the middle of the night

Melatonin production increases in the evening

Melatonin level falls to normal daytime low by early morning

Melatonim production (pg/ml)

Figure 1.40 The release of melatonin varies over a 24-h period, peaking during the night.

Answers to starter questions

1. Specific hormones, such as sex hormones in women, dramatically reduce over time (menopause). In contrast, the decline decline in male sex hormones with advancing age is more gradual, and whether men go through 'male menopause' is a controversial issue. Other hormones, such as growth hormone, also decline with age. There is also a slow decline in thyroid hormone, cortisol and insulin during the letter years. This decline is part of the aging process rather than being indicative of a disease state.

2. Physical stress from pain, illness or starvation can affect hormone balance, causing levels of cortisol, adrenaline and growth hormone to increase. Prolonged physiological stress leads to the body downregulating certain nonessential systems, such as the reproductive system. This is why menstruation stops in women during extreme physical or psychological hardship.

3. Hormone levels differ widely between individuals and there is no single correct concentration for any hormone. This can make interpreting test results complicated because hormone levels have to be interpreted in the context of the clinical situation. As the normal range for a hormone only covers 95% of the population, normal healthy individuals can still record an abnormal test result.

4. Iodine is essential for the synthesis of thyroid hormone which plays a vital role in the normal development of the fetal nervous system. Severe iodine deficiency in pregnancy (seen in endemic iodine deficient regions) is associated with severe neurological deficit in the offspring, called cretinism. There is evidence that even mild deficiency of dietary iodine during pregnancy is associated with low IQs in babies. Iodine is contained in dairy products, eggs and fish, and in some countries (e.g. the USA) salt is fortified with iodine.

5. Absence of parathyroid glands (congenital or from destruction by surgery), or non-functioning parathyroid glands (autoimmune or through exposure to radiotherapy) have a wide range of clinical effects. The initial symptoms of hypocalcaemia may be mild (such as, twitching or tetany) but these progress to severe neurological events (such as, seizures) or cardiac arrhythmias and, if left untreated, may progress to death.

6. Pigmented skin inhibits the passage of ultraviolet light preventing the synthesis of vitamin D. Individuals with dark skin are more likely to be vitamin D deficient in countries such as the UK where there is less sunlight (especially in winter).

7. Patients who have damage to their hypothalamus (e.g. by stroke, surgery or radiotherapy) lose their ability to control their body temperature, resulting hypothermia or hyperthermia . They therefore need to use behavioural methods of temperature regulation such as adjusting clothing, altering the ambient temperature of their environment or use of hot and cold drinks to regulate their body temperature.

8. Hypothalamic hormones have been developed (and are used for testing the pituitary function), but their short half-lives and expense limit their clinical use. End-organ hormones, e.g. oestrogen, progesterone, testosterone, are readily available and cheaper so are used instead. The exception is antidiuretic hormone, which is made in the hypothalamus and available as a tablet, spray or injection to treat cranial diabetes insipidus.

9. There are no clinical conditions caused by a prolactin deficiency in men. However, in some animals prolactin has actions in addition to lactation, such as regulating water and electrolyte balance, cell growth and proliferation, modifying behaviour, and effects on the immune system. It is possible that there is an unidentified syndrome with very subtle effects in men with prolactin deficiency.

Answers *continued*

10. The anterior pituitary gland receives venous blood from the hypothalamic-pituitary portal system via the median eminence rather than direct arterial blood. This blood contains the stimulatory and inhibitory hormones that control the anterior pituitary gland function. The posterior pituitary in comparison receives direct arterial blood from the superior hypophyseal artery.

11. Anterior pituitary hormones (including ACTH, gonadotrophins, TSH, prolactin and growth hormones) are secreted in pulses. The reasons for the pulsatile secretion are poorly understood, but in some cases the hormone's message to its target tissue is critically dependent on a pulsatile input, for example pulsatile secretion of ACTH is crucial for the normal physiological secretion of glucorticoids from adrenal cortex. Hormones can be replaced without the pulsatility (for example, in case of ACTH deficiency, non-pulsatile dose of hydrocortisone replacement is given), but it is possible that this lack of correlation with physiology can have subtle consequences on morbidity and mortality.

12. Patients with no adrenal glands are deficient in aldosterone produced by the glomerulosa cells of the adrenal cortex. Aldosterone stimulates the active uptake of sodium (salt) from the distal tubules of the kidney. Aldosterone deficiency leads to depletion of sodium in the body and a craving to replace it with salt.

13. Apart from adrenal medulla, adrenaline and noradrenaline are also produced by non-adrenal organs, in particular sympathetic nerves. Therefore, although levels of these hormones tend to be lower after bilateral adrenalectomy, replacement is not necessary as the body can adapt to life with lower levels of these hormones for the 'fight and flight' response. Other hormones, such as cortisol, can also mount a stress response and accommodate for the reduced level of adrenaline.

14. Glucose provides energy for cells in the body. It is also has key roles in glycogen, protein and fat synthesis. Neurones have an absolute requirement for a continuous supply of glucose; without it they will not survive.

15. If a normal person's blood glucose falls below 4.5 mmol/L, serum insulin concentrations fall. If it continues to fall below 3.8 mmol/L then the counter regulatory hormones (e.g. glucagon, catecholamines, cortisol, growth hormone) are secreted. Below 3.8 mmol/L, there are symptoms of hypoglycaemia (feeling of hunger, tremor, sweating) and below 2.6 mmol/L there is cognitive dysfunction (or confusion). The level of blood glucose at which symptoms develop is often different if someone has had longstanding diabetes and has frequent hypoglycaemic episodes..

16. When glucose is taken orally it stimulates the release of incretin hormones from the gut, which augment insulin secretion from the pancreas. However, when glucose is given intravenously, it bypasses the gut and therefore does not stimulate the incretin secretion. This phenomenon is known as the incretin effect.

17. There is no dramatic decline in testosterone in men like the female decline in oestrogen that causes menopause. However, there is a gradual decline in testosterone level in men seen in late middle-age. It is not known if this is a normal part of aging or a pathological hormone deficiency.

18. Temperature plays a key role in spermatogenesis. The testes are usually 2°C lower than the rest of the body. If someone has a low sperm count they are advised to wear loose fitting clothing and not sit down all day in an attempt to lower the temperature of the testes.

Answers *continued*

19. There is conflicting evidence on whether menstrual synchrony really exists. The positive studies could be compromised by the varying lengths of women's cycles (between 28 and 35 days) that mean cycles sync anyway. There have been no chemical signals (dubbed pheromones) discovered that would provide a physiological mechanism for menstrual synchrony.

20. Despite being in the centre of the brain, the pineal gland contains light-sensitive pinocytes. However, they do not detect light but instead convert autonomic signals from the retina into hormonal impulses in the form of melotonin. Through melatonin the pineal gland plays a role in the control of the sleep-wake cycle.

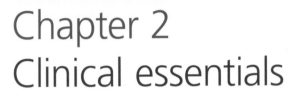

Chapter 2
Clinical essentials

Introduction

A principle in endocrinology, as in other clinical disciplines, is to make a clinical diagnosis from the history and examination of a patient before carrying out confirmatory blood tests and imaging studies to determine the nature of the abnormality and its pathological cause. This approach avoids the risk of misdiagnosis. It also reduces the cost of unnecessary investigations, as well as their potential harm, for example from the ionising radiation used in radiological studies.

All endocrine tests have an inherent false positive and false negative rate.

- A false positive is a positive test when the disease is absent
- A false negative is a negative test when the disease is present

Therefore tests must be done on the basis of the clinical diagnosis. Immediate imaging can cause confusion and harm by identifying incidental and irrelevant findings. Functioning endocrine tumours can be as small as 1 mm in diameter, so it is essential to know what lesion is being sought and where to look for it before carrying out an imaging study.

Common symptoms and how to take a history

Starter questions

Answers to the following questions are on page 143.

1. Why is an accurate drug history vital before performing endocrine investigations?
2. Why are endocrine conditions often diagnosed at a late stage?
3. How can you discuss issues patients don't want to talk about?
4. Why are employment and social habits the most relevant aspects of the social history for endocrinology?

The symptoms of endocrine disease occasionally develop acutely, so patients may present in an emergency setting. More commonly, endocrine symptoms develop gradually and there is a delay in diagnosis. This is especially so when the condition is rare or progresses slowly, for example in cases of acromegaly. Because of the non-specific nature of early symptoms of endocrine disease, patients are often seen by many other specialists before an endocrine referral is made and a diagnosis reached.

Symptoms of endocrine disease

Taking an endocrine history requires an understanding of patterns of symptoms that cluster to form a recognisable syndrome. For example, two patients who present with fatigue (tiredness or lethargy) may have entirely different endocrine (or non-endocrine) diseases depending on the nature of associated symptoms.

- Fatigue associated with thirst, urinary frequency and weight loss suggests diabetes mellitus
- Fatigue associated with weight gain, dry skin, constipation and cold intolerance suggests hypothyroidism

Take a thorough clinical history at the first meeting with the patient, even in cases of 'spot' diagnosis (a diagnosis, such as acromegaly, that can be made based on typical physical features). The history is the most sensitive diagnostic tool. (i.e. the tool most able to identify a condition correctly) Always remember the presenting complaint (e.g. carpal tunnel syndrome), because this is what the patient wants treated or explained. The presenting complaint is not just a diversion during investigation of the 'spot' diagnosis.

The symptoms of endocrine disease are commonly non-specific and of a type that could be caused by a wide variety of pathologies. Patients have often looked up their symptoms on the Internet and may have their own ideas about the cause. Therefore patients may have certain expectations at the time of presentation, and these must be handled sensitively if they prove incorrect.

Fatigue

Many endocrine and non-endocrine conditions cause fatigue (**Table 2.1**). It is one of the commonest complaints encountered in endocrinology. However, although fatigue is a significant indication of pathology, remember that it is also experienced in normal everyday life in the absence of pathology.

Identifying pathological fatigue can be challenging. A detailed history of the duration, nature and degree of fatigue is crucial, in addition to identification of other associated symptoms (**Table 2.2**). Lifestyle factors, such as poor bedtime routine or a change in personal circumstances, should be

Causes of fatigue	
Category	Disorder(s) or other explanation
Endocrine (see Table 2.2)	Diabetes mellitus
	Hyperthyroidism
	Hypothyroidism
	Cushing's syndrome
	Addison's disease
	Hypopituitarism
Malignant	All malignant solid and haematological tumours
Haematological	Anaemia
Infective	Viral or bacterial infections (including tuberculosis)
Biochemical	Electrolyte disturbance
Inflammatory	Chronic autoimmune conditions
Drug use	Use of prescribed or illicit drugs
Psychological	Depression
Organ system failure	Renal, cardiac, liver and respiratory failure
Other	Chronic fatigue syndrome, sleep disturbance and obstructive sleep apnoea

Table 2.1 Common causes of fatigue

Symptoms associated with fatigue with an endocrine cause	
Disorder	Other associated symptoms
Diabetes mellitus	Polyuria, polydipsia and weight loss
Hyperthyroidism	Weight loss, anxiety, sweats, tremor, palpitations and heat intolerance
Hypothyroidism	Weight gain, constipation, dry skin, hair loss and cold intolerance
Cushing's syndrome	Weight gain, bruising, weakness and depression
Addison's disease	Weight loss, weakness, vomiting and abdominal pain
Hypopituitarism	Symptoms of specific hormone deficiencies (cortisol, thyroid, sex hormones and growth hormone)

Table 2.2 Symptoms associated with fatigue caused by endocrine disease

excluded. It is helpful to develop a structured method for thinking about the causes of fatigue, to avoid missing potential pathologies (see **Table 2.1**).

Thirst

Excessive thirst (polydipsia) is the sensation of compulsion to drink. It can have a physiological cause (e.g diabetes mellitus or diabetes insipidus) or have a psychological basis (**Table 2.3**).

The following questions need to be considered for a patient who describes thirst:

- How much fluid is drunk in 24 h?
- Does the patient wake up during night to drink?
- Is there excessive fluid loss (from urination, diarrhoea, sweating, etc.)?
- Has the patient lost weight?

Thirst that wakes a patient at night is a stronger indicator of pathology than daytime thirst. In cases of diabetes insipidus, low circulating blood volume and concentrated plasma stimulate thirst at night; in contrast, psychogenic polydipsia is present only in the daytime.

Causes of thirst	
Category	Disorder(s) or other explanation
Normal response to fluid loss	Dehydration: gastrointestinal fluid loss, poor fluid intake, sweating and fever
Endocrine	Diabetes insipidus
	Diabetes mellitus
Biochemical	Hypercalcaemia
Pharmacological	Use of anticholinergic agents (e.g. oxybutynin), antidepressants (e.g. amitriptyline) or diuretics (e.g. furosemide)
Psychological	Psychogenic polydipsia

Table 2.3 Causes of thirst

Causes of high urine output	
Mechanism	Cause
Solute loss causing osmotic diuresis	Diabetes mellitus
Inability to concentrate urine	Diabetes insipidus
Physiological high output secondary to excessive water intake	Psychogenic polydipsia
Urogenital abnormality*	Urological abnormalities such as hypertrophy or cancer of the prostate, and gynaecological abnormalities
Pharmacological	Use of diuretics

*Urogenital abnormalities are more likely to increase urine output by increasing frequency of urination rather than volume of urine passed each time.

Table 2.4 Causes of high urine output

Excessive urination

Excessive urination (polyuria) can present as:

- frequent passage of small volumes of urine
- less frequent passage of large volumes of urine

The recording of frequency of urination and the amount of urine passed helps distinguish between the two presentations. Causes of high urine output are listed in **Table 2.4**.

Weight loss

Unintentional weight loss is always a worrying symptom. Loss of a large amount of weight or rapid weight loss is more commonly associated with severe pathology. The lists of potential causes (**Table 2.5**) and associated symptoms (**Table 2.6**) are long, so the priority is to exclude a malignant process.

Addison's disease causes weight loss because of cortisol deficiency. The condition can be associated with nausea, vomiting and abdominal pain, accompanied by reduced appetite. Therefore Addison's disease is commonly mistaken for a gastrointestinal disorder, creating a delay before the correct diagnosis is made.

Causes of weight loss	
Category	Disorder(s)
Endocrine (see Table 2.6)	Diabetes mellitus
	Addison's disease
	Hyperthyroidism
Malignant	Any solid organ or haematological malignancy
Infectious	Any acute or chronic infection (e.g. pneumonia, tuberculosis and HIV)
Malabsorption	Coeliac disease, pancreatic insufficiency, short bowel syndrome and bacterial overgrowth
Psychological	Anorexia nervosa, bulimia nervosa and depression
Neurological	Dysphagia secondary to stroke or Parkinson's disease

Table 2.5 Causes of weight loss

Symptoms associated with weight loss with an endocrine cause	
Disorder	Other associated symptoms
Diabetes mellitus	Polydipsia, polyuria, fatigue and blurred vision
Addison's disease	Fatigue, depression, weakness and darkening of the skin (hyperpigmentation)
Hyperthyroidism	Heat intolerance, sweating, tremor, anxiety, diarrhoea and palpitations

Table 2.6 Symptoms associated with weight loss caused by endocrine disease

Type 1 diabetes mellitus also causes weight loss. However, the classic symptoms of polydipsia and polyuria are more easily recognised, so diagnosis is usually swift.

Information about the speed of onset and degree of weight loss can help identify a cause.

- Rapid weight loss occurs in type 1 diabetes mellitus. Weight loss is also rapid when thyrotoxicosis is severe, compared to mild thyrotoxicosis when there is little or no weight loss.
- Patients with Addison's disease may present with a large amount of weight loss relative to their original weight but due to the often slow onset of Addison's disease, the weight loss occurs gradually.

Also consider the following associated features:

- Appetite: this is increased in thyrotoxicosis and often reduced in malignant diseases
- Gastrointestinal symptoms: increased stool frequency suggests thyrotoxicosis, and nausea and abdominal pain suggest Addison's disease
- Other localising symptoms: chest symptoms (e.g. cough and breathlessness) point to lung malignancy associated with an endocrine disease, such as syndrome of inappropriate ADH caused by ectopic antidiuretic hormone (ADH) secretion
- Anaemia: this suggests a pathological process rather than intentional weight loss

Weight gain

Because of the combination of easily available, low-price, highly calorific food and modern sedentary lifestyles, weight gain and obesity are rapidly increasing in prevalence in both the developed and developing world. However, rare pathological causes for weight gain and obesity exist. Distinguishing obesity with a pathological cause from lifestyle-related obesity is difficult and requires understanding of the patient's history and associated symptoms and signs (**Table 2.7**).

Features of obesity with a pathological cause	
Feature	**Example(s)**
A history of recent weight gain (rather than obesity gradually worsening from childhood) or weight gain not associated with life events such as pregnancy	Lifestyle-associated obesity
Abnormal distribution of weight	Central obesity in Cushing's syndrome
Associated symptoms that indicate a syndrome	Fatigue, constipation and cold intolerance: associated with hypothyroidism
	Hirsutism, irregular menstrual cycle and acanthosis nigricans: associated with polycystic ovary syndrome
Associated biochemical abnormalities	High blood glucose in diabetes mellitus

Table 2.7 Features that suggest obesity with a pathological cause rather than lifestyle-related obesity

There are a few genetic forms of obesity, such as autosomal recessive leptin deficiency. Leptin is released from adipose tissue and is involved in signalling satiety. The exact prevalence of such disorders is unknown, but leptin deficiency in common with other genetic syndromes is an extremely rare cause of obesity.

In the vast majority of cases, no pathological cause for weight gain can be identified. This can be a disappointment for some patients with obesity.

Palpitations

Palpitations are the sensation of being aware of your own heartbeat. Patients often describe a racing, thumping, fluttering or irregular heartbeat. Palpitations may be continuous or intermittent and sometimes have recognisable triggers (e.g. bending or lifting causes release of adrenaline in phaeochromocytoma). Endocrine causes of palpitations are determined by increased sympathetic tone (**Figure 2.1**).

Tremor

Tremor is when part of the body shakes uncontrollably. It has endocrine and non-

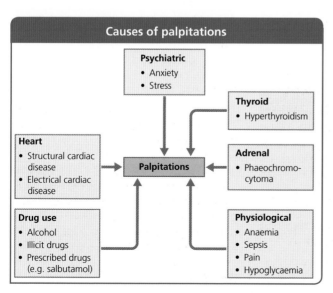

Figure 2.1 Causes of palpitations.

Causes of palpitations

Psychiatric
- Anxiety
- Stress

Thyroid
- Hyperthyroidism

Heart
- Structural cardiac disease
- Electrical cardiac disease

Palpitations

Adrenal
- Phaeochromo-cytoma

Drug use
- Alcohol
- Illicit drugs
- Prescribed drugs (e.g. salbutamol)

Physiological
- Anaemia
- Sepsis
- Pain
- Hypoglycaemia

endocrine causes (**Table 2.8**). Symptoms associated with tremor with an endocrine cause are listed in **Table 2.9**.

Goitre

A goitre is an enlarged thyroid gland or a lump in a thyroid gland. This may be noticed by the patient (e.g. seen or felt by an individual), a friend or relative, or another health care professional when palpating the neck.

Many goitres grow slowly, so they can go undetected for several years. Information about the symptoms associated with a goitre helps to identify the underlying pathology (**Table 2.10**).

Excessive sweating

Sweating is a normal feature of thermoregulation. However, when sweating becomes profuse (hyperhidrosis) it can become a distressing problem. Physiological sweating is more prominent in people who are overweight or obese.

Consider the following questions in cases of excessive sweating:

- Is the sweating constant or does it occur at night only? Night sweats may be caused by chronic infection (e.g. tuberculosis) or malignancy (e.g. lymphoma)
- Is it associated with other menopausal symptoms, such as amenorrhoea or oligomenorrhoea, flushing, vaginal dryness and mood swings?
- Is the sweating localised, for example to the palms, feet, face and axillae? Excessive sweating localised to specific areas of the body is known as primary idiopathic hyperhidrosis (which is treated symptomatically with antiperspirants)
- Are there signs of autonomic neuropathy or other neuropathies (which can occur in diabetes mellitus)? Profuse sweating precipitated by eating (gustatory sweating) occurs in diabetic autonomic neuropathy
- Is the sweating relieved by eating? This would indicate hypoglycaemia

Causes of tremor	
Category	Causes
Endocrine (see Table 2.9)	Thyrotoxicosis
	Phaeochromocytoma
	Hypoglycaemia
Neurological	Parkinson's disease, multiple sclerosis and cerebellar pathology
Drug use	Use of β agonists (e.g. salbutamol), and chronic alcohol use and withdrawal
Idiopathic	Benign essential tremor
Physiological	Fear and severe anxiety

Table 2.8 Causes of tremor

Symptoms associated with tremor with an endocrine cause	
Endocrine cause of tremor	Associated symptoms
Thyrotoxicosis	Weight loss, sweating, anxiety and heat intolerance
Phaeochromocytoma	Palpitations, anxiety and hypertension
Hypoglycaemia	Hunger, palpitations, sweating and confusion

Table 2.9 Symptoms associated with tremor caused by an endocrine disease

Features of a goitre	
Associated feature	Likely causes
Pain (spontaneous pain and tenderness on palpation)	Thyroiditis
	Haemorrhage into a cyst
Rapid growth (of part of or entire thyroid gland)	Malignancy
	Haemorrhage
Hoarse voice	Malignancy
Symptoms of thyrotoxicosis (see page 198)	Graves' disease
	Toxic nodular goitre
Breathlessness, stridor or difficulty swallowing	Large goitre compressing the trachea
Solitary nodule	Benign or malignant tumour

Table 2.10 Features of a goitre

Flushing

Flushing is a reddening and warming of the skin. It results from vasodilation of the subcutaneous capillaries. These capillaries are most superficial and numerous in the face, so this is the most commonly affected area. Flushing is a normal response to stress, embarrassment, anxiety and anger.

Pathological flushing is a result of dysfunction of autonomic sympathetic nerves to the skin or the presence of circulating hormonal mediators such as histamine.

The following cause flushing:

- Carcinoid syndrome (often stimulated by consumption of certain tyramine-containing foods; **Figure 2.2**): flushing associated with carcinoid syndrome is often referred to as 'dry flushing', because it is not associated with sweating although the skin does feel warm
- Alcohol: alcohol consumption leads to excessive flushing in people whose bodies have limited ability to metabolise alcohol (e.g. the many people of East Asian origin who lack the aldehyde dehydrogenase enzyme)
- Post-menopausal state
- Use of certain medications: calcium channel blockers, opiates, tamoxifen and bromocriptine are recognised causes of flushing

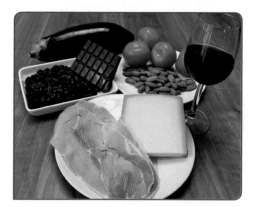

Figure 2.2 Foods that contain tyramine: smoked meat, mature cheese, alcohol, coffee, red wine, chocolate, nuts and certain vegetables (e.g. aubergine and tomatoes). Tyramine-containing foods stimulate flushing in patients with carcinoid syndrome.

Low libido

Libido (sex drive) is determined by multiple factors: hormonal, physical and psychosocial (**Figure 2.3**). Low libido is a distressing symptom that can affect men and women at any part of their adult lives. Exploring the duration, severity and context of the symptoms gives a clue to diagnosis. A detailed history of sexual development is vital (see page 77), because a developmental disorder may be responsible for low libido (see page 287).

Erectile dysfunction

Erectile dysfunction is the inability to obtain or maintain sufficient erection of the penis to enable sexual intercourse. The cause is commonly multifactorial. The presence of other symptoms of testosterone deficiency, such

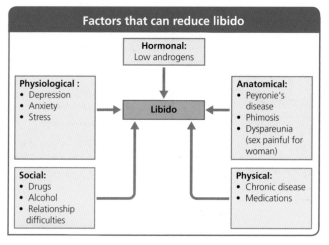

Figure 2.3 The multiple factors that can reduce libido.

as poor libido, fatigue and reduced muscle strength, may point to an endocrine cause.

Remember to ask about the occurrence of early morning erections, because these are often lost at an early stage in cases of hypogonadism. Preservation of early morning erections indicates a psychological cause for erectile dysfunction.

Diabetes mellitus can cause erectile dysfunction in various ways (**Figure 2.4**).

> In patients with diabetes mellitus, erectile dysfunction can be an early indicator of vascular disease. Diabetic patients with erectile dysfunction are at a higher risk of cardiovascular complications and death.

Menstrual irregularities

Categorisation of menstrual irregularities aids diagnosis.

- Primary amenorrhoea is the absence of menarche (the first occurrence of menstruation) by the age of:
  - 16 years in the presence of normal secondary sexual characteristics
  - 14 years in the absence of secondary sexual characteristics
- Secondary amenorrhoea is the absence of menstrual cycles for at least:
  - 3 months in women with previously normal menstrual cycles
  - 9 months in women with previous history of oligomenorrhoea
- Oligomenorrhoea is a state of infrequent menstrual bleeding, (fewer than nine cycles per year)

When discussing menstrual irregularities, it is helpful to ask the patient about other aspects of pubertal development, such as the development of breasts and pubic hair (see page 78).

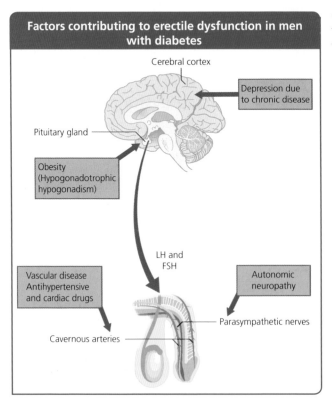

Factors contributing to erectile dysfunction in men with diabetes

Cerebral cortex

Depression due to chronic disease

Pituitary gland

Obesity (Hypogonadotrophic hypogonadism)

LH and FSH

Vascular disease Antihypertensive and cardiac drugs

Autonomic neuropathy

Parasympathetic nerves

Cavernous arteries

Figure 2.4 The multiple factors that contribute to erectile dysfunction in men with diabetes. FSH, follicle-stimulating hormone; LH, luteinising hormone.

Galactorrhoea

Galactorrhoea is inappropriate lactation, i.e. production of a milky secretion outside the peripartum or post-partum state (around the time of birth or after birth, respectively). The secretions are usually bilateral and small in volume. Physiological galactorrhoea often occurs on mechanical stimulation of the breast or nipple, but it can occur spontaneously.

Galactorrhoea can occur in men and women, and it has various causes (**Table 2.11**). Symptoms associated with pituitary causes are listed in **Table 2.12**.

Unilateral galactorrhoea or bloody discharge from the nipple and breast masses are concerning symptoms that raise the possibility of a breast pathology, such as infection or cancer. Referral to a breast surgeon is advisable.

In any woman of childbearing age presenting with amenorrhoea or galactorrhoea, the first step is to exclude pregnancy as a cause. A pregnancy test is needed even if the patient reports using adequate contraception.

Causes of galactorrhoea	
Category	Disorder(s)
Pituitary gland	Prolactinoma
	Compression of the pituitary stalk
Other endocrine	Hypothyroidism
Pharmacological	Antipsychotic agents (e.g. risperidone), antiemetic agents (e.g. metoclopramide), tricyclic antidepressants (e.g. amitriptyline) and the combined oral contraceptive pill
Other	Chronic renal impairment, chest wall trauma, overstimulation of nipple

Table 2.11 Causes of galactorrhoea

Symptoms associated with galactorrhoea caused by pituitary disorder	
Disorder	Associated symptoms
Prolactinoma	Amenorrhoea and oligomenorrhoea
Pituitary stalk compression	Bitemporal hemianopia and specific symptoms of functional pituitary tumours

Table 2.12 Symptoms associated with galactorrhoea caused by disorders of the pituitary gland

Delayed puberty

Delayed puberty is defined as follows.

- Males: testicles < 4 mL in volume, or the absence of testicular development, in boys of 14 years or older
- Females: the absence of breast development in girls of 13 years or older

Late-onset or incomplete puberty has a wide range of causes. These include:

- constitutional delay (usually inherited delay or no identified cause)
- chronic illness
- malnutrition
- medical treatments (e.g. steroids)
- pituitary or hypothalamic abnormality
- gonadal abnormality (testicular or ovarian failure)

Hirsutism

Hirsutism is defined as excessive growth of body hair in women. Hair grows in androgen-dependent areas of the face, neck, chest, abdomen, thighs and back.

Patients commonly complain when hair growth affects the face, because facial hair is harder to conceal than body hair. Dark hair is more noticeable and therefore more troublesome.

Infertility

Couples failing to conceive despite having regular unprotected sexual intercourse for ≥ 12 months are defined as having infertility.

- Primary infertility is diagnosed in couples who have never conceived together or

whose pregnancies have not resulted in a live birth (one member of a couple may have had a child before)
- Secondary infertility is diagnosed in couples who are unable to conceive a pregnancy resulting in a live birth despite having done so previously
- When a couple presents with infertility, it is necessary to consider both partners' histories of sexual development, because abnormal or delayed development may indicate an endocrine or a genetic cause (see pages 283 and 289).

Gynaecomastia

Gynaecomastia is unilateral or bilateral enlargement of breast tissue in men. The condition can occur as a normal part of pubertal development and usually resolves by the end of the teenage years.

A full developmental history is required in order to identify the rare cases of gynaecomastia with a syndromic cause (see page 289). Symptoms of testosterone deficiency (low libido, erectile dysfunction, weakness and reduced body hair) may be present.

Gynaecomastia occurs when there is an imbalance in the ratio of testosterone to oestrogen. Endocrine causes of gynaecomastia include conditions resulting in oestrogen excess, testosterone deficiency or androgen insensitivity. Non-endocrine causes of gynaecomastia may be identified from the history; these include:

- medications such as the potassium-sparing diuretic spironolactone, the cardiac drug digoxin and the antihypertensive agent methyldopa
- illicit drugs such as cannabis and opiates
- alcoholic liver disease
- food and herbal products containing plant oestrogens called phyto-oestrogens (e.g. soya beans and supplements containing phyto-oestrogens)

Anosmia

Anosmia is an absence of the sense of smell. The condition may be present in the congenital disorder Kallmann's syndrome (which is characterised by hypogonadotrophic hypogoinadism causing pubertal delay and inferiority) and in diabetes mellitus. Non-endocrine causes of anosmia include nasal conditions such as rhinitis, upper respiratory tract infections and frontal lobe or suprasellar tumours.

How to take an endocrine history

The principles of history taking in endocrinology are similar to those of general history taking. Depending on the complexity of the clinical scenario, 10-30 min may be needed for this part of the consultation.

The history should elicit the 'story' of the clinical problem, including:

- an accurate and detailed assessment of the significant symptom (or symptoms)
- how symptoms have evolved over time
- how severely symptoms are affecting the patient

It is also necessary to identify any relevant factors in the medical, social, drug, surgical and family history. Other symptoms may be uncovered that indicate additional concurrent clinical problems that affect the presenting complaint or require further investigation in their own right.

If a woman presents with a single complaint of primary amenorrhoea, then a full and detailed developmental and childhood history is useful. She may have a congenital disorder that causes other anomalies. For example, cases of Turner's syndrome are often associated with cardiac or renal abnormalities. In contrast, if a woman presents with a recent history of secondary amenorrhoea accompanied by sweating, weight loss, tremor and anxiety, a diagnosis of thyrotoxicosis is likely and a detailed developmental history is unnecessary.

To take an endocrine history, it is helpful to use a basic structure to prevent omission of relevant details. This structure will need to be modified according to the patient's presenting complaint. The key aspects of history taking are:

- presenting problem or symptoms
- history of presenting complaint
- medical history
- developmental and reproductive history
- drug history
- family history
- social history
- systems review

At the end of the history, it is good practice to summarise to the patient the information they have provided. This allows them to correct any aspects of the history that may have been misunderstood or misinterpreted. At this juncture, it is useful to ask the patient if there is anything else they would like to add. This affords the patient an opportunity to relay information that has not been mentioned during initial questioning.

Presenting problem

Start with the presenting problem or symptoms. Allowing the patient to describe their symptoms in their own words, without interruption, is a good technique to get the consultation started. Use an open question, such as:

'Your GP has asked me to see you, because you've been troubled by sweating. Please could you tell me a little about this?'

This encourages the patient to give a descriptive account of their symptoms and allows them to express their concerns for their health. It also ensures that their symptoms of concern match the referral.

Some patients come well prepared and have a list of symptoms. In such cases, it may be difficult to cover all aspects in the time allotted for an appointment, so the questions need to be more closed, such as:

'What are the three symptoms that concern you the most?'

If a symptom suggests a syndrome, the questions can become completely closed (requiring 'yes' or 'no' answers) to try to elicit other related symptoms; for example:

'Do you sweat with those flushes?'

Remember that patients may fail to mention symptoms that they feel are irrelevant, so direct questioning may be needed.

Symptoms and signs often develop over many years. Old photographs are useful for the diagnosis of conditions with slowly progressing physical changes, for example central obesity and intrascapular fat in Cushing's syndrome and prognathism and frontal bossing (protruding jaw and forehead respectively) in acromegaly.

Medical history

A medical history helps establish if the patient has any previously diagnosed conditions that may be part of a syndrome. It also alerts the clinician to any increased risk of developing associated conditions. Information about other endocrine diseases is particularly useful.

More details about the condition, such as the duration of diabetes mellitus and how well it has been controlled, give clues to the likelihood of complications. Ensure that details of previous medical, surgical and radio-therapeutic treatments are carefully documented as these are occasionally highly relevant in determining the aetiology of the current condition, e.g. previous radiotherapy to the nasopharynx to treat a cancer causing hypopituitarism in later life.

Developmental and reproductive history

In endocrinology, a developmental history may suggest a diagnosis, especially if the condition started in childhood or is a congenital syndrome.

A developmental history should answer the following questions:

- Were there any maternal illnesses in the intrauterine period (the time the patient spent in their mother's womb)? For example, the patient's mother may have had diabetes mellitus
- Was birth and early development normal? Did the patient achieve developmental milestones such as crawling, walking and talking at the usual ages? The patient's parents may need to provide this information
- Did the patient's growth in terms of height and weight progress normally? This information is not always known

by the patient so parents will need to be questioned for past height and weight progress.

■ Are any other associated features present? For example, patients with Turner's syndrome or Klinefelter's syndrome may have a mild degree of intellectual disability such as problems with language or numeracy or problems with social skills and hyperactivity.

■ Are atypical or ambiguous genitalia mentioned in the history?

■ Does the patient's family have a history of delayed puberty? A positive history may suggest hereditary pubertal delay

■ Is there a history of systemic illness, stress and malnutrition? These can also cause pubertal delay or pubertal arrest

The reproductive history focuses on the development of the reproductive organs, both structurally and functionally.

Questions to consider for male patients are as follows:

■ Are there any concerns with regard to the structure of the penis and testes? Was there cryptorchidism (undescended or hidden testes)? Cryptorchidism can occur in conditions such as Prader–Willi syndrome

■ Did puberty occur at a normal age (similar to their peers), and were the normal features of puberty present (pubic hair growth, deepening of the voice, testicular and penile enlargement and growth spurt)? Absence or delay points to hypogonadism

■ In sexually mature males, are there any symptoms of hypogonadism, such as fatigue, reduced muscle bulk, erectile dysfunction and poor facial hair growth?

In female patients, consider the following questions:

■ Was there normal development of secondary sexual characteristics (breast enlargement, pubic hair growth, growth spurt and menarche)?

■ Have periods been regular?

■ Are there any symptoms of androgen excess, such as hirsutism? Remember to ask how frequently hair is removed, because excess body or facial hair is unlikely to have been left to grow for clinical examination

■ Are there any symptoms of oestrogen deficiency, which would indicate the menopause? These climacteric symptoms include sweats, flushing, vaginal dryness, mood swings and amenorrhoea or oligomenorrhoea.

Drug history

The drug history includes details of any prescription drugs, over-the-counter preparations, hormone supplements (including the oral contraceptive pill) and non-prescribed medications the patient may have used. Include questions about herbal remedies and traditional medicines, which can contain hormones or other substances that affect hormone balance (e.g. iodine). Pharmaceutical products and alternative medicines are increasing available for sale on the internet, and many people self-prescribe therefore the drug list may be more extensive than it initially seems.

Family history

Many endocrine disorders are inherited, so a detailed family history is documented. The inheritance of an endocrine disease may be polygenic or monogenic.

■ In polygenic inheritance, a number of genes affect a person's susceptibility to the disorder; for example, type 2 diabetes mellitus is a strongly heritable polygenic disorder but a number of other factors (e.g. obesity) need to be present for a person to be affected

■ In monogenic inheritance, any person who inherits the defective gene will be affected by the condition; some forms of diabetes mellitus have this pattern of inheritance (such as HNF1-alpha diabetes, page 163)

Autoimmune endocrine conditions tend to cluster in an individual and families. Examples are autoimmune thyroid diseases, autoimmune Addison's disease and type 1 diabetes mellitus. Patients may not know exactly what family members died from, but a history of sudden death in members of the family of a patient with a suspected phaeochromocytomas may be relevant.

If a disorder runs in the patient's family, it is helpful to draw their family tree (**Figure 2.5**).

> **Taking a family history not only helps identify genetic conditions; it also explains patients' fears or their understanding of heritable disease.** 'Granddad was on insulin and look what happened to him'. 'I used to give the insulin to my Mum - it's not that bad'.

Social history

Take a social history to identify the effects that endocrine diseases and their associated complications or symptoms have on patients, their family and their carers.

Consider the following:

- The patient may need help with taking their medications at home, for example if they have:
  - visual disturbance
  - impaired manual dexterity (e.g. affecting their ability to give themselves insulin injections)
  - memory problems
- Some diagnoses have implications for employment
  - Night shifts may necessitate adjustments to medication

planning (e.g. dosing hydrocortisone replacement during night shifts with reversed diurnal patterns)
  - Patients who have started insulin therapy may need to make special arrangements if they drive certain vehicles professionally; for example, they may be required to provide evidence of glycaemic control to the national driver-licensing authority
  - Patients receiving insulin may be barred from certain jobs in the armed forces
- Lifestyle factors can influence assessment and treatment
  - Smoking is a synergistic risk factor for macrovascular disease in patients with diabetes mellitus
  - Excessive alcohol intake can give a clinical picture of pseudo-Cushing's syndrome, which resolves on abstinence from alcohol
  - A poor and unbalanced diet may make treating a condition, such as diabetes mellitus, more difficult
  - Excessive exercise may need to be carefully managed in patients with conditions such as type 1 diabetes mellitus, to avoid hypoglycaemic episodes. In Addison's disease, doses of steroid replacement will need to be increased before intense exercise
- Drug misuse can affect blood results; heroin can cause secondary

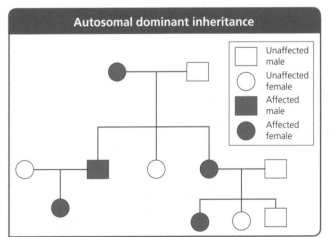

Autosomal dominant inheritance

Unaffected male
Unaffected female
Affected male
Affected female

Figure 2.5 Family tree showing autosomal dominant inheritance of multiple endocrine neoplasia type 1. The condition affects family members in all generations, which is typical for this pattern of inheritance.

hypogonadism, and cocaine affects increases metadrenaline (metanephrine).

> **Patients need to feel that the clinician is on 'their side' and not judging them.** The resulting trust encourages honesty when discussing aspects such as diet, smoking and alcohol intake. For example, agreeing that an occasional food 'treat' is acceptable, and avoiding demanding unrealistic outcomes, may encourage a patient to agree to making targets for changes to their lifestyle.

Systems review

A systems review involves asking questions about each system of the body in turn, to identify any missed or forgotten details. In endocrinology, a systems review is essential, because symptoms are multiple and are often not mentioned by patients unless direct questions are used. For example, the mention of a cough or diarrhoea may give a clue to the location of a tumour causing ectopic Cushing's syndrome.

To perform a systems review, consider the following systems and symptoms:

- Constitutional: fever, fatigue, weight loss, reduced appetite and malaise
- Cardiovascular: chest pain, peripheral swelling, palpitations, shortness of breath, dizziness and syncope
- Respiratory: cough, haemoptysis (coughing up blood) and wheeze
- Gastrointestinal: nausea, vomiting, diarrhoea, constipation, abdominal pain and blood in the stool
- Urogenital: urinary frequency, urinary incontinence and haematuria (blood in the urine)
- Neurological: headaches, visual disturbances, limb weakness and fits
- Psychological: anxiety, depression and hallucinations

Common signs and how to examine a patient

Starter questions

Answers to the following questions are on page 143.

5. Why are old photographs of patients helpful when diagnosing endocrine conditions?
6. Can endocrine conditions be diagnosed on sight?
7. How can an adolescent's parents help with an examination?

The history obtained from the patient is used to guide a targeted endocrine examination. For example, symptoms typical of hyperthyroidism (weight loss, sweats and palpitations) prompt the clinician to examine the thyroid to look for signs of this condition, such as thyroid eye disease (which occurs only in Graves' disease). Certain manoeuvres may be necessary only in patients in whom a specific disease is suspected, for example testing for lid lag in cases of suspected hyperthyroidism.

Physical examination is not only used for diagnosis; it also has a vital role in screening for long-term complications in chronic endocrine diseases. For example, regular examination of the feet of patients with diabetes mellitus identifies those at risk of ischaemia, neuropathy and infection.

Signs of endocrine disease

In many cases, endocrine examination is normal, so the diagnosis is made on the basis of history alone. When signs of endocrine disease are present, they are often subtle and non-diagnostic. However, in combination, they often reveal a pattern that points strongly to a clinical diagnosis.

Clinical signs also vary with the severity of the disease. For example, a person with mild biochemical hyperthyroidism, with only a slight excess of thyroxine (T_4), may have no clinical signs (e.g. tremor, tachycardia and lid lag) but still have symptoms (e.g. heat intolerance, tiredness and anxiety). Conversely, someone with marked biochemical hyperthyroidism (with very high circulating T_4 levels) usually has many of the classic signs of hyperthyroidism (see Table 5.4).

Hand signs

It is helpful to start the examination routine in the same place with every patient. The hands are a good place to start as a variety of endocrine signs are seen there.

Clubbing

This is a loss of nail fold angle and increased longitudinal curvature of the nails (**Figure 2.6**). The only endocrine condition that causes clubbing is Graves' disease, in which case it is termed thyroid acropachy (see Figure 5.2b). The following are more common, non-endocrine causes of clubbing.

- Gastrointestinal causes: inflammatory bowel disease and primary biliary cirrhosis
- Pulmonary causes: cancer, fibrosis, bronchiectasis, empyema and cystic fibrosis
- Cardiac causes: subacute bacterial endocarditis and congenital cyanotic heart disease
- Familial clubbing

Enlarged hands

Enlargement of the hands (and feet) is a feature of acromegaly; it is caused by tissue overgrowth. Palpate for a 'doughy' enlargement of the soft tissue of the hands. Rings may have to be resized, and shoes may no longer fit. Because of median nerve compression at the wrist, carpal tunnel syndrome or scars from carpal tunnel decompression surgery may also be present.

Cardiac signs

Endocrine diseases can affect the cardiovascular system, resulting in clinical signs.

Tachycardia

This is a heart rate of > 100 beats/min. This sign is found in hyperthyroidism, and intermittently in phaeochromocytoma.

Bradycardia

This is a heart rate of < 60 beats/min. Bradycardia occurs in hypothyroidism.

Hypertension

High blood pressure (hypertension) is diagnosed on the basis of repeated blood pressure measurements > 140/90 mmHg. Hypertension is a risk factor for cardiovascular disease and renal failure in people with diabetes and other metabolic disturbances.

For causes of hypertension, see **Table 7.4**.

Hypotension

Abnormally low blood pressure (hypotension) is common in patients with adrenal

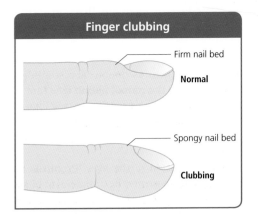

Finger clubbing

Firm nail bed

Normal

Spongy nail bed

Clubbing

Figure 2.6 Finger clubbing.

Causes of postural hypotension	
Category	Conditions
Neurogenic	Autonomic neuropathy (secondary to diabetes mellitus, excessive alcohol consumption, etc.)
	Multisystem atrophy ('Parkinson plus' syndromes)
Dehydration or intravascular depletion	Poorly controlled diabetes
	Addison's disease
	Other conditions causing fluid loss (e.g. vomiting, diarrhoea, bleeding, sepsis and use of diuretic agents)
Cardiovascular	Bradycardia
	Cardiac failure

Table 2.13 Causes of postural hypotension

Cardiac signs in endocrine diseases	
Condition	Cardiac defect
Turner's syndrome	Bicuspid aortic valve
	Coarctation of the aorta
	Aortic stenosis
	Multisystem atrophy ('Parkinson plus' syndromes)
Noonan's syndrome	Pulmonary artery stenosis
	Atrial septal defects
Hyperdynamic states (hyperthyroidism and phaeochromocytoma)	Aortic systolic flow murmur

Table 2.14 Cardiac signs in endocrine diseases

insufficiency. A significant decrease in blood pressure (systolic, >20mmHg; diastolic, >10mmHg) when changing posture from a lying to standing position is called postural hypotension. This clinical sign may be present in several endocrine disorders, such as Addison's disease, secondary adrenal insufficiency and diabetic autonomic neuropathy (**Table 2.13**).

Cardiac murmurs

These are caused by turbulent blood flow across a heart valve that is structurally abnormal, narrowed or incompetent (leaky). Cardiac murmurs are associated with a small number of endocrine conditions. They are a common feature of Turner's and Noonan's syndromes (**Table 2.14**). A systolic flow murmur (a consequence of high-volume blood flow across the aortic valve) may be audible in patients with hyperthyroidism; it is caused by the hyperdynamic circulation.

Facial signs

Facial signs associated with endocrine diseases may provide the clinician with a 'spot' diagnosis on first sight of the patient. This is especially true of the facial features of acromegaly and Cushing's syndrome (see Figures 6.2 and 6.8).

Enlarged tongue

In acromegaly (see Figure 6.3b), soft tissue overgrowth may enlarge the tongue (macroglossia). Because the enlarged tongue is confined to a fixed oral cavity, its lateral borders may be inadvertently damaged by biting. Macroglossia is also rarely associated with severe hypothyroidism.

Increased interdental spacing

This sign is the result of gum overgrowth in acromegaly. Teeth often become loose and fall out. The presence of dentures in patients with other features of acromegaly informs the clinician of previous loss of teeth.

Prognathism

This term describes protrusion of the mandible to produce an underbite. This sign occurs in acromegaly (see Figure 6.2).

Rounded facies

Previously known as 'moon face', rounded facies refers to the round, plump face that is a feature of Cushing's syndrome (see Figure 6.8). The face is often plethoric (red).

Proptosis

This is protrusion of the eyes. Proptosis in thyroid eye disease may be unilateral or bilateral, and is often asymmetrical. Proptosis is

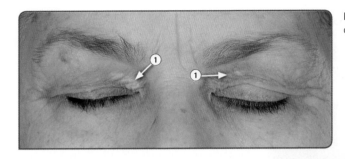

Figure 2.7 Bilateral xanthelasma on the upper eyelids ①.

most apparent when looking at the eyes from above the patient.

Xanthelesma

Xanthelesmas are circumscribed, yellowish plaques of skin on the eyelids resulting from cholesterol deposit (**Figure 2.7**). They are often associated with hypercholesterolaemia (see page 168).

Skin signs

The skin can be affected by endocrine conditions locally (e.g. the loss of skin pigment in vitiligo) or more generally (e.g. the thin, easily bruised skin of patients with Cushing's syndrome).

Thin skin

Thinning of the skin occurs in states of excess corticosteroids, either endogenous (e.g. Cushing's syndrome) or exogenous (e.g. prolonged treatment with steroids in conditions such as chronic obstructive pulmonary disease or rheumatoid arthritis). The skin appears translucent, and veins are easily visible.

Bruising

Easy or low-trauma bruising occurs in patients with Cushing's syndrome (**Figure 2.8**), as well as in those receiving corticosteroid therapy. It may also occur in patients with haematological conditions such as clotting or platelet disorders.

Hyperpigmentation

Excessive pigmentation (see Figure 7.4) can be difficult to distinguish from natural skin pigmentation caused by sunlight exposure. Abnormal pigmentation may be more easily

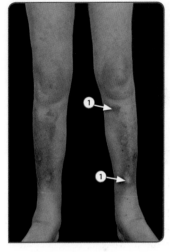

Figure 2.8 Multiple bruises ① in a man with Cushing's syndrome. He also has proximal muscle wasting (in the thigh muscles) and ankle oedema, which are other signs of the syndrome.

identifiable in areas not exposed to sunlight, and it is more likely to occur in surgical scars.

Pigmentation in palmar creases or on buccal mucosa points to melanocyte-stimulating hormone excess, which occurs in Addison's disease and Nelson's syndrome (**Figure 2.9**). Both these conditions cause excessive secretion of ACTH, and melanocyte-stimulating hormone is secreted as a by-product of ACTH production.

Abdominal striae

These are linear markings on the abdomen. Pink abdominal striae are commonly referred to as stretch marks and are seen in women whose abdomen has expanded to accommodate a growing baby, as well as in the overweight and obese. Purple striae are a sign of Cushing's syndrome.

Vitiligo

This depigmentation of the skin is often bilaterally symmetrical. Vitiligo is common in patients who are prone to autoimmune

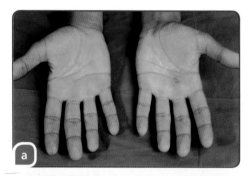

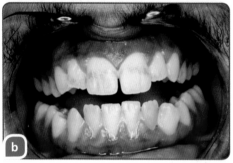

Figure 2.9 Hyperpigmentation palmar skin creases (a) and buccal mucosa (b) in Addison's disease.

diseases, such as Addison's disease and type 1 diabetes mellitus.

Acanthosis nigricans

This appears as velvety hyperpigmented patches of skin on the neck or under the axillae (**Figure 2.10**). It is a sign of insulin resistance and occurs in type 2 diabetes mellitus and polycystic ovary syndrome.

Acne

This is characterised by red pimples, which are the result of blocked sebaceous glands. Acne occurs as part of normal puberty.

However, it is also a common symptom of polycystic ovary syndrome and Cushing's syndrome.

Pretibial myxoedema

Also known as thyroid-associated dermopathy, pretibial myxoedema is a skin abnormality caused by deposition of hyaluronic acid in the skin. This causes patches of non-pitting oedema usually over the tibial area (Figure 5.2c).

Pretibial myxoedema can develop in patients with Graves' disease. It is also rarely associated with autoimmune hypothyroidism.

Peripheral oedema

This is swelling of the feet and ankles. In severe cases, it can extend further up the lower limbs. Peripheral oedema is characteristically bilateral in systemic disorders.

- If compression by a finger leaves an imprint, this is called pitting oedema; pitting oedema can occur in obesity, hypothyroidism and Cushing's syndrome (**Figure 2.6**)
- If the oedema is not compressible, it is termed non-pitting (lymphoedema); lymphoedema may be present in Turner's syndrome

Other signs

Specific signs in endocrine disease may not fit into a classic systems approach.

Proximal myopathy

This refers to wasting and weakness of the proximal muscles, namely those of hip and knee extension and the shoulder girdle (see **Figure 2.8**). A simple test for proximal

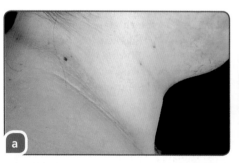

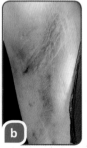

Figure 2.10 Darkened, velvety skin change of acanthosis nigricans on the neck (a) and axilla (b) of a woman with type 2 diabetes mellitus.

myopathy is to ask the patient to rise from a chair without the aid of their arms. They can also be asked if they can climb stairs. Proximal myopathy is present in Cushing's syndrome and hyperthyroidism.

Galactorrhoea

This term describes the secretion of a milky discharge from the nipples at times other than during pregnancy, the postnatal period or breastfeeding. Patients can often demonstrate the galactorrhoea themselves for confirmation of this sign.

Signs of hypocalcaemia

Patients with hypocalcaemia may have hyper-reflexia (brisk reflexes) on neurological examination. When examining a patient with hypocalcaemia, two additional specific clinical signs are sought: Trousseau's sign and Chvostek's sign.

To look for Trousseau's sign, apply and inflate the cuff of a sphygmomanometer to a pressure greater than systolic blood pressure. Leave the cuff inflated for 3 min. Patients with hypocalcaemia may develop spasm in the muscle of that arm, causing flexion of the wrist and clawing of the fingers (positive Trousseau's sign).

To look for Chvostek's sign, tap on the facial nerve at the angle of the jaw. In hypocalcaemia, this may cause the muscles to contract, causing a twitch at the ipsilateral side of the mouth (positive Chvostek's sign).

Examination sequence

The endocrine examination is tailored to the clinical scenario. The history often provides a likely diagnosis and therefore guides the examination. Not all parts of the examination are required for each patient. For example, if the clinical history points towards a diagnosis of Addison's disease, the clinician carries out a general examination but also looks for features such as postural hypotension, skin pigmentation and features of other autoimmune disease (e.g. vitiligo). In this scenario, examination of the visual fields would not be indicated, although this procedure would be essential if pituitary pathology were suspected from the history.

The examination is done to look not only for signs of an endocrine disease but also for the presence of complications of the disease. For example, examination of a patient with diabetes mellitus would also include a search for specific complications of the disease, such as peripheral neuropathy, vascular disease and retinopathy.

Examination methodology

Although it is necessary to tailor examinations to the clinical scenario and condition of individual patients, it is also helpful to maintain a consistent methodological approach. The examination is done in the following manner.

- Check basic measurements: weight, height, blood pressure and heart rate
- Carry out a brief general inspection, looking for striking signs of endocrine disease
- Examine the hands, face and skin (see pages 81–83)
- Carry out a systems examination, as indicated by the history and other clinical findings; systems that may be examined are:
  - the cardiovascular system
  - the thyroid
  - the eyes (include visual field testing)
  - the gastrointestinal system
  - the respiratory system
  - the neurological system
  - the joints
- Look for specific signs of certain conditions, such as hypocalcaemia (see page 85), as indicated by the history
- Look for signs of complications of diabetes mellitus (diabetes assessment)

An endocrine examination usually requires exposure of the patient's whole body. Verbal consent must be obtained before examination. A chaperone is offered to patients (as recommended by local guidelines), especially during sensitive (e.g. breast and genital) examinations. Be sensitive to the fact the patients from certain cultural backgrounds may find all physical examination unacceptable (especially when a male clinician is examining a woman).

Basic measurements

It is essential to have an accurate record of weight, height, blood pressure and heart rate, because changes to these variables over time are clinically significant. For example, insulin treatment may cause progressive weight gain in patients with diabetes mellitus.

Weight

Use accurate weighing scales to measure the patient's weight; use special bariatric scales if they are morbidly obese. In the UK, it is common practice is to record weight in kilograms (kg). However, many patients think of their weight in stones, pounds and ounces, so it is helpful to have a conversion table available.

Weight is measured after the patient has removed their shoes and heavy outer garments. Measurements are best done at the same time of day to minimise variation caused by temporal fluctuation in body weight.

Height

Measurements done with a wall-fixed meter are the most accurate and reproducible. Height is best measured after the patient has removed their shoes and socks. The patient stands with their heels, buttocks, shoulders and head touching the wall.

Height is best expressed in meters (m) and centimetres (cm). However, values can be converted to feet and inches for the patient's benefit, if necessary.

Body mass index

This is an expression of a person's weight in relation to their height.

Body mass index $(kg/m^2) =$ weight $(kg)/height^2 (m^2)$

Body mass index is used to categorise a patient's body weight (**Table 2.15**). The use of body mass index to define overweight and obesity has attracted criticisms. For example, very muscular persons may be categorised as overweight or obese despite having very little body fat. Other means of assessment, such as estimation of fat mass and measurement of waist circumference, are sometimes used. However, in most situations body mass index provides a simple, useful and representative classification of body weight.

Blood pressure

An accurate blood pressure reading is an essential part of any examination. The patient should be lying down (supine) or in a seated position, and is ideally left undisturbed for 15 min before their blood pressure is measured. Ask the patient to refrain from speaking during the procedure. Clothing is removed to expose the upper arm, which should be supported and relaxed (**Figure 2.11**).

It is vital to use the correct-sized cuff.

■ If the cuff is too small, the blood pressure measurement may be falsely high
■ If the cuff is too large, it may be falsely low

An electronic or a manual sphygmomanometer (blood pressure meter) is used.

Body mass index and body weight categories	
Body mass index (kg/m²)	Category
< 18.5	Underweight
18.5-25	Healthy weight
25-30	Overweight
30-35	Grade 1 obesity
35-40	Grade 2 obesity
> 40	Grade 3 obesity

*World Health Organization classification.

Table 2.15 Definition of body weight categories by body mass index*

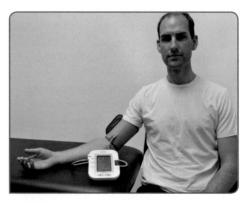

Figure 2.11 Measuring blood pressure.

The blood pressure reading must be interpreted in the context of the situation in which it was obtained. Many patients are nervous or feel stressed at clinic visits, so the reading may not truly reflect their actual blood pressure. Furthermore, blood pressure fluctuates greatly during any given day as a result of normal physiological mechanisms. Therefore a single reading is difficult to interpret.

With the increasing availability of 24-h blood pressure monitors and good quality home blood pressure monitors, a more accurate assessment of blood pressure may be made once the patient has left the endocrine clinic.

> **Large variations in blood pressure or nocturnal hypertension may be a sign of endocrine disease.** For example, these findings are characteristic of phaeochromocytoma.

Lying and standing blood pressure

This is measured by asking the patient to lie down for 5 min. With the patient in the supine position, their blood pressure is measured. The patient is then asked to stand for 3 min, and their blood pressure is measured again. The normal response is for the blood pressure to increase on standing.

A decrease in systolic blood pressure of >20 mmHg is diagnostic of postural hypotension. Be aware of any symptoms experienced during this procedure, for example light-headedness and fainting. There are a number of endocrine causes for postural hypotension (**Table 2.15**).

Heart rate

This is assessed by palpating an artery, typically the radial artery at the wrist, and recording the number of beats per minute. The rhythm may be irregular, which indicates possible arrhythmias, such as atrial fibrillation. In such cases, it is preferable to use an electrocardiogram to assess the heart rate, because not all cardiac depolarisations lead to a palpable peripheral pulse. Without a reliable palpable peripheral pulse, manual measurement may underestimate the true heart rate.

General inspection

This part of the consultation provides an overall impression of the patient. It is helpful to have a few questions in mind when first inspecting the patient.

- Does the patient look generally well or unwell?
- Are they generally overweight, underweight or of normal weight?
- Is their sexual development appropriate for their age?
- What is their emotional state? Patients with hyperthyroidism or phaeochromocytoma may be agitated or hyperactive (the converse may be true in those with hypothyroidism or hypopituitarism)
- Are there any classic syndromic features? For example, does the patient have the typical facial appearance of those with acromegaly, or the short stature and webbed neck of those with Turner's syndrome?
- Are there any skin signs?

The initial inspection may provide clues to a diagnosis, or it may prove diagnostic if the patient has a classic syndrome.

> **Be clear, specific and tactful when describing signs.** Remember that clinic letters are copied to patients, who may feel sensitive about their appearance as well as emotionally vulnerable. Use appropriate medical terms. For example, 'buffalo hump' is better described as an interscapular fat pad, and 'moon face' as rounded facies. Use emotionally neutral language and avoid words that could be interpreted as judgemental. For example, in the history it is better to say that patients 'described' symptoms rather than 'complained of' them.

Examination of patients with suspected thyroid disease

The aim in doing a thyroid examination is to answer the following questions.

- Is the patient clinically euthyroid, hyperthyroid or hypothyroid?

- Is there evidence of a goitre or thyroid mass? If yes, are there:
  - signs or symptoms of compression of the trachea (breathlessness and stridor) (see Figure 5.10)?
  - signs of malignancy, such as lymphadenopathy and hoarseness of the voice (caused by recurrent laryngeal nerve compression or invasion)?
  - signs of a cause of thyroid disease (e.g. signs of autoimmunity, such as vitiligo)?
- Is thyroid eye disease present?

Inspection of the thyroid gland

On general inspection, observe whether the patient is fidgety, agitated or sweaty, suggesting hyperthyroidism. In hypothyroidism, the patient is withdrawn; their skin may be dry and their hair thin and fragile.

The neck

Is there an obvious goitre? If a goitre or central neck mass is present, ask the patient to swallow; a goitre or thyroid mass will elevate on swallowing (**Figure 2.12a**). Then ask them to stick out their tongue;a thyroglossal cyst will elevate on tongue protrusion (**Figure 2.12b**). Are there any scars from previous thyroid surgery?

The hands

Is clubbing present? In rare instances, this is caused by Graves' disease and is termed thyroid acropachy. Rarely, onycholysis of the nails (their detachment from the nail bed), is present in cases of hyperthyroidism. Onycholysis occurring in thyrotoxicosis is termed Plummer's nails. Onycholyisis occurs in other non-endocrine conditions such as psoriasis or neoplasia.

Look and feel the palms. Patients with hyperthyroidism may have warm and sweaty palms or palmar erythema (reddening of the skin of the palm).

Ask the patient to hold their hands outstretched. Look for the fine tremor associated with hyperthyroidism; this can be accentuated by placing a piece of paper on top of the hands (**Figure 2.13**).

The eyes

Signs of thyroid eye disease may be present in patients with autoimmune thyroid disease. Do the patient's eyes show the obvious changes of thyroid eye disease, such as periorbital swelling or redness, conjunctival redness, proptosis and squint (see Figure 5.2a)? If any of these signs are present, specifically assess:

- visual acuity
- lid lag
- lid retraction
- eye movement

A Snellen chart is used to formally assess visual acuity. However, it can be assessed

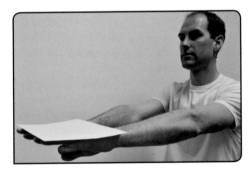

Figure 2.13 Detection of tremor. A piece of paper placed on the patient's outstretched hands makes tremor more pronounced.

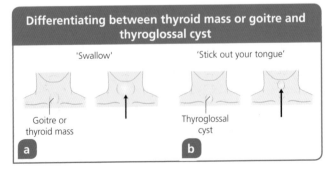

Differentiating between thyroid mass or goitre and thyroglossal cyst

'Swallow'   'Stick out your tongue'

Goitre or thyroid mass   Thyroglossal cyst

a   b

Figure 2.12 Differentiating between a thyroid mass or goitre and a thyroglossal cyst. (a) Ask the patient to swallow. A goitre or thyroid mass will rise on swallowing. (b) Ask the patient to stick out their tongue. A thyroglossal cyst will rise, but a goitre or thyroid mass will not.

more quickly by asking the patient to count how many fingers are being held up or by asking them to read some text.

Lid lag is a sign of hyperthyroidism of any cause. Ask the patient to look at a finger held about 30 cm away from them above the eye line. Ask them to keep their head still, then move the finger in an arc in front of them (**Figure 2.14**). When following the finger, the eyes may move earlier and the eyelids 'lag' behind in their movement.

The eyelids may be retracted in hyperthyroidism and thyroid eye disease. Lid retraction leaves white sclera visible above and below the eye.

To assess the movements of the eyes, ask the patient to look at a finger held in front of them. Move the finger in an enlarged 'H' across their visual field. Look for failure of movement in any direction of either eye (gaze palsy). Also, ask the patient if they experience double vision.

> **In thyroid eye disease, the retro-orbital tissues and extraocular muscles become inflamed.** This inflammation causes proptosis (forward displacement of the eyeballs), reduced eye movement and double vision (gaze palsies), corneal dryness and ulceration and, most seriously, compression of the optic nerve. Corneal damage and optic nerve compression may reduce visual acuity.

Palpation of the thyroid gland

The thyroid gland is best examined while standing behind the seated patient. Place one hand on either side of the gland, and palpate systematically around the neck (**Figure 2.15**). The normal thyroid gland is difficult to palpate. Ask the patient to swallow a sip of water during palpation; the thyroid will rise in response.

If a nodule or multiple nodules are felt, determine the following characteristics.

- Site: which lobe of the thyroid is palpable, and in which region?
- Size: roughly what is the diameter of the mass?
- Character: is the mass soft (a cyst), firm (a nodule) or hard and irregular (often malignancy)?
- Tenderness: tender nodules suggest recent haemorrhage, infection or inflammation (thyroiditis)
- Fixation: if the nodule is not freely mobile, this suggests fixation and raises the suspicion of malignancy
- Lymphadenopathy: enlargement of the cervical lymph nodes associated with thyroid nodules can be caused by infection or malignant spread

If the entire thyroid gland feels enlarged, try to establish answers to the following questions.

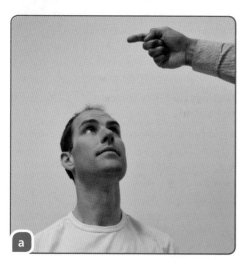
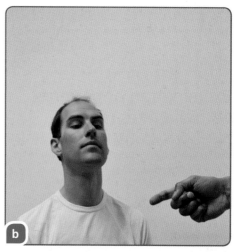

Figure 2.14 Examination for lid lag. (a) The clinician asks the patient to look at a finger held above the eye line. (b) Keeping the head still, the patient follows the movement of the clinician's finger. The movement of the patient's eyelids may lag behind that of the eyes.

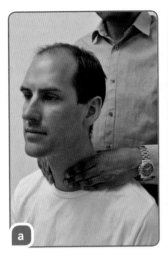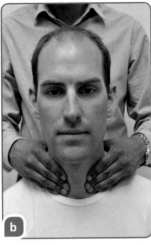

Figure 2.15 Examination of the thyroid gland. This is best done while standing behind the patient.

- Is the goitre symmetrical?
- Is it smooth (Graves' disease) or nodular (multinodular goitre)?
- How large is the goitre?
- Does the goitre extend behind the sternum (retrosternal extension)?
- Is the goitre tender (suggesting a thyroiditis)?
- Is the goitre causing obstruction of the thoracic inlet? Ask the patient to raise both arms; in cases of thoracic inlet obstruction, they develop facial plethora (positive Pemberton's sign; see Figure 5.9).

Auscultation of the thyroid gland

A stethoscope is used to auscultate the thyroid. A thyroid bruit (audible blood flow in the thyroid gland) may be heard if the thyroid is hypervascular; this finding indicates hyperthyroidism.

Examination of patients with diabetes mellitus

The diagnosis of diabetes mellitus is based on history and the results of biochemical investigations (see page 151) rather than clinical examination.

- Examination of the newly diagnosed patient with diabetes may give clues as to the cause of their diabetes
- Patients with previously diagnosed diabetes require regular review and

examination to ensure the early recognition and treatment of any complications

Newly diagnosed diabetes mellitus

Diabetes mellitus, especially type 2, is often asymptomatic at diagnosis. A history of polyuria, polydipsia, lethargy, blurred vision and weight loss is typical at presentation of type 1 diabetes mellitus. The following aspects of the examination can also be used to help distinguish between type 1 and type 2 diabetes mellitus.

Type 1 diabetes is associated with other autoimmune disorders, so look for signs of:

- vitiligo, which is associated with type 1 diabetes mellitus and other autoimmune disorders (e.g. Addison's disease)
- goitre, thyroid eye disease and signs of hyper- or hypothyroidism, all signs of autoimmune thyroid disease

Findings that may indicate type 2 diabetes mellitus are:

- acanthosis nigricans, a sign of insulin resistance
- obesity, which increases the risk of developing type 2 diabetes

Signs of dehydration may be apparent in both types of diabetes, because of osmotic fluid loss in the urine:

- dry tongue
- reduced skin turgor

- tachycardia
- postural hypotension

Cardiovascular system
Cardiovascular disease is the commonest cause of death in patients with diabetes mellitus. Therefore a full cardiovascular examination is done at diagnosis. This examination includes:

- inspection for signs of cardiac failure (elevated jugular venous pressure, peripheral oedema and crepitation at the lung bases)
- auscultation of the heart (a 3rd heart sound indicates cardiac failure)

Examination of patients with newly diagnosed diabetes must also include the features examined in the annual review of patients with existing diabetes, as outlined below.

Annual review of patients with diabetes
The multisystemic effects of diabetes mellitus mean that a thorough examination is required at regular intervals, at least annually. The annual review incorporates clinical examination and biochemical tests (**Table 2.16**)

> **In the UK, the annual diabetes review is carried out in primary care.** It is usually done by practice nurses who have received training in the assessment and management of chronic disease.

Eye examination
Microvascular damage from hyperglycaemia is responsible for diabetic retinopathy (see Chapter 4). Annual examination of the

Aspect of examination	Purpose
Blood pressure measurement*	To check for hypertension and assess cardiovascular risk
Weight* and height measurement	To determine body mass index, which is used to identify and monitor overweight or obesity
Examination of feet*	To identify peripheral vascular disease and peripheral neuropathy, and thus reduce the risk of serious diabetic foot problems
Palpation of pulses and determination of ankle-brachial pressure index	To identify peripheral vascular disease
Determination of urinary albumin:creatinine ratio (see page 104)*†	To identify microalbuminuria (an early sign of diabetic nephropathy)
Eye examination, including retinal photography*‡	To assess diabetic retinopathy
Examination of insulin injection sites	To assess for lipohypertrophy or lipoatrophy
Asking about smoking status*	To give smoking cessation advice and support, if required
Urinalysis with a urine dipstick (see page 103 and Table 2.20)	To identify proteinuria
Determination of estimated glomerular filtration rate*	To assess renal function
Measurement of cholesterol lipids concentration (total cholesterol, LDL and HDL cholesterol and triglyceride)*	To check for hyperlipidaemia and assess cardiovascular risk
Determination of haemoglobin A1c value*	To monitor glycaemic control

*These make up the key aspects assessed in primary care in the UK

†A more sensitive and quantitative test for detecting small amounts of albumin in the urine than urinalysis with the urine dipstick.

‡This has replaced direct ophthalmoscopy for examination of the retina.

Table 2.16 Annual examination for all patients with diabetes mellitus

retina (with pupil dilation), is required for all patients with diabetes mellitus.

For examination of the retina, digital retinography (photography of the retina) has superseded direct ophthalmoscopy (examination with an ophthalmoscope). Visual acuity testing with a Snellen chart is done at the time of retinal screening to detect deterioration in vision.

> In the UK, a free nationwide retinal screening programme is provided for patients with diabetes. The patient is directed to a hospital ophthalmology department or to an optician for digital retinal photography. The retinal photographs are then sent for specialist assessment, and the presence and degree of retinopathy is recorded.

Foot examination

The feet must be examined thoroughly at the annual review. Foot examination is also necessary when patients are admitted to hospital, to identify patients at high risk of developing foot ulceration while immobile.

The following are assessed during foot examination:

- the shape of the feet
- the skin
- vascular supply to the feet
- the nervous supply to the feet

Peripheral neuropathy may cause deformities of foot shape. Unopposed extension of the toes causes clawing of the toes. Charcot's foot can develop as a complication of neuropathy. The joint destruction and joint subluxation associated with this condition results in a misshapen and deformed foot (see Figure 4.11). This causes abnormal weight distribution across the plantar aspect of the foot. Abnormal loading and peripheral neuropathy commonly result in ulcer formation.

Skin examination

Examine the skin; is it intact or damaged? Look for the presence of any skin lesions associated with diabetes (see page 83). Is there erythema of the skin that might be associated with infection of inflammation

(see Figure 4.12)? If the skin has an ulcer, check for and record the following features.

- Size and depth: large ulcers are more serious but small ulcers (even 1mm diameter) can be serious if deep and probing down to bone (which means a high likelihood of underlying osteomyelitis)
- Position: ulcers over pressure areas are likely to be neuropathic; deep ulcers in other areas are likely to have been caused by impaired blood supply
- Ulcer base: are there any signs of granulation (healing) tissue?
- Infection: is pus being discharged? Is this pus malodorous? Is the ulcer surrounded by cellulitis?

Look between the toes for signs of fungal infections (e.g. athlete's foot). Fungal infections cause a break in the skin and are a portal for secondary bacterial infection. Also assess the toenails; these should be long enough to avoid the risk of causing lacerations to the toes.

Vascular examination

Diabetes is a strong risk factor for peripheral vascular disease, especially in combination with hypertension, hypercholesterolaemia and smoking. Peripheral vascular disease causes morbidity and mortality.

When examining the feet, check whether they are red and well perfused with arterial blood, or pale or blue? Palpate the feet, assessing their warmth; cool feet indicate poor blood supply. The adequacy of blood flow is also assessed by capillary refill time. Compress the skin on the big toe for 5 s. The toe will appear pale once pressure is applied. If blood flow is normal, the colour will return within 2 s. Slow capillary refill indicates inadequate blood flow.

Palpate the foot pulses to ensure their presence.

- Dorsalis pedis artery pulse: palpate just lateral to the extensor hallucis longus tendon on the dorsum of the foot
- Posterior tibial artery pulse: palpate just posterior to the medial malleolus

If arteries are impalpable, a handheld Doppler ultrasound scanner can be used to detect arterial blood flow (**Figure 2.16**).

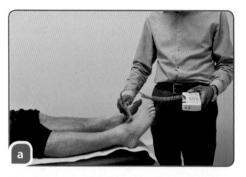
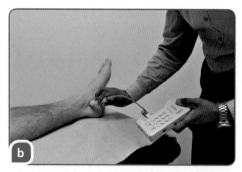

Figure 2.16 Examination by Doppler ultrasound. (a) Right dorsalis pedis pulse. (b) Left posterior tibial pulse.

Ankle-brachial pressure index

The relationship between ankle and brachial blood pressure is assessed by determining the ankle-brachial pressure index (ABPI). ABPI is measured by inflating a sphygmomanometer at the ankle, and using Doppler ultrasound to detect the pressure at which the artery is occluded.

Under normal circumstances, ankle blood pressure is greater than brachial blood pressure (ABPI >1). However, in peripheral vascular disease, ankle blood pressure may be reduced.

In patients with diabetes, the ankle pressure may be falsely increased because of arterial calcification and non-compressible arteries in the lower limb. For this reason, ABPI should be interpreted with caution in patients with diabetes.

> **Always ask patients with diabetes mellitus if they examine their feet.** Ideally, patients should examine their feet daily, looking for any skin damage, redness or ulceration. Reminders from health care professionals highlight to the patient the importance of looking after their feet, wearing appropriate footwear and reporting problems promptly.

Neurological examination

Diabetes mellitus can cause peripheral neuropathy. This affects the longest sensory nerve fibres first, i.e. the fibres supplying the feet and hands. Therefore sensory neuropathy tends to results in a 'glove and stocking' distribution of sensory loss (**Figure 2.17**).

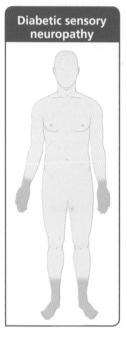

Diabetic sensory neuropathy

Figure 2.17 The 'glove and stocking' distribution of diabetic sensory neuropathy.

A number of techniques may be used to assess peripheral neuropathy (the Ipswich touch test, the monofilament test and neurothesiometer). The simplest is the Ipswich touch test, which can be carried out by health care professionals and patient's relatives.

1. Ask the patient to close their eyes and to say 'yes' when they feel a touch on their toes
2. Lightly touch one of their 1st (big) toes with a finger
3. Repeat by touching the 3rd (middle) and 5th (little) toe of the same foot, then the 1st, 3rd and 5th toes of the other foot

4. Calculate a score out of 6 for the number of times they correctly said 'yes' in response to a touch
5. A score of 4 or less indicates significant sensory neuropathy

Two simple reproducible tests can be done in the clinic setting:

■ the monofilament test, which is used to detect increased risk of ulceration (**Figure 2.18**)
■ vibratory sensory threshold determination with a neurothesiometer which is less widely available (**Figure 2.19**)

> **Check the footwear of patients with diabetes.** Poor-fitting footwear can rapidly lead to ulceration in those with existing neurovascular compromise. Do the shoes provide appropriate protection? If a foot deformity is present, does the shoe accommodate this? Orthotic shoes (specially made footwear) can be designed to fit an individual patient's feet and to relieve pressure on the deformed areas.

Injection sites

Examine the injection sites of patients who inject insulin, checking for:

■ lipohypertrophy (fatty lumps)
■ lipoatrophy (areas of fat loss)

Lipohypertrophy and lipatrophy are particularly likely to develop if the patient does not rotate injection sites. These findings are clinically significant, because injection into these areas causes variable absorption of insulin and therefore unpredictable swings in blood glucose.

Examination of patients with abnormalities of sexual development

Examination of the external genitalia and assessment of sexual development and pubertal stage must be carried out sensitively

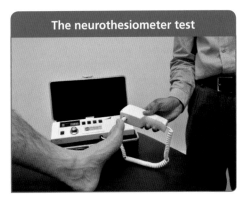

Figure 2.19 The neurothesiometer test to detect sensory neuropathy. The neurothesiometer is placed on the pulp of the 1st toe and produces a vibratory stimulus to test the large sensory fibres. Vibration amplitude is increased until the patient detects the vibration. A result of > 25 mV indicates an increased risk of neuropathic foot.

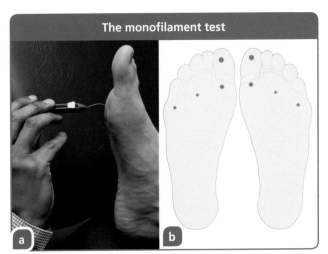

Figure 2.18 The monofilament test. (a) The monofilament, a thin nylon wire, is pushed against the plantar aspect of the feet on the 1st (big) toe and over the 1st, 3rd and 5th metatarsophalangeal joints. (b) Pressure is applied until the nylon buckles, representing 10 g of pressure, and the patient is asked if it can be felt. Inability to detect the pressure at any of the four sites on either foot means that the foot is at increased risk of ulceration.

and sympathetically. Formal assessment of pubertal state is done by a process named Tanner staging. This repeatable assessment allows objective recording of an individual patient's stage of puberty.

Tanner staging is in two parts. Pubic hair development is graded in a similar manner for males and females (**Tables 2.17** and **2.18**). Then for males, the sexual organs (penis, scrotum and testes) are assessed, and for females, breast development is graded. The Tanner stage is finally expressed, for example as G2/P3 in a male patient or B4/P3 in a female patient.

Examination of the male patient

Listen to the patient's voice to assess whether it has broken. In males, testosterone-dependent hair growth characteristically occurs in the armpits, in the beard area, on the chest, below the umbilicus on the abdomen, and on the back and limbs, in addition to in the genital region.

Palpate the testes. A Prader orchidometer is used to assess testicular size (**Figure 2.20**). The orchidometer is a series of fixed-volume oval beads on a string. The size of the testicle is compared with the size of the bead and the testicular volume described in millilitres (mL). If the testes are not palpable in the scrotum, palpate up the inguinal ligament to assess for maldescent.

Assess the penis. Does it show normal development? Is it an appropriate size? The term micropenis is used to describe a stretched penile length that is 2.5 standard deviations below the mean for age.

Tanner staging: male patients		
Genital stage	**Pubic hair stage**	**Features**
G1 Childlike penis, scrotum and testes	P1 No pubic hair	
G2 Enlargement of testes (> 4 mL) and coarsening of scrotal skin	P2 Sparse, straight, downy hair over at the base of the penis	
G3 Increased size of the penis, testes and scrotum	P3 Hair becomes darker and coarser but is still sparse around the pubic region	
G4 Further increase in length and circumference of the penis, and darkening of scrotal skin	P4 Pubic hair of adult type but no spread to inner thighs	
G5 Full development of sexual organs with adult appearance	P5 Adult quantity and distribution of pubic hair extending to inner thighs	

Table 2.17 Tanner staging for male patients

Tanner staging: female patients			
Breast stage	Features	Pubic hair stage	Features
B1	Childlike breasts	P1	No pubic hair
B2	Breast buds, each an elevated areola and papilla on a small mound	P2	Sparse, straight, downy hair over and along the labia majora
B3	Great enlargement of the breasts and areolae without contour development	P3	Hair becomes darker and coarser but is still sparse around the pubic region
B4	Further enlargement of breast tissue and areolae, with development of contour above the breast	P4	Pubic hair of adult type but no spread to inner thighs
B5	Adult breasts: recession of the areolae to the mound of the breast	P5	Adult quantity and distribution of pubic hair extending to inner thighs

Table 2.18 Tanner staging for female patients

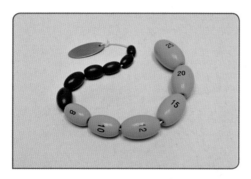

Figure 2.20 The Prader orchidometer.

Small testes are a feature of conditions in which there is primary hypogonadism or a prepubertal or long-standing deficiency of gonadotrophins (luteinising hormone and follicle-stimulating hormone). Primary hypogonadism occurs in Klinefelter's syndrome. Gonadotrophin deficiency occurs in Kallmann's syndrome and hypogonadotrophic hypogonadism (secondary gonadal failure). Patients have some pubertal hair development and penile growth through the actions of adrenal androgens, but the testes remain small.

Examination of the female patient

In addition to determining the Tanner stage, obtain a history of menstruation, because this provides information about sexual development. Examine the patient for other signs of abnormal sexual development.

Clitoromegaly

This is abnormal clitoral enlargement caused by androgen excess. If present at birth, it is the result of virilising congenital adrenal hyperplasia. Clitoromegaly that develops later in life is caused by androgens secreted from adrenal tumours.

Ambiguous genitalia

Exposure of the fetus to its own androgens (and rarely to exogenous androgens taken by the mother) determines the development of female or male external genitalia. The term ambiguous genitalia denotes an intermediate state between clitoromegaly and penis formation. This occurs in congenital adrenal hyperplasia, Turner's syndrome, Klinefelter's syndrome and other rare chromosomal abnormalities.

Examination of the visual fields in patients with hypothalamopituitary disease

Pituitary macroadenomas (tumours of the pituitary gland > 1 cm in diameter) and hypothalamic lesions can compress the optic chiasm. Pituitary macroadenomas create a specific visual field defect called bitemporal hemianopia (**Figure 2.21**). This defect is demonstrated by carrying out visual field testing by confrontation.

Visual field testing by confrontation

In this examination, the clinician systematically compares their own visual field with that of the patient (**Figure 2.22**).

1. Sit opposite the patient with your eyes at the same height and about 60 cm apart
2. Ask the patient to cover their right eye with their right hand, and cover your left eye with your left hand
3. Look at the patient's uncovered eye, and ask them to look into your uncovered eye
4. To assess the temporal field, hold a red hatpin equidistant between you and the patient, and move it from the superior right-hand corner of the (patient's) field of vision into the centre, asking the patient to say 'yes' when they can see the pin and when it looks bright red; compare the point at which the patient first sees the pin to your own field of vision, assessing whether you see the pin before the patient does
5. Repeat the procedure from the inferior right-hand corner of the patient's temporal field of vision
6. Assess the nasal field to determine the extent of any visual field defects (nasal field defects are uncommon in pituitary pathology unless the tumour is very large); to assess the nasal field, place your right hand over your left eye and ask the patient to remain with their right hand over their right eye
7. Move the pin from the superior and inferior left corners using the left hand, and again compare the patient's point of perception with your own

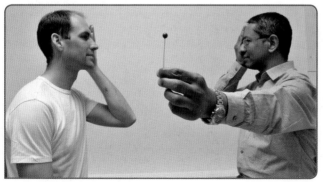

Figure 2.22 Examination of the visual fields by confrontation.

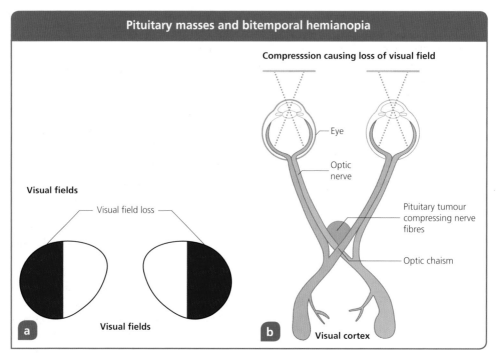

Pituitary masses and bitemporal hemianopia

Compresssion causing loss of visual field

Eye

Optic nerve

Visual fields

Visual field loss

Pituitary tumour compressing nerve fibres

Optic chaism

Visual fields

a

b   Visual cortex

Figure 2.21 The effect of a large pituitary mass on a patient's vision. (a) Bitemporal hemianopia, the specific visual field defect caused by pituitary macroadenomas. (b) The sensory visual nerve fibres from the temporal fields of each eye cross at the optic chiasm and travel to the opposite visual cortex. Bitemporal hemianopia occurs when the chiasm is compressed by a pituitary mass of sufficient size.

8. Repeat the procedure for the patient's right eye (asking them to cover the left eye with the left hand)

Patients with bitemporal hemianopia are unable to perceive the pin in the temporal visual fields of both eyes.

Visual field testing by confrontation is not highly sensitive; it does not detect subtle visual field defects. Therefore a test should be confirmed by formal visual field testing (see Figure 6.6).

Investigations

Starter questions

Answers to the following questions are on page 144.

8. Why are stimulation and suppression tests useful in endocrinology?
9. Does a normal 'negative' test result rule out an endocrine condition?
10. What are incidentalomas?
11. Why are investigation protocols used especially frequently in endocrinology?

Investigation of endocrine disease requires a methodical approach, because most endocrine tests are not part of regular screening and so have to be considered specifically in certain contexts. The few exceptions in the UK include thyroid function tests for congenital hypothyroidism and digital retinal photography for diabetic retinopathy.

The history and examination provide a differential diagnosis that helps guide which additional tests are likely to be diagnostic. Investigations for endocrine disorders are done in the following order:

■ biochemical tests
■ imaging studies
■ cytological and histological investigations

Deviation from this order of investigation can lead to diagnostic confusion, because abnormalities in the endocrine gland can be extremely small and therefore invisible or confused for artefact on a scan. On the other hand, an abnormality visible on a scan can be an incidental (non-significant) finding. Small cysts or adenomas are commonly found in the pituitary gland, thyroid gland, adrenal gland and pancreas and may be of no consequence. For this reason, imaging is usually carried out after a biochemical diagnosis is made.

> **Do not assume that a given diagnosis in the patient record is correct.** Patients with endocrine conditions are often followed lifelong in clinic, and seeing a patient for the first time is an opportunity to scrutinise and confirm the original diagnosis. Endocrine assays have become more accurate, and definitions of the underlying condition change, so it is useful to reassess the diagnosis from time to time.

Introduction to biochemical tests

Biochemical tests in endocrinology are carried out in different samples, including blood, urine, saliva and tissue fluid.

Endocrine conditions lead to a range of biochemical abnormalities. The abnormalities may be:

■ directly diagnostic of the condition (e.g. an extremely high serum prolactin concentration indicates prolactinoma)
■ indirectly diagnostic as a consequence of an endocrine diagnosis (e.g. anaemia in chronic kidney disease resulting from diabetic nephropathy)

Biochemical tests often need to be done in several stages, before diagnosis is complete. For example, a high serum glucose concentration confirming diabetes mellitus sometimes needs to be followed up with further testing, for example measurement of C-peptide concentration (in urine or plasma) or specific antibodies (in serum) to confirm or exclude type 1 diabetes mellitus.

The results of individual biochemical tests often need to be interpreted as part of a group of test results. The simplest example of this is serum thyroid-stimulating hormone (TSH) concentration, which usually needs to be interpreted alongside serum T_4 concentration, as a low TSH alone may be due to several different conditions (e.g. thyrotoxicosis, secondary hypothryoidism or sick euthyroid). Therefore, the two are often done together.

Many endocrine glands secrete hormones in a periodic pattern (see page 31). Therefore the result of a single hormone blood test is rarely enough to reach a diagnosis, so further dynamic and invasive tests are often needed to confirm abnormal secretion of that hormone.

The biochemical tests used to investigate endocrine disorders are categorised as follows.

■ Basal tests (see page 102): one-off 'spot' or a series of blood or urine tests done in an unstimulated state to diagnose abnormal hormone secretion or to guide further testing
■ Dynamic tests (see page 105): tests on blood samples taken over various time periods, often with administration of a drug, to show stimulation or suppression of the hormone tested

- Multiple invasive sampling tests (i.e. samples taken during the same procedure) (see page 110): arterial or venous samples are taken from different anatomical sites to identify the source of the excess hormone

Interpreting biochemical test results: general considerations

In the last 20 years, new endocrine assays have been developed and existing assays updated, giving more reliable results. Studies done using older, less sensitive or specific assays, need to be repeated with modern assays to reach more accurate conclusions. Various matters are considered when interpreting the results of biochemical endocrine tests:

- assay reliability
- normal range
- assay interference
- timing of the test
- feedback loops for hormone secretion

Assay reliability

Modern biochemical assays are very reliable and reproducible, but there is always some variability in results. A laboratory can provide information on the variability in results from multiple tests on the same sample (interassay variation).

Interassay variation is usually so small as to make no difference to the interpretation of the results. However, when the diagnosis of an endocrine condition is based on a fixed biochemical result (e.g. 48 mmol/mol as a cut-off point of HbA1c for the diagnosis of diabetes mellitus), repeating the test can lead to a marginally different result that may mean that the patient avoids a diagnostic label with widespread implications, for example for insurance premiums. Therefore borderline results should be repeated.

Normal range

The normal range of the results of a biochemical test is determined by the assay's manufacturers. Biochemistry laboratories may also state a normal range according to the local population, i.e. a value that lies within 2 standard deviations of the mean value for that population. This range encompasses 95% of the population; 2.5% of the normal population would be below the lower end of the normal range, and 2.5% above it (**Figure 2.23**). Therefore bear in mind that a result lying outside the normal range for a test is not necessarily abnormal; it may be normal for that individual patient. If a patient has no symptoms or has previous results that are very similar, it may be more appropriate to repeat the test in a few months rather than to immediately start treatment.

Assay interference

Some tests are based on the binding between an antibody (the component of the assay) and the molecule being tested, for example a hormone the antibody specifically recognises. The presence of endogenous autoantibodies (called heterophile antibodies) or human anti-animal antibodies can interfere with the reaction between the hormone being tested in the sample and reagent antibodies in the immunoassay. This is termed assay interference and can produce false results.

For example, if a patient's blood contains antibodies against the animal whose antibodies are used in the assay (e.g. because they have a pet rabbit), these can compete with the assay antibodies and bind to the molecule

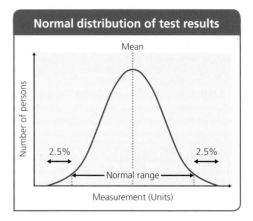

Figure 2.23 Normal distribution of test results, with a normal range encompassing 95% of the population around the mean.

being tested, leading to false positive results. This phenomenon may occur when measuring serum TSH, because the antibodies used in this biochemical assay are synthesised from animal antibodies.

Diagnostic confusion can also arise from the use of certain drugs that interfere with biochemical tests. For example, if a woman is taking the oral contraceptive pill, her test results may show a high concentration of serum cortisol even in the absence of abnormal cortisol secretion. This is because the oral contraceptive pill can increase the concentration of cortisol-binding globulin. This, in turn, increases the amount of cortisol bound to the cortisol-binding globulin (this bound cortisol is metabolically inactive). Therefore the total serum cortisol concentration may be high even if the concentration of free or unbound (and therefore metabolically active) cortisol is normal.

A thorough drug history and awareness of drug interference with hormone assays helps prevent misinterpretation of some tests. If a drug directly alters the concentration of a hormone, then use of the drug may need to be temporarily suspended to enable accurate measurement of the concentration of that hormone. For example, angiotensin-converting enzyme inhibitors can affect renin and aldosterone levels, so these drugs must be stopped for a few weeks before measurement of the concentration of these hormones.

Timing of the test

As described in Chapter 1, most hormones are released in pulses, and secretion of many hormones also shows a circadian rhythm. Therefore the result for a hormone concentration may be affected by the timing of the test. **Figure 2.24** shows this effect for testosterone: samples drawn at two different times may yield two very different concentrations of serum testosterone.

Similarly, because of diurnal variation in cortisol secretion, the serum concentration of this hormone measured in a sample taken in the afternoon will be lower than that in an early morning sample. Measuring an undetectable midnight cortisol excludes active Cushing's syndrome (when the diurnal variation is lost and cortisol is secreted throughout

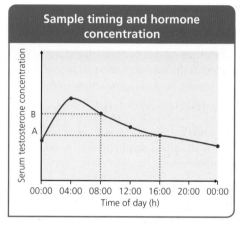

Figure 2.24 Effect of sample timing when hormones have a diurnal pattern of release. In a normal healthy man, testosterone concentration peaks before dawn. A sample taken at 16:00 (A) would be erroneously interpreted as indicating testosterone deficiency if judged against the same criteria as a 08:00 sample (B).

the day). Therefore a record of the timing of sampling is necessary when interpreting the results of hormone tests. Normal ranges usually reflect the most appropriate time for testing, for example the early morning for testosterone.

Apart from diurnal variation in hormone secretion, other physiological events may affect hormone levels. For example, secretion of luteinising hormone and follicle-stimulating hormone varies at different stages of the menstrual cycle. Therefore luteal phase, follicular phase and post-menopausal reference ranges are needed to help interpret test results for these hormones.

Feedback loops for hormone secretion

Identification of the hormone whose levels are abnormal is often not enough to ascertain the cause of the patient's symptoms. It is necessary to differentiate between two explanations:

- a primary disorder of the endocrine gland secreting the hormone
- a secondary problem arising from disorder of other endocrine glands involved in the feedback loop controlling secretion of that hormone

Consider a man with symptoms of hypogonadism and low serum testosterone concentration. The pathology could lie in the testes (primary hypogonadism) or in the hypothalamus or pituitary (secondary hypogonadism). To determine which of these two scenarios is the case, it is necessary to measure the serum gonadotrophins (luteinising hormone and follicle-stimulating hormone), which stimulate production of testosterone from the testes.

- Increased gonadotrophin concentrations suggest that feedback from the pituitary is working well and sending a hormonal message to try to stimulate the testes to produce testosterone, therefore the problem is in the testes (i.e. primary hypogonadism)
- Decreased gonadotrophin concentrations suggest that the hormonal message from the pituitary or the hypothalamus to the testes to produce testosterone is insufficient (i.e. secondary hypogonadism)

In this way, the results of biochemical tests can be used not only to diagnose hormone deficiency (hypogonadism in this case) or excess but also to determine the anatomical site of the pathology (the testis, pituitary or hypothalamus).

Understanding endocrine disease requires understanding of hormonal feedback systems. This is a frequent topic in examinations, so be sure to learn the feedback loops for all hormones, especially those for hormones secreted by the hypothalamus, pituitary and end organs (i.e. thyroid, adrenal and gonads).

Biochemical tests in endocrinology

Most of the biochemical endocrine tests are carried out in a basal or unstimulated state. Examples of these basal biochemical endocrine tests are shown in **Table 2.19**.

Blood tests

Biochemical tests in endocrinology, including measurements of hormone concentration, are most commonly carried out on blood. Blood may be drawn from a peripheral vein or from a specific vein close to the endocrine gland of interest. For example, blood samples are taken from the adrenal vein in investigations of aldosterone-secreting adenoma.

Basal biochemical endocrine tests: examples		
Endocrine system	Test(s)	Disorder(s)
Thyroid	TSH, free T_3 and free T_4	Hypothyroidism (primary and secondary)
		Hyperthyroidism
Male reproductive	Testosterone, luteinising hormone and follicle-stimulating hormone	Hypogonadism (primary and secondary) and infertility
Female reproductive	Oestradiol, luteinising hormone and follicle-stimulating hormone	Hypogonadism (primary and secondary)
Prolactin	Prolactin	Hyperprolactinaemia
Renin-angiotensin-aldosterone	Aldosterone:renin ratio	Hyperaldosteronism
Parathyroid	Parathyroid hormone and calcium	Hyperparathyroidism
		Hypoparathyroidism
Glycaemic control	Capillary and plasma blood glucose, HbA1c	Diabetes mellitus

T_3, -tri-iodothryonine; T_4, thyroxine; TSH, thyroid-stimulating hormone.

Table 2.19 Examples of basal biochemical tests in endocrinology

Hormone concentrations are measured in serum and plasma, samples of which are obtained by centrifugation of blood.

- Plasma is stored in tubes containing an anticoagulant and therefore contains clotting factors and fibrinogen
- Serum is allowed to clot, so it does not contain clotting factors and fibrinogen

Capillary blood samples are occasionally used for biochemical tests in endocrinology. The commonest example is blood glucose monitoring using portable blood glucose monitors in patients with diabetes mellitus which are extensively used by patients. Biochemical tests for diabetes diagnosis and degree of control include determination of the haemoglobin A1c value (**Figure 2.25**).

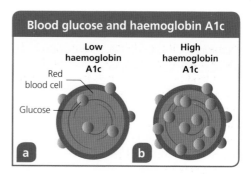

Blood glucose and haemoglobin A1c

Figure 2.25 The degree of glyclation of red blood cells determines haemoglobin A1c value. (a) If blood glucose concentration is low, less haemoglobin in red blood cells becomes glycated, giving a low haemoglobin A1c value. (b) If blood glucose concentration is high, more haemoglobin becomes glycated, giving a high haemoglobin A1c value.

Capillary and venous blood glucose concentrations differ when they are measured simultaneously. Glucose concentration in capillary blood is higher than that in venous blood because:

- capillary blood has yet to deliver its glucose to tissues and is therefore glucose-rich
- venous blood has delivered its glucose to the tissues while passing through them and is therefore glucose-depleted

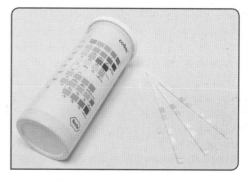

Figure 2.26 The urine dipstick test.

Urine tests

Urine tests are common in endocrinology. Many hormones are excreted by the kidneys, so they or their metabolites can be measured in the urine. A urine sample may be taken as a 'spot' one-off sample, or samples can be collected over a period of time (e.g. 24-h urine collection for the measurement of cortisol concentration in investigations of Cushing's syndrome).

Tests on 'spot' urine samples

The urine dipstick test is done by briefly dipping a test strip into a urine sample. The test strip has various chemical reagents bonded to it (**Figure 2.26**), and these change colour in response to different test substances in the urine.

After the test strip is removed from the urine, the strip is held horizontally (to avoid chemical reagents cross contaminating) and the colours of each reagent are compared with those on a colour reference chart (after defined time periods of 30–60 s). The intensity of each colour reflects the urine concentration of the test substance reacting with each reagent.

Table 2.20 lists the substances tested by most urine dipstick tests and the relevance of positive results. Certain combinations of results suggest specific diagnoses, for example the presence of glucose and ketones indicates diabetic ketoacidosis (the presence of ketosis alone can be caused by fasting).

Urine dipstick results		
Test item	Result	Clinical significance
Glucose	Negative	Normal
	Positive	Diabetes mellitus or renal glycosuria
Ketones	Negative	Normal
	Positive	Uncontrolled diabetes, or fasting or starved state
Protein	Negative	Normal
	Positive	Diabetic nephropathy or renal disorders
Specific gravity	Low	Normal
	High	Dehydration, glycosuria or syndrome of inappropriate antidiuretic hormone
Haemoglobin	Negative	Normal
	Positive	Haematuria, haemoglobinuria and myoglobinuria, or menstrual bleeding
White blood cells	Negative	Normal
	Positive	Urinary tract infection or sterile pyuria
Nitrites	Negative	Normal
	Positive	Urinary tract infection

Table 2.20 Interpretation of urine dipstick results

Glycosuria (the presence of glucose in the urine) is not always caused by diabetes mellitus. The condition occurs when blood glucose is so high that the renal tubules are unable to reabsorb it all. The so-called renal threshold has been reached, and the excess glucose leaks into the urine.

However, if the renal threshold is reduced, as it is in pregnancy, glycosuria can occur despite normal blood glucose levels. This condition is called renal glycosuria.

Other examples of 'spot' urine tests include the test for microalbuminuria (the presence of small abnormal amounts of albumin in the urine) in a patient with diabetes mellitus to investigate for diabetic nephropathy. Urinary

sodium and osmolality are useful tests for investigation of the syndrome of inappropriate antidiuretic hormone (**Figure 2.27**) and diabetes insipidus. Urine osmolality and sodium will be high in syndrome of inappropriate antidiuretic hormone, yet urine osmolatity will be low in diabetes insipidus.

Tests on 24-h urine samples

Collection of urine over a set time period enables the daily excretion of a hormone or chemical substance to be calculated. The success of this investigation relies on the cooperation of the patient; a low urinary volume suggests that urine collection is incomplete. Several tests are done on samples collected over 24 h, including measurement of:

- free cortisol
- adrenaline (epinephrine), noradrenaline (norepinephrine) and their breakdown products metadrenaline (metanephrine) and normetadrenaline (normetanephrine)
- 5-hydroxyindole acetic acid
- calcium

24-h urinary free cortisol

This test is used to detect oversecretion of cortisol and is commonly used to screen for Cushing's syndrome. However, there are several causes of false positive results, including depression, chronic alcoholism and polycystic ovary syndrome.

24-h urinary adrenaline, noradrenaline, metadrenaline and normetadrenaline

Excessive production of the hormones adrenaline (epinephrine) and noradrenaline (norepinephrine) is a classic indication of phaeochromocytoma. Evidence for excessive adrenaline and noradrenaline production is also provided by a high concentration of their breakdown products, metadrenaline (metanephrine) and normetadrenaline (normetanephrine).

Certain medications, such as tricyclic antidepressants, can cause false positive results. Therefore use of these drugs are temporarily suspended before urine collection.

24-h urinary 5-hydroxyindole acetic acid

This test is carried out in investigations of carcinoid syndrome. Some foods, such as

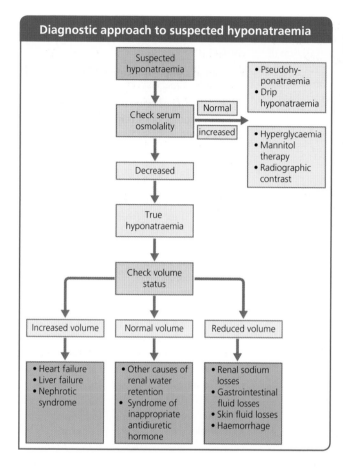

Figure 2.27 The diagnostic approach to suspected hyponatraemia.

avocados, walnuts, bananas, tomatoes and aubergines (eggplants), contain precursors of 5-hydroxyindole acetic acid; their consumption can produce false results showing increased 5-hydroxyindole acetic acid concentration. Therefore patients should avoid eating these foods in the 3 days before the test.

24-h urinary calcium

The results of this test give a measure of urinary calcium excretion. Causes of high urinary calcium (hypercalciuria) include primary hyperparathyroidism, excess calcium or vitamin D intake or replacement, sarcoidosis and renal tubular acidosis. Hypercalciuria increases the risk of formation of renal stones.

Saliva tests

Occasionally, hormone concentration is measured in saliva. For example, measurement of midnight salivary cortisol concentration

is a useful test in investigations of Cushing's syndrome. The sample for this test can be collected by the patient at home during the night, after waking from sleep.

Tests on tissue fluid

Biochemical tests are sometimes carried out on tissue fluid. An example is the continuous glucose-monitoring system. This system includes a small indwelling cannula that sits under the skin and measures glucose concentration in the interstitial tissue fluid every few minutes. The cost of this system limits its everyday use in patients with diabetes.

Dynamic biochemical tests

Dynamic tests are needed in investigations of a few endocrine conditions. These tests require a series of blood and occasionally urine samples to be taken at different intervals over time, often with administration of a drug, to show stimulation or suppression of the hormone tested.

Dynamic endocrine tests are broadly divided into the following categories:

- Hormone stimulation tests
- Hormone suppression tests
- Restriction (deprivation) tests

Hormone stimulation tests

Hormone stimulation tests are used to detect hormone deficiency. In these tests, drugs that enhance hormone secretion from the endocrine gland are administered and the gland's response to this stimulation assessed. The results determine whether the low concentration of a hormone in the blood, as measured by basal testing, reflects physiological variation or a deficiency.

The three most commonly used hormone stimulation tests are:
- the short Synacthen test
- the insulin stress test
- the glucagon test

Other tests, with other drugs stimulating hormonal production, are also used, particularly in paediatrics. However, these are beyond the scope of this chapter and are rarely performed.

Short Synacthen test

In this commonly used test for adrenal insufficiency, synthetic ACTH (tetracosactide, Synacthen) is used to stimulate cortisol secretion from the adrenal cortex. This simple test is easily carried out in both inpatient and outpatient settings.

Patients who take hydrocortisone tablets should not take any on the day of the test, because, as a corticosteroid, this drug can interfere with the result. Longer-acting corticosteroids, such as dexamethasone and prednisolone, need a longer 'washout' period. Patients are advised to stop taking oestrogen-containing medications 6 weeks before the test as this increases the cortisol-binding globulin leading to a falsely elevated cortisol result.

The short Synacthen test usually starts at 9 a.m to capture the early morning peak in cortisol.

1. A blood sample is taken to measure serum cortisol concentration at baseline
2. Next, 250 µg of Synacthen is injected intravenously or intramuscularly
3. Blood samples are taken 30 and 60 min later for repeat measurements of serum cortisol

In subjects without adrenal insufficiency, serum cortisol concentration will have increased to >550 nmol/L at 30 min after Synacthen injection (this threshold may differ between assays used in different laboratories). A failure of serum cortisol to increase to >550 nmol/L within 30 min indicates adrenal insufficiency.

The short Synacthen test does not reliably distinguish between primary and secondary adrenal failure, because the results can also be abnormal in chronic secondary adrenal failure. This condition develops when loss of ACTH production from the pituitary gland causes atrophy of the adrenal cortex. After an extended period of ACTH deficiency, the adrenal gland becomes unable to respond to Synacthen administration, therefore the peak cortisol concentration measured in the test will be reduced.

Insulin stress test

This test, also known as the insulin tolerance test, is used to detect:

- cortisol deficiency caused by hypothalamic or pituitary failure, i.e. secondary adrenal insufficiency
- growth hormone deficiency

The test exploits that fact that, ordinarily, an episode of hypoglycaemia causes a surge in cortisol and growth hormone secretion. Therefore if cortisol and growth hormone concentrations fail to adequately increase in response to artificially induced hypoglycaemia, the deficiency of these hormones is confirmed.

The insulin stress test is carried out as follows.

1. Venous blood samples are drawn for measurement of glucose, cortisol and growth hormone concentrations at baseline

2. Hypoglycaemia (blood glucose concentration < 2.2 mmol/L) is induced by infusing rapid-acting insulin through an intravenous cannula
3. Serial blood samples are drawn at 30, 60, 90 and 120 min for measurement of glucose, cortisol and growth hormone concentration; the test is terminated early if adequate hypoglycaemia is achieved before 120 min

In a healthy subject, adequate hypoglycaemia (i.e. blood glucose concentration < 2.2 mmol/L) is induced (usually after 30 min), causing serum cortisol concentration to increase to > 550 nmol/L. Failure to reach this threshold serum cortisol concentration indicates adrenal insufficiency.

An increase in growth hormone concentration to > 6 µg/L after adequate hypoglycaemia is a normal response. However, growth hormone concentration < 3 µg/L indicates growth hormone deficiency severe enough to warrant growth hormone replacement in an adult.

As an example, **Table 2.21** shows insulin stress test results for a patient with hypopituitarism. The plasma blood glucose concentration of 2.1 mmol/L at 30 min shows that the test produced adequate hypoglycaemia. Cortisol and growth hormone deficiency are shown by the lack of an appropriate increase in the concentration of either hormone in response to this hypoglycaemia.

The insulin stress test is unsuitable for patients with epilepsy, because the severe hypoglycaemia required for the test may precipitate a seizure. Similarly, the test should not be taken by patients with ischaemic heart disease, in whom hypoglycaemia can cause angina.

The induced hypoglycaemia produces symptoms that are often unpleasant for patients. These include tremor, profuse sweating and feelings of hunger.

Glucagon test

This test is used to investigate growth hormone deficiency when the insulin stress test is contraindicated, for example in patients with epilepsy or ischaemic heart disease.

The glucagon test is carried out as follows.

1. A venous sample is drawn for measurement of baseline growth hormone concentration
2. Next, 1 mg of glucagon is injected subcutaneously
3. Serial blood samples are drawn at 30, 60, 90 and 120 min for further measurement of growth hormone

As in the insulin stress test, an increase in growth hormone concentration to > 6 mg/L after the challenge is a normal response in adults.

> **The gold standard test for assessing for growth hormone deficiency** is the insulin stress test. However, because of the potential risks with hypoglycaemia, this test is not performed in all hospitals and never in general practice.

Hormone suppression tests

Hormone suppression tests are used to diagnose excessive hormone secretion. These tests involve giving drugs that suppress secretion of specific hormones; inadequate suppression suggests abnormally high levels of hormone secretion.

The 3 most commonly used hormone suppression tests are:

- the overnight dexamethasone suppression test
- the low-dose dexamethasone suppression test
- the oral glucose tolerance test

Example insulin stress test results			
Time (min)	Plasma glucose concentration (mmol/L)	Plasma cortisol concentration (nmol/L)	Plasma growth hormone concentration (mg/L)
0	4.3	132	0.9
30	2.1	157	1.9
60	4.0	141	1.6
90	4.2	122	1.6
120	4.2	119	1.2

Table 2.21 Insulin stress test results for a patient with hypopituitarism

Overnight dexamethasone suppression test

This is a screening test for Cushing's syndrome. It is commonly used to exclude excessive cortisol secretion in patients incidentally discovered to have adrenal nodules on abdominal computerised tomography (CT) or magnetic resonance imaging (MRI).

The test involves the following steps.

1. Check that the patient is not taking exogenous steroids or enzyme-inducing or enzyme-inhibiting drugs
2. At 11 p.m., the patient takes 1 mg of oral dexamethasone
3. At 9 a.m. the following day, a serum cortisol sample is taken

The normal response is for the morning serum cortisol concentration to be suppressed to <50 nmol/L. Failure of overnight dexamethasone to adequately reduce serum cortisol suggests cortisol hypersecretion (Cushing's syndrome), however there are many false positives with this test.

Low-dose dexamethasone suppression test

This test is used to screen for Cushing's syndrome, especially if the results of other screening tests (e.g. 24-h free urinary cortisol and 1 mg overnight dexamethasone suppression test) are contradictory.

The procedure is as follows.

1. At 9 a.m., a blood sample is drawn for measurement of baseline serum cortisol concentration
2. Next, 0.5 mg of dexamethasone is administered orally every 6 h for 48 h
3. At 48 h, so again at 9 a.m., another blood sample is drawn to measure serum cortisol

A normal response is suppression of serum cortisol concentration to <50 nmol/L at 9 a.m. on day 2. Inadequate suppression of serum cortisol suggests cortisol hypersecretion (Cushing's syndrome).

Oral glucose tolerance test

The oral glucose tolerance test is occasionally used as a stimulation test to diagnose diabetes mellitus (by measuring a rise in glucose). However, it is also used to assess excessive growth hormone secretion in patients with suspected acromegaly. Growth hormone secretion is normally inhibited by glucose.

The test is carried out as follows.

1. Confirm that the patient has fasted overnight
2. A blood sample (at baseline, time 0) is taken to measure glucose and growth hormone concentration
3. Next, 75 g of oral glucose solution is administered
4. Blood samples are taken at 30, 60, 90 and 120 min for measurement of glucose and growth hormone concentration

In a healthy subject, growth hormone concentration is suppressed to <0.6 µg/L after the glucose load. Failure to suppress growth hormone concentration to <0.6 µg/L after the glucose load confirms a diagnosis of acromegaly. A glucose level >11.1 mmol/L at 120 min is diagnostic of diabetes mellitus.

Restriction (deprivation) tests

Some endocrine tests involve a series of blood (and urine) tests after restriction of fluid or food. Two examples of such tests are:

- the water deprivation test for investigation of diabetes insipidus
- the supervised 72-h fast for investigation of spontaneous hypoglycaemia

Water deprivation test

This test is used to investigate diabetes insipidus. In a healthy subject, fluid restriction increases serum osmolality, which stimulates release of antidiuretic hormone from the posterior pituitary. The effects of the antidiuretic hormone are to concentrate the urine and decrease urinary output.

However, patients with diabetes insipidus continue to produce large amount of dilute urine despite water deprivation. There are two explanations for this.

- Cranial diabetes insipidus: lack of synthesis or release of antidiuretic hormone as a result of disorders of the hypothalamus or posterior pituitary gland
- Nephrogenic diabetes insipidus: insensitivity of the kidneys to antidiuretic hormone

The water deprivation test is carried out as follows.

1. The patient stops drinking tea, coffee, alcohol, and other fluids, and refrains from smoking, from midnight on the day before the test. If the symptoms are severe (such that a patient would struggle to stop fluid overnight) the fluid is only restricted in the morning of the test.
2. At the start of the test the following morning, the patient is weighed, and basal blood and urine samples are taken for determination of serum and urine osmolality, respectively
3. Water and food are withheld for up to a further 8 h
4. Urine and serum osmolality are measured at regular intervals (between 1 and 3 hourly)
5. If weight loss exceeds 3% of the initial body weight, or if serum osmolality is > 305 mOsm/kg, the test is stopped and synthetic antidiuretic hormone (desmopressin acetate) is administered (see page 128); otherwise the test continues for a further 8 h
6. If urine fails to become concentrated (urine osmolality < 750 mOsm/kg) after 8 h of water deprivation, desmopressin is given by intranasal spray or intramuscularly and the patient is allowed to drink; blood

and urine samples (for serum and urine osmolality) are monitored for a further 4 h

Table 2.22 outlines the interpretation of the results of the water deprivation test. In healthy subjects, restriction of fluid intake causes the release of antidiuretic hormone. The effect of this hormone is to reduce urine output and thus increase urine osmolality (to > 750 mOsm/kg) while maintaining normal serum osmolality.

In cranial diabetes insipidus (antidiuretic hormone deficiency), the body is unable to concentrate urine. Therefore urine osmolality remains < 750 mOsm/kg despite water deprivation. However, administration of desmopressin restores the body's ability to concentrate urine.

In nephrogenic diabetes insipidus (antidiuretic hormone insensitivity), the body fails to concentrate urine when deprived of fluids, and administration of desmopressin has no effect.

Supervised 72-h fast to investigate spontaneous hypoglycaemia

Spontaneous hypoglycaemia may be caused by excessive insulin secretion from an insulinoma, an insulin-producing tumour arising from pancreatic beta cells. A supervised 72-h fast is carried out to investigate insulinoma in patients presenting with symptoms of spontaneous hypoglycaemia (see Chapter 10).

The supervised 72-h fast is carried out as follows.

1. The patient is admitted to hospital, and food is withheld for up to 72 h (the patient is permitted to drink water freely)
2. If the patient experiences symptoms of hypoglycaemia, a blood sample is drawn

Interpretation of water deprivation test results			
Condition	Urinary volume	Post-water deprivation urine osmolality (mOsm/kg)	Post-desmopressin urine osmolality (mOsm/kg)
Normal	Decreases	> 750	*
Cranial diabetes insipidus	Remains high	< 300	> 750
Nephrogenic diabetes insipidus	Remains high	< 300	< 300

*These patients do not receive desmopressin, because their urine osmolality is > 750 mOsm/kg after water deprivation.

Table 2.22 Interpretation of results of the water deprivation test

for measurement of plasma glucose concentration

3. The test is terminated as follows.
   - If plasma glucose decreases to less than 2.2 mmol/L, another blood sample is taken for measurement of insulin and C-peptide concentration, and the patient is allowed to eat
   - If plasma glucose concentration remains > 2.2 mmol/L after the 72-h fast, the test is terminated and the patient is allowed to eat

If hypoglycaemia does not occur after a 72-h fast, the diagnosis of insulinoma is highly unlikely.

The insulin and C-peptide concentrations measured at the time of hypoglycaemia (blood glucose < 2.2 mmol/L) during the test are interpreted as follows.

- Increased concentrations of insulin and C-peptide suggest endogenous insulin overproduction (e.g. by an insulinoma)
- Increased insulin concentration but undetectable C-peptide suggests that the patient is taking exogenous insulin and is factitiously inducing hypoglycaemia (to induce symptoms of an illness).

> **If blood glucose is low during a 72-h fast test, the urine or blood must be screened for sulfonylureas.** Sulfonylureas are a class of drugs used to treat type 2 diabetes mellitus by stimulating insulin production in the pancreas. Therefore hypoglycaemia associated with sulfonylurea use is associated with increased insulin and C-peptide (as in cases of insulinoma). Screening for sulfonylureas excludes factitious illness (e.g. Munchausen's syndrome).

Invasive biochemical tests

Occasionally, invasive investigations are necessary to localise the origin of excess hormone secretion. In invasive tests, hormone concentrations are measured in blood samples from blood vessels close to the endocrine gland rather than from the peripheral circulation.

The two most commonly performed invasive endocrine tests are:

- inferior petrosal sinus sampling
- adrenal vein sampling

Other tests include parathyroid sampling, to locate a parathyroid adenoma not seen on imaging or pancreatic sampling, to locate a small neuroendocrine secretory tumour of the pancreas.

Inferior petrosal sinus sampling

This investigation is done to distinguish between pituitary-dependent Cushing's disease and Cushing's syndrome caused by an ACTH-secreting non-pituitary tumour (ectopic ACTH syndrome) (see Chapter 6). It is a useful investigation when other biochemical and imaging studies fail to conclusively differentiate between these two conditions.

Inferior petrosal sinus sampling is available only at specialist centres. It is carried out as follows.

1. On each side of the body, an intravenous catheter is fed through the femoral vein to reach the inferior petrosal sinus (**Figure 2.28**)
2. Blood samples are drawn simultaneously from both sides of the inferior petrosal sinus, as well as a peripheral vein, for measurement of baseline ACTH concentration
3. Next, 100 µg of corticotrophin-releasing hormone is administered intravenously

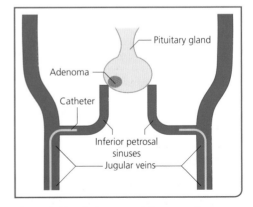

Figure 2.28 Inferior petrosal sinus sampling.

4. A series of blood samples are taken simultaneously from each of the catheters in the inferior petrosal sinus and the peripheral vein for measurement of ACTH

The results of the test are interpreted as follows.

- If ACTH concentration (basal or after stimulation with corticotrophin-releasing hormone) in the blood samples from the inferior petrosal sinus are higher than those from the peripheral vein, this implies a pituitary source for the excess ACTH causing Cushing's syndrome
- If ACTH concentration in the blood samples from the inferior petrosal sinus and the peripheral vein are similar, this suggests an ectopic (i.e. non-pituitary) source of ACTH as the cause of Cushing's syndrome

Adrenal vein sampling

This invasive test is used to measure hormonal secretion from each adrenal gland before adrenalectomy is considered. Imaging studies (e.g. CT or MRI) may miss a small secretory nodule, or they may detect an incidental nodule that is not responsible for the excessive hormonal secretion. Therefore adrenal vein sampling is used to confirm that the site of excessive secretion correlates with the position of the anatomical abnormalities visible on the scan.

An intravenous catheter is fed through each femoral vein to reach the adrenal veins. The two catheters are then used to take blood samples from both adrenal veins for the measurement of adrenal hormones such as cortisol, aldosterone and metadrenaline (metanephrine) concentration.

Adrenal vein sampling is used to compare hormone secretion on each of the two sides. It is a technically demanding procedure, because cannulation of the right adrenal vein is often difficult (see Chapter 1). Therefore this test is done in specialist centres only.

Imaging studies

These have an essential role in investigations of endocrine disorders. Imaging studies are carried out to identify or localise structural and functional abnormalities in endocrine organs.

In endocrinology, imaging studies are ideally done after clinical history, physical examination and biochemical tests. However, incidental abnormalities are sometimes found when a scan is done for another reason and the history, exam and biochemical investigations are done in reverse. A wide variety of imaging modalities are available; diagnosis depends on selection of the correct ones.

Plain X-ray

Despite the introduction of more sophisticated imaging techniques, the plain X-ray remains a valuable study in endocrinology. Plain X-rays are particularly useful for identifying bony abnormalities and calcified lesions. For example, they are commonly used in the investigation of diabetic foot disease to identify bone destruction from Charcot's arthropathy and osteomyelitis. Other uses of plain X-rays in endocrinology include identification of the following:

- calcium-containing renal stones in primary hyperparathyroidism
- calcification of the adrenal glands in Addison's disease resulting from tuberculosis (see Figure 7.2)
- delayed or accelerated bone age in assessment of pubertal development
- generalised reduction in bone density and crush fracture of vertebral bodies in severe osteoporosis, although dual-energy X-ray absorptiometry (DEXA) scan is the imaging of choice to diagnose osteoporosis (see page 112)
- Shortened 4th and 5th metacarpal bones in pseudohypoparathyroidism (type 1a)
- Expansion of the pituitary fossa on a skull X-ray in cases of large pituitary tumour; however, skull X-rays are no longer routinely used to assess pituitary tumours now that more detailed imaging modalities (such as MRI and CT) for pituitary lesions are readily available

Computerised tomography

Computerised tomography is a sensitive modality for showing abnormalities in the soft tissues. Therefore it is especially useful in investigations of lesions in the adrenal glands (**Figure 2.29**), pancreas, liver and small endocine tumours in the lung. Contrast can be used to improve differentiation between tissues.

Avoid injudicious use of CT. This technique exposes patients to a high dose of ionising radiation, which increases their risk of developing cancer in the future.

Magnetic resonance imaging

Magnetic resonance imaging provides excellent differentiation between tissues, and contrast is often used to enhance tissue contrast, for example gadolinium in pituitary imaging.

- MRI does not use radiation, so it is ideal for the repeated imaging studies required for long-term follow-up of slow-growing tumours such as pituitary adenomas or screening in patients with a genetic mutation predisposing them to endocrine tumours
- MRI is unsuitable for patients with metallic implants such as intracranial aneurysm clips, cardiac pacemakers and some coronary artery stents because of the magnetic field

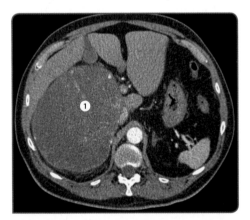

Figure 2.29 Computerised tomography scan showing a large right adrenal tumour ① in a patient with a phaeochromocytoma.

Magnetic resonance imaging machines are noisy and cramped. Patients with claustrophobia may require sedation, especially for head and neck scans when, for example, scanning the pituitary gland (even though pituitary MRI is quick). Options for patients who are unable to tolerate MRI with a standard closed MRI scanner are use of an open MRI scanner, MRI under anaesthetic or, occasionally, CT instead.

Magnetic resonance imaging is the imaging modality of choice for lesions in the pituitary gland. It is also useful for imaging studies of the adrenal glands and pancreas as an alternative to CT. MRI is occasionally used to identify deep-seated infection in diabetic foot disease.

Ultrasound

The sensitivity of ultrasound depends on the experience of the operator. Furthermore, the procedure can be difficult to carry out on patients who are overweight or obese. However, ultrasound has the advantages of involving no ionising radiation and having no contraindications.

Ultrasound is the first-line imaging modality for the thyroid gland. Fine-needle aspiration and cytological investigation under ultrasound guidance is the investigation of choice for patients presenting with a thyroid nodule (see Chapter 5). Ultrasound is also often used for the parathyroid glands.

This technique is less sensitive than CT or MRI for imaging intra-abdominal endocrine organs. However, endoscopic ultrasound is useful for detecting small pancreatic endocrine tumours that are not visible on the cross-sectional images provided by CT and MRI.

Dual-energy X-ray absorptiometry

Dual-energy X-ray absorptiometry scans ('bone density scans') are produced by a special X-ray technique that measures bone mineral density in investigations of osteoporosis.

In DEXA, a dedicated specialist X-ray machine sends two low-dose X-ray beams with different energy peaks through the bones being examined.

- One of the X-ray beams is absorbed by the soft tissues
- The other X-ray beam is absorbed by the bone

The DEXA machine has specialised software that computes bone mineral density by subtracting the energy absorbed by the soft tissues from the total energy absorbed. The femoral head, radius and lumbar spine are the bones in which bone mineral density is most commonly assessed.

The DEXA scan generates two scores as measurements of bone mineral density (see Figure 8.4).

- The T-score denotes the bone mineral density compared with that of a healthy young adult whose bones are at peak mass
- The Z-score denotes the bone mineral density compared with that of a typical adult of the same age and sex

The World Health Organization classification of osteoporosis is based on T-scores (see Table 2.23).

Bone mineral density, measured by DEXA, on its own is a poor predictor of future fractures. Although patients with osteoporosis are at increased risk of fractures, those with normal bone mineral density may still be at high risk if other risk factors for fracture are present.

FRAX is an online tool that provides an accurate estimate of the 10-year probability of fractures. It calculates this risk by integrating data on bone mineral density with those for other clinical variables, including:

- history of previous fracture
- family history of hip fracture
- body mass index
- steroid use
- presence of secondary causes of osteoporosis
- daily alcohol intake
- smoking status

Scintigraphy

In scintigraphy (radioisotope imaging), a radioisotope is injected into the body and absorbed preferentially by specific tissues. The radioisotope emits radiation, which is detected by a gamma camera next to the patient.

Areas of high radioisotope uptake emit more radiation than areas of low uptake, and therefore appear as bright areas on the image (**Figure 2.30**). In this way, scintigraphy visualises areas of high metabolic activity, such as tumours or autonomous hyperfunctioning nodules.

Scintigraphy is widely used to investigate disorders of the thyroid, parathyroid and adrenal glands. For example:

- thyroid scintigraphy using technetium-99m, iodine-123 or iodine-131 is used to determine different causes of thyrotoxicosis (see Figure 5.3)
- scintigraphy using iodine-131 is used to detect metastatic deposits after thyroidectomy and radioiodine ablation treatment for thyroid carcinoma
- parathyroid scintigraphy using technetium-99m (called a sestimibi scan) is used to detect parathyroid adenoma causing primary hyperparathyroidism (Figure 8.3b)
- scintigraphy using iodine-131 meta-iodobenzylguanidine (MIBG) (a MIBG scan; **Figure 2.31**) is useful for the detection of adrenal and extra-adrenal phaeochromocytoma (see Chapter 7)

Classification of osteoporosis by T-score	
T-score	Diagnosis
> -1 (i.e. within 1 SD of the mean)	Normal
-1 to -2.5 SDs (i.e. 1-2.5 SDs below the mean)	Osteopenia
< -2.5 SDs (i.e. more than 2.5 SDs below the mean)	Osteoporosis
< -2.5 SDs below the mean plus fragility fracture	Severe osteoporosis
SD, standard deviation.	

Table 2.23 World Health Organization classification of osteoporosis

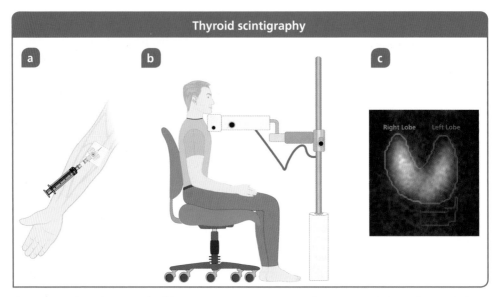

Thyroid scintigraphy

Figure 2.30 Thyroid scintigraphy. (a) Step 1: intravenous injection of a tracer containing radioactive iodine (iodine-131). (b) Step 2: detection of radioactive emission by a gamma camera. (c) Step 3: radioisotope uptake by the thyroid gland is demonstrated on the final image.

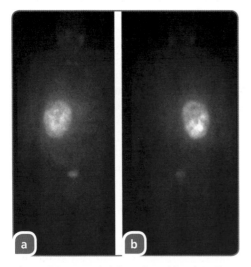

Figure 2.31 Meta-iodobenzylguanidine (MIBG) scans, 24 h after radioisotope injection, showing a large area of radioisotope uptake in the right adrenal area. (a) Anterior view. (b) Posterior view.

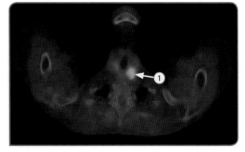

Figure 2.32 Positron emission tomography scan showing abnormal uptake of the radioactive tracer fluorine-18 fluorodeoxyglucose in the left lobe of the thyroid gland ①.

Positron emission tomography

Positron emission tomography (PET) produces detailed three-dimensional images, in contrast to the two-dimensional images produced by scintigraphy.

In PET, a positron-emitting radioactive tracer is injected into a peripheral vein and becomes concentrated in areas of the body with high metabolic activity. (The tracer most commonly used is fluorodeoxyglucose (FDG), a glucose analogue containing the radioisotope fluorine-18.) A radiosensitive camera is then used to visualise these areas with greater uptake of tracer.

This imaging modality enables the anatomical nature of a tumour to be correlated with its functional nature (**Figure 2.32**). In endocrinology, PET scans are generally used for identification of primary or metastatic endocrine tumours, when other imaging modalities have shown inconclusive results.

Cytological and histological investigations

Cytology and histology are diagnostic modalities in endocrinology used to secure the diagnosis suspected on biochemistry and imaging. Cytology looks at individual cells that have been aspirated from the concerning tissue usually using a needle and syringe (which disrupts the architecture). These cells are put on a glass slide. Histological samples are larger, whole pieces of tissue or organs (maintaining their architecture). The samples are stained and examined under a microscope.

Fine-needle aspiration and cytological examination is the investigation of choice for a patient presenting with a thyroid nodule to assess for malignancy as it is simple to perform and easy to interpret (see Chapter 5). This investigation is occasionally used to assess masses in other endocrine glands, for example confirmation of metastases in the adrenal glands , the result of which will influence the decision of whether to remove the gland or not.

Histological examination, of either a biopsy or a surgical specimen, normally confirms the diagnosis. For example, clinical and biochemical suspicions of acromegaly are confirmed by histological examination with immunochemistry after a pituitary resection by identifying a growth hormone-staining pituitary adenoma. Likewise, histological examination of a thyroid lump determine the type of thyroid cancer, with implications for management and prognosis.

Chromosomal and genetic tests

Several endocrine disorders are caused by chromosomal disorders resulting from addition, loss or rearrangement of a part of a chromosome. The two commonest examples of endocrine diseases resulting from chromosomal disorders are Klinefelter's syndrome and Turner's syndrome (see Chapter 9).

Diagnosis of chromosomal disorders is made by chromosomal analysis (karyotyping). Karyotyping examines the chromosomes in a sample of cells to identify abnormalities in numbers or structure, such as in Turner's syndrome or Klinefelter's syndrome. It is usually carried out on a venous blood sample; however, other cells or tissue from the body can be used instead such as buccal (cheek) smears.

Many endocrine conditions are caused by a single-gene defect (mutation), so they follow a simple Mendelian pattern of inheritance. These mutations are detected by direct DNA sequencing. Detection of a mutation not only confirms the molecular diagnosis of the condition; it can also have important implications for its management and prognosis. Identifying the mutation can help predict the likely manifestations of a syndrome and guide the screening programme. It can also help to predict whether a disease such as a phaeochromocytoma may be benign or malignant

An example of an endocrine condition arising from a single-gene defect is 21-hydroxylase deficiency congenital adrenal hyperplasia, which can be caused by different types of mutation in the same gene (the *CYP21A2* gene). The severity of the condition varies from classic salt-losing congenital adrenal hyperplasia to atypical congenital adrenal hyperplasia with minimal symptoms.

The results of genetic investigations can also prompt predictive testing for family members. For example, medullary thyroid cancer is sometimes associated with a mutation in the *RET* gene (see Chapter 5). Identification of a mutation of the *RET* gene in a patient with medullary thyroid cancer means that genetic screening can be offered to members of the patient's family to determine if they carry the same mutation. If the *RET* gene mutation is found, prophylactic thyroidectomy is offered, because over 90% of people with this genetic error develop medullary thyroid cancer.

Management options

Starter questions

Answers to the following questions are on page 144.

12. Should all patients with type 1 diabetes have a pancreas transplantation?
13. Can management do more harm than good?
14. What is the best way to communicate a management plan to patients and family?
15. Is having a long-term doctor-patient relationship beneficial?

Endocrine conditions often involve lifelong treatment, which may change with age and with intercurrent illness. For this reason, patients need to be masters of their condition; this requires self-management and often the education of others so that they can help in times of difficulty. For example, patients with type 1 diabetes need to know how to self-administer insulin, and their family and friends may need to know how to treat a severe hypoglycaemic episode resulting in unconsciousness.

To prevent deterioration, patients with some endocrine conditions need to be able to change doses of medication when they are unwell. For example, patients receiving steroid replacement therapy may need to increase their dose of hydrocortisone to prevent an adrenal crisis.

Ageing can also necessitate changes to treatment. Elderly patients with diabetes mellitus may need to have their blood glucose targets relaxed (increased) to avoid the consequences of hypoglycaemia, which could, for example, precipitate a fall.

To achieve the lifelong care commonly required for endocrine conditions, a holistic approach combining different management tools is needed. These tools include:

- patient education and counselling, including education of carers and relatives
- diet and lifestyle management
- psychological interventions
- drug treatment (hormone replacement or suppression of excessive hormone secretion)
- surgery
- radiotherapy
- organ and tissue transplantation

Multiple modalities are commonly used to treat a single condition, and often different approaches (surgical and non-surgical) can be equally effective. Treatment plans have to be individualised in collaboration with the patient. Furthermore, management of many endocrine conditions demands input from a multidisciplinary team comprising an appropriate combination of dietician, specialist nurse, psychologist, endocrinologist, general practitioner (GP), surgeon, radiologist, pathologist and oncologist. Endocrine conditions are commonly chronic, so a long-term relationship between patient and health care provider offering individual support, guidance and sharing of up-to-date information is essential.

Guidance and evidence-based therapies

Many endocrine conditions are rare, so large-scale clinical trials of treatments for them may not be possible. Consequently, guidance for the management of such conditions often consists of expert opinion and is therefore not truly evidence-based.

Diabetes mellitus is an exception. It is a common condition, so large-scale randomised controlled clinical trials are more feasible and provide robust evidence to show the effectiveness of treatment.

Guidance on the management of endocrine conditions is available from government-funded organisations (e.g. the National Institute for Health and Care Excellence in the UK), as well as from independent professional organisations (e.g. Diabetes UK and the Society for Endocrinology).

> **Some treatments for endocrine conditions are restricted on grounds of cost.** Growth hormone replacement is expensive, so in the UK its use is limited to patients who have symptoms, biochemical evidence of deficiency and poor quality of life despite adequate treatment of other pituitary hormone deficiencies. A specific quality of life assessment, the Quality of Life - Assessment of Growth Hormone Deficiency in Adults, is used to confirm continuing need.

Patient education and counselling

The diagnosis of an endocrine disease may feel like a crossroad in the patient's life. They experience great relief to have a diagnosis after what may have been a long time with unrecognised symptoms. However, they often have problems accepting the huge impact a chronic disease will have on their future. For example, the diagnosis of type 1 diabetes mellitus obligates the patient to a lifetime of blood glucose monitoring, daily insulin injections and regular appointments with health care professionals. The diagnosis has wide implications on both physical and psychological health, as well as on social well-being, with effects on interpersonal relationships and employment.

Patient education is central to the treatment of many endocrine conditions, because they require a high degree of self-management. Patients may obtain information about their condition and its management through:

- direct consultations with health care providers

- patient education leaflets and internet resources , e.g. medical society literature or public health documents
- professional organisations
- group education courses (e.g. carbohydrate-counting courses for patients with type 1 diabetes)
- charitable patient support groups and societies, and 'buddy systems' where patients are paired with other people with the same condition, in a similar situation.
- patient self-help groups and online blogs and chatrooms

Patients need to understand their disease well enough to be able to change the doses of their medication according to the situation.

- During intercurrent illness, patients with diabetes need to monitor their blood glucose more frequently and increase their insulin doses accordingly, and patients with steroid deficiency may need to be admitted to hospital for parenteral steroid therapy if they have diarrhoea and vomiting
- Travel is more problematic if drugs such as growth hormone or insulin need to be stored in cool conditions, or if needles and syringes need to be taken into an aeroplane cabin; furthermore, insurance can be more expensive for patients with certain endocrine conditions
- Pregnancy can be complicated by many endocrine disorders, including commonly thyrotoxicosis and hypothyroidism, and more appointments many be required during antenatal care

Diet and lifestyle management

Healthy lifestyle changes, such as making dietary modifications, introducing exercise and stopping smoking can affect morbidity and mortality associated with endocrine conditions. It can be introduced as first-line treatment prior to medication (such as with type 2 diabetes mellitus) or in parallel to medical treatment (such as in type 1 diabetes mellitus). In some cases of type 2 diabetes this can be sufficient to avoid or delay any medical or surgical intervention.

Dietary modification

Changes in weight are a common feature of many endocrine diseases and also form part of plans for their management.

Weight loss is typically seen before diagnosis in cases of type 1 diabetes, thyrotoxicosis, Addison's disease and endocrine cancers. When these conditions are treated, weight is restored. This weight gain may be unwelcome, so patients may need to modify their diet during treatment to accommodate this effect.

Other conditions, such as Cushing's disease, hypothyroidism and growth hormone deficiency, are associated with weight gain. Treatment helps patients reduce weight, but advice on a healthy diet is also necessary.

Conditions such as obesity and type 2 diabetes are directly associated with weight gain. For patients with these conditions, dietary advice is the cornerstone of treatment.

Calorie restriction is essential for patients with obesity, as well as for many with type 2 diabetes. For patients with type 2 diabetes, dietary advice is usually about losing weight and limiting sugar intake. However, patients with type 1 diabetes mellitus require a detailed understanding of their diet, because carbohydrate intake determines insulin requirement. Protein and fat have less of an effect on insulin requirement, but they may affect the speed of absorption of carbohydrate.

Dietary modification to reduce salt intake helps improve blood pressure in patients with hypertension.

Dietary advice can be delivered individually or in a group setting. Information can also be given to patients in written or electronic form.

Exercise

Many endocrine conditions reduce muscle mass and strength. For example:

- Cushing's syndrome, diabetes mellitus and thyrotoxicosis can cause proximal muscle wasting and weakness (proximal myopathy)
- growth hormone deficiency is associated with reduced muscle mass

It is wise to avoid exercise in the acute phase of such conditions. However, exercise should form part of the recovery programme and focus on affected muscles, such as the proximal muscles in Cushing's syndrome and thyrotoxicosis. Also, fatigue is a common feature in many endocrine conditions, for example hypothyroidism, and graded exercise programmes in addition to thyroxine replacement may help address this symptom.

In patients with type 1 and 2 diabetes mellitus, exercise improves blood glucose control independently of weight loss. Prescribed exercise courses and exercise counselling benefit motivated patients who are keen to improve fitness and lose weight. Doses of some medications, such as insulin and steroids, may need to be adjusted if patients are doing prolonged exercise such as marathon training.

Smoking cessation

Smoking poses a health risk in any condition. However, the risks of smoking are particularly enhanced in patients with other risk factors for atherosclerotic disease, such as diabetes mellitus. Smoking also increases the risk of certain endocrine disorders, such as Graves' disease and thyroid eye disease.

Various methods of support are available to patients wanting to stop smoking:

- community health service or GP advice with self-help material
- individual or group behavioural therapy
- pharmacotherapy (nicotine replacement therapy; nicotine receptor agonists, e.g. varenicline or treatments reducing nicotine cravings, e.g. bupropion)
- telephone helplines or mobile phone applications
- mass media and government campaigns

Nicotine replacement therapy comes in various forms, including gums, inhalators, lozenges and nasal sprays.

Psychological interventions

Chronic endocrine diseases are difficult for patients to come to terms with (**Table 2.24**). Patients can experience a period of denial and isolation at diagnosis, followed by times

Indications for psychological support	
Common associated problem	Endocrine conditions often associated
Appearance	Acromegaly
	Cushing's syndrome
	Obesity
	Thyroid eye disease
	Turner's syndrome
Accepting chronic diagnosis	Type 1 diabetes mellitus
Accepting treatment	Type 1 diabetes mellitus
	Type 2 diabetes mellitus requiring insulin therapy
Need for behaviour modification and acceptance of personal responsibility	Diabetes mellitus
	Obesity
Feeling of isolation	Rare syndromes (e.g. acromegaly)
Feeling of guilt	Genetic syndromes (e.g. multiple endocrine neoplasia)

Table 2.24 Common indications for the need for psychological support

of anger and depression, similar to the stages of bereavement. Patients whose disease is diagnosed in childhood often go through periods of resentment about their condition, particularly during adolescence.

The ability of patients to prioritise their health and manage their condition effectively can fluctuate over time, because of the effects of other life events, such as a change of job or relationship breakdown. This can manifest as missed appointments and non-adherence to treatments, which can lead to increased hospital admissions. Many patients, particularly those with obesity and type 2 diabetes mellitus, suffer from low self-esteem, feelings of shame and high levels of self-criticism.

Recognition of the emotional effects of endocrine conditions on patients and their families has a vital role in optimising treatment outcomes.

Psychological support is part of the treatment framework for many conditions and is key to successful outcomes, so help from a psychologist is an integral part of the service. For example, in the obesity service, patients need to tackle underlying dysfunctional eating behaviours, such as binge-eating disorder, before being referred for bariatric surgery; this approach results in better post-surgical outcomes in the long term.

Different techniques are used, depending on the type of psychological stress the patient is experiencing. Those with emotional eating and binge eating disorder often receive a combination of cognitive behavioural therapy, along with interpersonal therapy and dialectical behavioural therapy.

- Cognitive behavioral therapy acknowledges that certain thoughts cannot be easily manipulated; it addresses these dysfunctional emotions and maladaptive behaviours by developing action plans to replace them with positive ones (e.g. a patient with obesity would have a brief period of exercise instead of eating a snack)
- Interpersonal psychotherapy aims to empathise with the patient, helping them feel understood; this type of support can encourage patients to regain control of their mood and functioning usually over a a few months
- Dialectical behavioural therapy is designed to help patients discontinue harmful patterns of behaviour, mainly by learning to recognise triggers for such behaviours and how to apply coping skills to improve their emotional and cognitive responses to such events

Newer strategies include 'mindfulness' eating, which encourages patients with obesity to control the urge to overeat and to avoid 'mindless' eating. Patients are advised to:

- savour every bite
- sit at a dining table rather than in front of the television or fridge
- avoid multitasking, so that their minds are focused on eating
- plan meals
- put the fork down and drink water between mouthfuls
- rate their hunger before eating

'Motivational interviewing' is another strategy that involves facilitating and engaging a patient's inner motivation to make a behaviour change by helping to resolve ambivalence. This is useful in all conditions that rely on self-management.

Group psychotherapy helps to identify maladaptive behaviours in a supportive social setting, and addresses emotional difficulties through feedback from members of the group. This approach is ideally suited to conditions such as obesity; supportive psychotherapy provides an explanation for the condition, reassurance and ideas for resolving difficulties in everyday life.

Drug treatment

A wide range of drug treatments are available to manage endocrine hyposecretion, hypersecretion and tumours, both benign and malignant.

Hyposecretion of hormones is generally managed with physiological hormone replacement. The deficient hormones, which are normally made inside the body (endogenous), are instead provided by hormones synthesised outside the body (exogenous). The aim is for the exogenous hormone to 'replace' the missing endogenous hormone, mimicking it in terms of both concentration and secretory profile, and thus recreate its physiological actions.

Other types of drug treatment can be used to:

- suppress the production or release of a hormone
- block the actions of a hormone at its receptor or receptors
- treat the symptoms or complications of hormone excess

Secretory endocrine cancers tend to be treated similarly to non-secretory cancers, with a combination of surgery, chemotherapy and radiotherapy. However, the excessive secretion of hormones may require additional treatment, for example alpha blockade to block the effects of adrenaline (epinephrine) before adrenalectomy for a phaeochromocytoma.

As an endocrine condition is treated, the resulting reduction in the concentration of hormone can progress to deficiency. For example, radiotherapy to the pituitary gland in a patient with acromegaly can eventually lead to growth hormone deficiency when the initial problem was growth hormone excess.

Over the last 20 years, more drugs have been developed to treat endocrine diseases, and drug treatments can obviate the need for a surgical solution. For example, the calcimimetic agent cinacalcet acts on the parathyroid glands to reduce parathyroid hormone secretion and can be used to treat hypercalcaemia in patients with hyperparathyroidism, so parathyroidectomy is not always necessary (if a patient is unfit for an operation or if an operation is unlikely to achieve a cure). However, drug treatments are often expensive and needed over the long term, so their cost-effectiveness must be considered.

Treatment of hormone insufficiency

Hormone insufficiency can arise in three ways:

- the hormone is partially absent
- it is totally absent
- the hormone is present but ineffective

Treatment can be enhanced by stimulating additional secretion of the hormone or by augmenting its effects. Hormone replacement is used if the hormone is no longer produced by the body, because the gland producing it has either failed permanently or been surgically removed. For example:

- permanent failure of the pancreatic beta cells necessitates insulin administration in patients with type 1 diabetes mellitus
- total thyroidectomy necessitates T_4 replacement therapy

Occasionally, hormones have indications for 'treatment' even when there is no deficiency requiring hormone replacement. The indications are based on much higher, pharmacological concentrations rather than physiological ones. **Table 2.25** shows when hormones are used as replacement therapy

Indications for hormone replacement and hormone treatment		
Hormone	Replacement indication (physiological doses)	Treatment indication (supraphysiological doses)*
Oestrogen	Hormone replacement therapy	Contraception (oral contraceptive pill) Polycystic ovarian syndrome
Progesterone	Hormone replacement therapy	
Glucocorticoid	Hypopituitarism Addison's disease Congenital adrenal hyperplasia	Thyroid eye disease Thyroid storm Inflammatory diseases (e.g. rheumatoid arthritis)
Desmopressin	Cranial diabetes insipidus	Mild haemophilia A von Willebrand's disease (stimulates release of factor VIII and von Willenbrand's factor)
Testosterone	Primary hypogonadism Secondary hypogonadism	No treatment indication but misused in sports (to increase muscle mass)
Growth hormone	Growth hormone deficiency	Short stature not caused by growth hormone deficiency (also misused in sports to increase muscle mass)
Erythropoietin	Haemoglobin synthesis in renal failure	No treatment indication but misused in sports to increase oxygen transfer capacity by increasing red blood cell count
Vitamin D	Rickets Osteomalacia	Osteoporosis
Fludrocortisone	Aldosterone deficiency (Addison's disease)	Postural hypotension in the elderly
*Hormone therapy administered in the absence of deficiency.		

Table 2.25 Endocrine hormones and their indications at physiological and pharmacological concentrations

and when they are used at supraphysiological doses as 'treatment'.

Introduction to hormone replacement

Some hormones are essential to life; others improve quality of life (well-being) or prevent morbidity. For some hormones, such as prolactin, there is no clear role for replacement therapy in cases of deficiency.

If an endocrine gland is non-functional, single-hormone replacement (e.g. T_4 therapy in hypothyroidism) or multiple-hormone replacement (e.g. cortisol and aldosterone therapy in Addison's disease) may be needed.

A number of factors complicate hormone replacement:

- degree of hormone deficiency
- clinical necessity for hormone replacement

- availability of a synthetic, human or animal hormone for replacement therapy
- mode of hormone delivery
- timing of hormone replacement
- pharmacokinetics of the hormone
- choice of replacement hormone
- interactions with other drugs
- the physiological state of the patient
- dosing and monitoring

Degree of hormone deficiency

Patients with partial hormone deficiency may be asymptomatic on a day-to-day basis but need hormone replacement when unwell. For example:

- in early type 1 diabetes mellitus, adequate insulin levels are present until an intercurrent illness occurs and the person becomes unwell and may develop diabetic ketoacidosis

- in mild hypocortisolism, a stressful event can lead to an adrenal crisis and metabolic collapse, but the patient can manage without routine daily cortisol replacement

Complete hormone deficiency requires a full hormone replacement regimen, for example testosterone replacement therapy in patients with primary testicular failure.

Clinical necessity for hormone replacement

Insulin and glucocorticoids are essential to life. In cases of complete deficiency, metabolic collapse and death ensue without appropriate hormone replacement. Replacement of other hormones prevents morbidity but is not life-saving. Examples of such hormones are growth hormone, oestrogen and testosterone, which support or are necessary for bone formation, muscle strength, vitality and fertility.

Availability of a synthetic, human or animal hormone for replacement therapy

When insulin was first discovered, it was extracted from pigs and cows, and porcine and bovine insulin remain in use by a minority of patients. However, now most insulin is synthetic.

Before 1985, growth hormone was extracted from pituitary glands from cadavers. Supplies were limited and dosing often suboptimal with frequent drug-free periods. Therefore growth hormone was expensive, and its use was restricted to the treatment of children with deficiency to increase their final adult height. Now that synthetic growth hormone is widely available, it is used to treat adults as well as children. Also, it is safer than extracted human growth hormone as each injection of cadaveric growth hormone contained several human pituitaries with a subsequent risk of transmission of diseases, such as Creutzfeldt-Jacob disease, even 15 years after treatment.

Porcine thyroid extract is available. However, it has a lower ratio of levothyroxine to liothyronine compared with that secreted by the human thyroid and is therefore not recommended for T_4 replacement therapy.

Mode of hormone delivery

Many hormones have more than one mode of delivery. Hormone replacement is most commonly oral; however, certain circumstances can affect absorption:

- diarrhoea and vomiting
- failure of enteral (intestinal) absorption (e.g. in cases of coeliac disease)
- interaction with other drugs (e.g. calcium supplements reduce the absorption of oral levothyroxine if the two are taken together)

If diarrhoea is suspected to be causing malabsorption, hormone replacement (e.g. with hydrocortisone) is administered parenterally, either intramuscularly or intravenously as an infusion.

Hormones such as insulin and growth hormone are destroyed by stomach acid so cannot be given orally. Therefore they are given subcutaneously by self-administration.

Nasal preparations provide rapid absorption of a hormone for a quick response. An example of a nasal preparation is desmopressin spray, which is used to treat cranial diabetes insipidus. Insulin has been developed as an inhaled preparation. However, inhaled insulin is not on the market, because of concerns about variability in its absorption.

Patches or gels are used for transdermal delivery of hormones such as oestrogen and testosterone. However, this route of administration sometimes causes skin reactions.

Timing of hormone replacement

In healthy people, cortisol levels are highest in the morning and peak just before waking. To replicate this circadian rhythm, the daily dose of cortisol replacement therapy is given in fractions, with the largest dose on waking. Insulin injections are often timed with food.

Pharmacokinetics of the hormone

The half-life of some hormones, such as insulin and growth hormone, is naturally short. Therefore their chemical structure is altered to create formulations that are absorbed or metabolised more slowly.

Some drugs used in endocrinology have long half-lives. Levothyroxine is an example; its long half-life means that patients on T_4

replacement therapy do not develop symptoms of hypothyroidism after missing a dose.

A drug with a short half-life can be useful in helping replicate physiology. For example, administration of hydrocortisone first thing in the morning and at lunchtime can match normal diurnal variation in cortisol, a hormone whose levels are lowest overnight.

Some drugs are contraindicated in hepatic or renal failure, because they accumulate in the body if they are inadequately metabolised or excreted by these organs. Other drugs can be used instead, but their dose may need to be adjusted. Insulin doses may need to be significantly reduced, because of reduced renal clearance in renal failure potentiating the effects of a single dose of insulin.

Choice of replacement hormone

Patients can choose from different formulations of hormones according to their lifestyle; this is particularly true for insulin. What suits one person may not suit another. For example, someone who does significant amounts of exercise and has variable mealtimes may require multiple daily insulin injections to achieve good blood glucose control. In contrast, an elderly person with fixed mealtimes may benefit from a simpler insulin regimen. Different formulations of insulin are discussed in detail in Chapter 3.

Interactions with other drugs

Certain drugs, such as antiepileptic agents, induce cytochrome P450 enzymes. These increase the metabolism of other drugs, including those used in hormone therapy. This action may:

- necessitate higher doses of replacement hormones (e.g. corticosteroids)
- reduce the reliability of the treatment because of increased hormone metabolism (e.g. of oestrogen in the oral contraceptive pill)

Conditions of hormone excess can also increase the metabolism of certain drugs. For example, thyrotoxicosis increases metabolism of beta-blockers. Consequently, higher doses are needed to achieve the same effect.

The physiological state of the patient

Higher doses of replacement corticosteroids and insulin are required during periods of stress or illness. Patients must understand the 'sick day rules', which explain how to adjust their treatment at these times. Other endocrine conditions may become decompensated (a functional deterioration when previously stable) when a patient is unwell. For example, if a patient with hypercalcaemia (resulting from hyperparathyroidism) has diarrhoea and becomes dehydrated, they can become increasingly symptomatic as the calcium increases; this may lead to renal failure and life-threatening hypercalcaemia.

Dosing and monitoring

Ways in which the effectiveness of hormone replacement is monitored are shown in **Table 2.26**. Levels of hormones such as insulin-like growth factor 1, which is used as a measure of growth hormone, decline with age. Therefore age-related reference ranges are used.

Blood tests measure either the total hormone (bound and unbound) or the free hormone (unbound); knowing whether results are for total or free hormone helps when interpreting the test. The concentration of bound hormone can vary without significant physiological effect. For example, use of the oral contraceptive pill can increase the amount of cortisol-binding globulin. The effect of this is to increase total cortisol concentration, but the concentration of active free cortisol remains the same.

The aim of hormone replacement is to achieve a concentration of hormone that is within the normal range. Therefore adverse effects are limited unless the hormone is over- or under-replaced.

Hormone replacement

Glucocorticoid replacement

Glucocorticoids are most commonly used in medicine for anti-inflammatory and immunomodulatory effects; however, recognition and replacement of deficiency (adrenal or pituitary) can be life-saving.

Hormone replacement: aims and monitoring of effectiveness		
Hormone or drug used	Aim	Method(s) of monitoring success
Insulin	To achieve glycaemic control in patients with diabetes mellitus	Measurement of capillary blood glucose concentration and determination of haemoglobin A1c value
Hydrocortisone	To provide minimum amount to ease symptoms of cortisol deficiency	Clinical judgement
		Serial measurements of serum cortisol concentration throughout the day (day curve)
Levothyroxine	To ease symptoms of hypothyroidism by maintaining a healthy concentration of thyroxine	Primary hypothyroidism: measurement of serum thyroid-stimulating hormone concentration
		Secondary hypothyroidism: measurement of serum thyroxine concentration
Fludrocortisone	To ease symptoms of postural hypotension and fatigue in patients with adrenal insufficiency or idiopathic postural hypotension	Measurement of postural blood pressure
		Measurement of serum sodium and plasma renin activity
Growth hormone	Children: to normalise height by increasing growth	Measurement of serum insulin-like growth factor 1 concentration
	Adults: to improve well-being, e.g. initiative and drive	Assessment of psychological improvement using disease specific questionnaires
Desmopressin	To control polyuria and maintain water homeostasis in patients with cranial diabetes insipidus	Measurement of urinary volume and serum sodium concentration
Oestrogen (hormone replacement therapy)	To ease symptoms of menopause	Assessment of symptomatic benefit on self-reporting
	To prevent osteoporosis and increase energy levels in cases of premature oestrogen deficiency (< 51 years)	
Testosterone	To ease symptoms and maintain bone density in cases of testosterone deficiency	Measurement of serum testosterone concentration

Table 2.26 Hormone replacement: aims and methods used to monitor effectiveness

Actions Glucocorticoid receptors are present in almost every cell in the body. Glucocorticoids have immunological, metabolic and homeostatic functions.

Indications At physiological doses, glucocorticoids are essential to life, so hormone replacement can be life-saving in cases of deficiency. At pharmacological doses, glucocorticoids are used mainly for their anti-inflammatory action and for immunosuppression. Therefore the indications for glucocorticoid replacement can be categorised as follows.

- Replacement: pituitary or adrenal deficiency
- Treatment: multiple indications, including asthma, autoimmune conditions (e.g. rheumatoid arthritis), malignancy (e.g.

lymphoma or cerebral metastases) and skin conditions (e.g. eczema)

Routes Glucocorticoids are administered through the following routes:

- oral
- subcutaneous
- intramuscular
- intravenous
- transdermal
- inhaled
- intraarticular

Adverse effects The aim of glucocorticoid replacement is to mimic normal physiology. Therefore the adverse effects of this type of therapy are minimal. Doses need to be increased when the patient is ill, because glucocorticoid replacement at an insufficient dose can precipitate an addisonian crisis (see page 315).

Glucocorticoids used pharmacologically are given at much higher, supraphysiological doses. Therefore this type of therapy can cause acute adverse effects, which include hyperglycaemia and psychological disturbances. In chronic use, glucocorticoids can:

- lead to the development of iatrogenic Cushing's syndrome (see Chapter 6)
- suppress endogenous cortisol secretion

In patients using non-steroidal anti-inflammatory drugs, glucocorticoid treatment increases the risk of gastric ulcer formation.

Factors affecting choices The main glucocorticoids are as follows.

- Hydrocortisone: the first choice in cortisol replacement, this short-acting (half-life, 8 h) glucocorticoid can replicate normal physiology if doses are taken two or three times daily; it has minimal growth-suppressing effects in children
- Prednisolone: this is the most commonly used oral glucocorticoid pharmacologically for adults and has a half-life of 16-36 h. It is used as a second line treatment for cortisol replacement (after hydrocortisone), particularly if compliance with multiple daily dosing is a problem
- Dexamethasone: this potent glucocorticoid has a long half-life (36-54 h) and minimal mineralocorticoid effects, so it is less likely to cause hypertension
- Methylprednisolone: this potent anti-inflammatory drug is given intravenously, has little mineralocorticoid effect, and is used in pulsed doses in conditions such as multiple sclerosis and thyroid eye disease

Thyroid hormone replacement

Thyroid hormone is essential to life. The predominant use is as a replacement for absent or diminished thyroid hormone. However, at higher doses, thyroid hormone can act as a tumour suppressant in thyroid cancer by suppressing TSH (which acts as a growth factor in certain thyroid cancers).

Actions Thyroid hormones are responsible for regulating metabolism and are essential to life (see Chapter 1).

Indications Thyroid hormone replacement is indicated for:

- hypothyroidism (primary or secondary)
- subclinical hypothyroidism (especially in pregnancy)

Routes Thyroid hormones can be given orally or intravenously.

Adverse effects The dose is individualised to maintain thyroid hormone concentrations within normal reference ranges. Thyroxine replacement after removal of the thyroid in certain thyroid cancers aims to suppress the TSH. Thyroid hormone replacement replicating physiology this way should not be associated with adverse effects. However:

- excess thyroid hormone replacement with levothyroxine causes symptoms resembling those of hyperthyroidism
- insufficient levothyroxine causes symptoms resembling those of hypothyroidism
- levothyroxine given to patients with undiagnosed Addison's disease can precipitate an addisonian crisis (see page 315)

Factors affecting choices Thyroid hormone replacement is with levothyroxine (T_4) or occasionally liothyronine (T_3).

- Levothyroxine (T_4) is the only type of thyroid hormone replacement recommended for the treatment of hypothyroidism; it is long-acting, with a half-life of 7 days
- Liothyronine (T_3) is used as follows:
  - to treat myxoedema coma (see page 317), because it can be given intravenously and its actions are rapid
  - in the treatment of thyroid cancer; it is useful in the short term while the patient is awaiting radioactive iodine therapy (T_3 has a short half-life, so it can be withdrawn rapidly to allow TSH concentration to increase sufficiently for the radiotherapy to be effective)

Some patients report a benefit to receiving T_3 or a combination of T_3 and T_4. However, these effects have not been conclusively shown by the results of randomised clinical trials.

Interactions Remember to advise patients to take levothyroxine on an empty stomach, because food can reduce its absorption. Certain drugs and supplements, for example colestyramine, calcium, iron and aluminium hydroxide, can also interfere with levothyroxine absorption. Therefore they must be taken at least 4 h before or after levothyroxine.

Insulin replacement

Since the discovery of insulin in the 1920s, millions of lives of patients with type 1 diabetes have been saved. However in recent years with the explosion of type 2 diabetes, a substantial part of the market for insulin is for patients with type 2 diabetes, who are unable to be controlled by tablets alone.

Actions Insulin is a key hormone in the regulation of glucose and is essential to life (see Chapter 1).

Indications It is used in the insulin stress test to investigate growth hormone and cortisol deficiency. Insulin is also used to treat both types of diabetes mellitus.

- Type 1 diabetes mellitus:
  - insulin deficiency
- Type 2 diabetes mellitus:
  - suboptimal glycaemic control on first-line agents
  - failure to tolerate or contraindication to oral agents
  - signs of insulin deficiency (e.g. weight loss, ketonuria and low C-peptide concentration)
  - acute illness, sepsis or treatment that increases blood glucose (such as prednisolone therapy)
  - perioperative management

Routes The routes of administration for insulin are:

- subcutaneous
- intravenous
- inhaled (in development)

Adverse effects The aim of insulin therapy is to maintain euglycaemia by trying to reproduce the physiological pattern of insulin production. However, this can be difficult to achieve, and the main potential adverse effects are:

- weight gain
- hypoglycaemia (see Chapter 4)
- lipoatrophy (thinning of subcutaneous fat)
- lipohypertrophy (excessive deposition of fat;), which can occur at sites of insulin injection and change the hormone's absorption time (patients are advised to rotate their injection sites to avoid this problem)

Factors affecting choices A wide variety of insulins are available, offering different durations of action and insulin release profiles (see Figure 3.4). Most patients use a pen device to self-administer insulin (see Figure 3.5).

- Rapid-acting insulin usually has peak action within minutes; it counteracts the rapid rise in blood glucose at mealtimes and its effects usually last up to 6 h (this type of insulin is also used in insulin pumps and intravenous insulin infusions)
- Isophane insulin is intermediate-acting, with an onset of action over hours and a typical duration of action of 14-20 h; it is usually given once or twice daily to provide a basal ('background') level of insulin
- Long-acting analogue insulin has a slow onset and long duration of action (>18 h); it produces fewer peaks and troughs of insulin concentration, and therefore patients whose blood glucose is tightly controlled are less likely to experience hypoglycaemia with this option
- Animal insulin, the first insulin to be used, was extracted from the pancreas of pigs (porcine insulin) and cows (bovine insulin), and can be short- or long-acting; animal insulin is used less frequently now, its use having been superseded by that of human insulin

Insulin regimens are tailored to meet the patient's needs. Patients can choose mixed insulin, with rapid-acting and intermediate-acting insulin premixed in the same preparation. Alternatively, they can use a basal-bolus regimen, in which longer-acting insulin is administered once or twice a day, with shorter-acting insulin at mealtimes. The latter allows much greater flexibility, so is used particularly in those with less predictable lifestyles or variable mealtimes. Patients with type 2 diabetes usually start with a basal (once- or twice-daily) injection of intermediate-acting insulin in combination with oral hypoglycaemic agents.

Oestrogen replacement

Since the development of the oral contraceptive pill in the 1960s, oestrogen treatment (to prevent ovulation and pregnancy) and replacement (to treat deficiency and prevent menopausal symptoms) are commonly prescribed medications. Their popularity has been influenced by growing recognition of complications, such as increased risk of breast and endometrial cancer, but oestrogen (combined with progesterone) remains one of the most commonly used methods of contraception today.

Actions Oestrogen is responsible for regulating menstrual cycles but also has many other physiological effects (see Chapter 1).

Indications The indications for oestrogen are:

- short-term (ideally 2–5 years) relief of menopausal symptoms, through post-menopausal hormone replacement therapy
- premature menopause or hypogonadotrophic hypogonadism, to improve well-being and protect the bones from osteoporosis
- contraception (when combined with progesterone)
- polycystic ovary syndrome, to reduce androgen levels (see Chapter 9)

Routes Oestrogen is available in various formulations:

- oral (the commonest and cheapest route)
- transdermal (the most physiological route, because it avoids the first-pass metabolism in the liver that occurs with the enteral, intestinal, route)

- vaginal (as a topical treatment for post-menopausal dryness)
- implant (a rarely used form of contraception; progesterone implants are more commonly used)

Adverse effects Patients can experience nausea, breast tenderness and weight gain (the extra weight is mainly from fluid). Trials in post-menopausal women suggest that the prolonged use over decades, rather than years, of oestrogen can increase the risk of venous thromboembolism, endometrial and breast cancer, and stroke.

Contraindications to oestrogen replacement and the oral contraceptive pill include a history of endometrial or breast cancer, venous thromboembolic disease or known clotting disorder, migraine with focal neurological symptoms, a recent episode of ischaemic heart disease, and uncontrolled hypertension. Oestrogen replacement and the oral contraceptive pill are also unsuitable for heavy smokers over 35 years old.

Factors affecting choices Patients who have a uterus require cyclical progesterone to prevent hyperplasia of the endometrium and potential transformation to endometrial cancer. Progesterone is unnecessary for patients who have had a hysterectomy.

Interactions Certain drugs, such as antibiotics, can induce enzymes that metabolise oestrogen and therefore reduce the effectiveness of contraception. Therefore other methods of contraception may be necessary to avoid this effect.

> **Testosterone is under development for use as a male contraceptive.** Supplementing elderly patient with low testosterone levels was also hoped to slow aging, but the lack of evidence for this means is not routinely used.

Testosterone replacement

Testosterone is used in replacement for those with established deficiency.

Actions Testosterone acts on testosterone receptors throughout the body, as described in Chapter 1.

Testosterone is used to:

- treat erectile dysfunction and low libido
- maintain bone density
- restore muscle mass
- normalise erythropoiesis

Indications Testosterone replacement is used in hypogonadism to treat:

- testicular failure in primary hypogonadism
- pituitary failure in secondary hypogonadism

Routes Testosterone is available in the following forms.

- Intramuscular testosterone:
  - testosterone enantate and testosterone propionate are short-acting preparations, so injections are required every 2-4 weeks
  - testosterone undecanoate as a long-acting preparation requiring injections every 10-14 weeks
- Transdermal testosterone (gel or patch): this provides a stable serum testosterone concentration, needs to be applied daily, and carries a small risk of skin irritation and transfer to the partner
- Oral testosterone (testosterone undecanoate): this is of limited use because of variable absorption and the need for multiple doses daily
- Sublingual testosterone: this form of testosterone is absorbed rapidly, but daily doses are needed and there is a small risk of local irritation
- Testosterone implant: these are small pellets inserted under the skin using local anesthetic which last between 3 to 5 months

Adverse effects Testosterone replacement has the following adverse effects:

- polycythaemia
- increased risk of prostate cancer
- aggression and emotional lability
- excessive libido

Patients treated with testosterone require regular monitoring of their serum testosterone concentration (to ensure the correct dose of testosterone), serum prostate specific antigen (for early diagnosis of prostate carcinoma) and haematocrit (to identify polycythaemia). Testosterone is contraindicated in patients with prostate cancer, breast cancer and polycythaemia.

Factors affecting choices The use of intramuscular testosterone undecanoate tends to produce a steady testosterone concentration, so is an increasingly popular choice. Some men prefer to self-administer testosterone gel at home. Implants are becoming less popular, because minor surgery is required to insert the implant.

Growth hormone replacement

Growth hormone can be given only by subcutaneous injection. In children, growth hormone is given to help them achieve a final height closer to the average for their age and mid-parental height. Growth hormone in adulthood, after the bones have fused, improves psychological well-being, increases muscle mass and maintains bone density.

Desmopressin

This is a synthetic antidiuretic hormone analogue. It binds to receptors in the kidneys to cause increased reabsorption of water by these organs and thus concentrates the urine. Administration is subcutaneous, nasal or oral.

- In cranial diabetes insipidus, which is a deficiency in antidiuretic hormone, desmopressin almost instantly switches off urine output
- Desmopressin is also used to treat enuresis (bedwetting) in children

Clinical symptoms and serum sodium concentration are monitored so that the dose can be adjusted accordingly. Excessive doses can lead to hyponatraemia.

Nephrogenic diabetes insipidus tends to be resistant to treatment with desmopressin.

Fludrocortisone

This is an aldosterone analogue that helps regulate salt and water retention in the kidneys. Its main use is in adrenal insufficiency (e.g. Addison's disease, bilateral adrenalectomy and congenital adrenal hyperplasia), but it is occasionally also given to patients to treat postural hypotension of unknown cause.

Fludrocortisone is administered orally. It can cause oedema, hypertension and headaches when used in excess.

Vitamin D

Most of the body's vitamin D is produced photochemically in the skin; only a small proportion is obtained from the diet. Deficiency arises from: inadequate exposure to sunlight (in most cases) or conditions leading to malabsorption (e.g. coeliac disease)

Certain medications, such as the antiepileptic drug phenytoin, cause accelerated catabolism of vitamin D. Infants obtain insufficient vitamin D from breast milk alone.

Vitamin D supplementation is indicated in:

- vitamin D deficiency
- pregnancy
- osteoporosis
- hypocalcaemia secondary to hypoparathyroidism (activated vitamin D increases serum calcium concentration)
- end-stage renal failure (activated vitamin D)

Parathyroid hormone activates 25-OH vitamin D to 1,25-OH vitamin D in the kidney, so vitamin D needs to be replaced in the active 1,25 form if there is no parathyroid hormone or functioning kidney. Severe deficiency leads to rickets in children, which presents as bowing of the legs, and osteomalacia in adults, which presents as a poorly mineralised skeletal matrix.

Large doses of vitamin D continue to be prescribed for a wide range of diseases other than vitamin D deficiency, despite little scientific evidence for their efficacy.

Vitamin D is available in several preparations. In patients with normal kidney function, treatment with calciferol (unhydroxylated vitamin D) is indicated. Calciferol is given orally at a high dose for around 4 weeks, and then at a maintenance dose (800 IU/day). Alternatively, it can be given by injection once every 3 months, particularly for patients with malabsorption or in cases of poor adherence to treatment. Some patients require vitamin D supplementation only in the winter months, when there is insufficient sunlight.

Patients with chronic kidney disease or hypoparathyroidism require activated vitamin D in the form of calcitriol. Serum calcium concentration is monitored in these patients to ensure that hypercalcaemia does not develop.

Hormone augmentation

Conditions that are the result of partial rather than complete hormone deficiency are treated using one of two strategies:

- stimulation of release of the hormone
- augmentation of the effects of the hormone

For example, type 2 diabetes mellitus results from a partial insulin deficiency and resistance of the body to the effects of insulin. These two pathologies are targeted by stimulation and augmentation with two commonly used oral medications.

- Stimulation: sulfonylureas increase pancreatic secretion of insulin, thus reducing hyperglycaemia
- Augmentation: biguanides and thiazolidinediones increase the body's sensitivity to insulin to help reduce blood glucose

Biguanides

Metformin is the only biguanide currently available and is considered a cornerstone of treatment of type 2 diabetes. The other drugs in this class have been withdrawn due to the risk of lactic acidosis, which can be fatal.

Actions Metformin augments the actions of insulin by decreasing hepatic gluconeogenesis and increasing glucose uptake and metabolism in muscles.

Indications Metformin has the following indications:

- type 2 diabetes mellitus (first-line therapy after lifestyle changes and weight loss)
- gestational diabetes

- improvement of insulin sensitivity (e.g. in polycystic ovary syndrome)

Routes Only oral metformin is available.

Adverse effects Half of patients may have gastrointestinal adverse effects, such as diarrhoea, bloating and epigastric discomfort, but these are often transient. Metformin is relatively contraindicated in patients with renal, hepatic and cardiac failure, because of the rare risk of lactic acidosis.

Factors affecting choices Metformin is available in standard or slow-release formulations. Slow-release metformin is more expensive, but it is associated with more tolerable gastrointestinal adverse effects.

Metformin is first-line therapy (after lifestyle and dietary modification) for type 2 diabetes mellitus, because it is cheap and does not cause weight gain. It also reduces cardiovascular risk independently of changes in blood glucose.

Sulfonylureas

Sulfonylureas are the oldest group of antidiabetic drugs, but are no longer first-line for the majority of patients with type 2 diabetes.

Actions Sulfonylureas act by binding to ATP-dependent potassium channels on the surface of pancreatic beta cells to stimulate insulin release.

Drugs Tolbutamide, gliclazide and glibenclamide are currently available.

Indications Sulfonylureas are used:

- as second-line therapy after metformin in patients with type 2 diabetes mellitus
- instead of metformin in patients with type 2 diabetes mellitus who are intolerant to metformin, especially if they are not overweight
- in some forms of monogenic diabetes, including neonatal diabetes and diabetes caused by HNF1α and HNF4α gene mutations

Route These drugs are available for oral administration only.

Adverse effects The main adverse effects of the sulfonylureas are weight gain and hypoglycaemia. Hypoglycaemia is more likely with the longer-acting sulfonylurea preparations.

Factors affecting choices Longer-acting preparations, such as glibenclamide, are used in cases of limited concordance (the sharing of treatment decisions between patient and clinician) where a once-daily preparation may be more tolerable to patients.

Sulfonylureas are well-established treatments for diabetes. They have been used to control hyperglycaemia for many decades, but there is limited evidence that these agents, acting independently, improve long term morbidity and mortality.

Thiazolidinediones

Thiazolidinediones, also known as glitazones, were part of a new wave of treatments for diabetes that first became available in the 1990s. Since their launch, several drugs have been wtihdrawn due to safety concerns.

Actions Thiazolidinediones increase insulin sensitivity by their interaction with peroxisome proliferator-activated receptor-γ. Peroxisome proliferator-activated receptor-γ is a nuclear receptor that regulates many genes to reduce hepatic glucose production and increase peripheral glucose uptake.

Drugs Pioglitazone is the only drug in this class that is currently licensed.

Indications Pioglitazone is indicated for type 2 diabetes mellitus as:

- second-line therapy after metformin (if the risk of hypoglycaemia is significant)
- third-line therapy after metformin and sulfonylurea (if preferable to insulin)

Routes Only oral pioglitazone is available.

Adverse effects Pioglitazone:

- can cause weight gain
- may be associated with bladder cancer and increased risk of osteoporotic fractures
- is contraindicated in patients with cardiac failure as it can cause fluid retention

Factors affecting choices Pioglitazone produces modest glucose reduction. It may also improve cardiovascular outcomes and is used as a second- or third-line agent.

Glucagon-like peptide-1 analogues

Glucagon-like peptide-1 analogues and dipeptidyl peptidase 4 inhibitors are a group of drugs targeted at the incretin hormones, which are gastrointestinal hormones that lead to a reduction in blood glucose (see Chapter 1). Glucoagon-like peptide-1 analogues have only been available as a treatment in the last 10 years.

Actions These drugs are similar to the incretin hormone glucagon-like peptide-1, which is usually broken down by dipeptidyl peptidase 4 (see page 49). They:

- increase insulin secretion
- inhibit glucagon secretion
- delay gastric emptying, thus slowing glucose absorption and producing early satiety

These effects cause patients to reduce their meal sizes, because they feel full earlier and often feel nauseous if they continue to eat past this point. Consequently, glycaemic control improves and weight loss is facilitated.

Drugs There are two glucagon-like peptide-1 analogues:

- exenatide (standard and long-acting)
- liraglutide

Indications Glucagon-like peptide-1 analogues are used as third-line therapy for type 2 diabetes mellitus if:

- body mass index is > 35 kg/m^2
- body mass index is < 35 kg/m^2 and insulin therapy would have significant occupational implications, or weight loss would benefit other significant obesity-related comorbidities

Routes Glucagon-like peptide-1 analogues are given by injection twice daily, daily or weekly, depending on the preparation.

Adverse effects Recently, the concern has been raised that glucagon-like peptide-1 analogues may increase the risk of pancreatitis and pancreatic cancer. This possibility is being investigated using data from post-marketing surveillance.

Factors affecting choices For patients who have difficulty adhering to treatment, their practice nurse can administer glucagon-like peptide-1 analogue once weekly. This therapy is expensive, so its effectiveness needs to be proved to justify continuation of its use beyond 6 months.

Dipeptidyl peptidase 4 inhibitors

Dipeptidyl peptidase inhibitors, commonly known as gliptins, target the incretin hormones (along with glucagon-like peptide 1 analogues). They help the body produce more insulin only when it is needed.

Actions Dipeptidyl peptidase 4 inhibitors (gliptins) act by blocking the actions of the enzyme dipeptidyl peptidase 4. Thus dipeptidyl peptidase 4 inhibitors prevent the breakdown of glucagon-like peptide-1, which results in increased insulin release.

Drugs Many dipeptidyl peptidase 4 inhibitors are available, but sitagliptin, vildagliptin and saxagliptin were the first to be marketed.

Indications The dipeptidyl peptidase 4 inhibitors are used as:

- second-line therapy after metformin (if the risk of hypoglycaemia with a sulphonylurea is significant)
- third-line therapy after metformin and sulfonylurea (if preferable to insulin)

Routes Dipeptidyl peptidase 4 inhibitors are only administered orally.

Adverse effects The adverse effects are similar to those of glucagon-like peptide-1 analogues and include nausea and diarrhoea.

Factors affecting choices Dipeptidyl peptidase 4 inhibitors have no effect on weight, reduce blood glucose modestly and are safe to use in patients with renal failure. They are a good choice when a modest reduction in haemoglobin A1c is needed, as well as in patients who wish to avoid injectable therapy.

Treatment of hormone excess

Hypersecretion of a range of hormones can be treated in multiple ways by regulating various steps in their signalling pathways (**Figure 2.33**).

Inhibition of the stimulus to produce the hormone

Excess production of a hormone can be limited by blocking the stimulus for the endocrine cells to produce it. This method is used in the treatment of prostate cancer: the production of testosterone, which is a growth factor for prostate cancer, is inhibited by goserelin. Goserelin is a gonadotrophin-releasing hormone agonist that stimulates the anterior pituitary gland to produce excessive amounts of luteinising hormone and follicle-stimulating hormone in a non-pulsatile manner. This non-physiological production of the gonadotrophins causes suppression of testosterone production from the gonads.

Augmentation of inhibition of hormone production

The production of some hormones is controlled by tonic inhibition. For example, prolactin production is inhibited by dopamine. In hyperprolactinaemia caused by a prolactinoma (a prolactin-producing pituitary adenoma), a dopamine agonist such as cabergoline is used to inhibit the excessive production of prolactin (**Figure 2.34**).

Dopamine agonists

Dopamine agonists revolutionised treatment of prolactinomas in the 1970s. Prior to their introduction, prolactinomas were treated surgically or with radiotherapy with frequent complications.

Actions Dopamine agonists mimic the action of dopamine, which in turn inhibits growth hormone and prolactin secretion from the pituitary gland.

Drugs The dopamine agonists are:

- cabergoline
- bromocriptine
- quinagolide

Indications Dopamine agonists are used to treat:

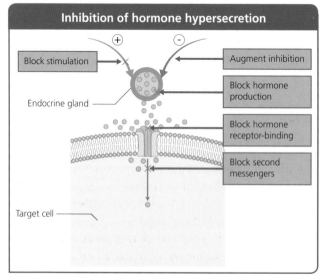

Inhibition of hormone hypersecretion

Block stimulation

Endocrine gland

Augment inhibition

Block hormone production

Block hormone receptor-binding

Block second messengers

Target cell

Figure 2.33 Drug therapies can inhibit hormone hypersecretion at multiple steps in the hormone-signalling pathway.

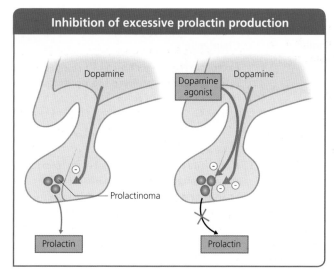

Figure 2.34 Inhibition of excessive prolactin production. (a) Excessive production of prolactin by a prolactinoma is uncontrolled, because of insufficient inhibition from dopamine secreted from the hypothalamus. (b) Dopamine agonist drugs activate dopamine receptors to inhibit prolactin production by the prolactinoma.

- prolactinomas
- acromegaly
- Parkinson's disease (in high doses)

Routes Dopamine agonists are for oral administration only. Cabergoline has a long half-life, so it can be given at a low dose once or twice a week to treat endocrine disorders.

Adverse effects Nausea or depression can sometimes limit the use of dopamine agonists.

Factors affecting choices Cabergoline is most commonly used, because it is potent and reasonably well tolerated. However, there is more experience of bromocriptine use in pregnancy.

Somatostatin analogues

Somatostatin analogues have provided an alternative to surgery for treatment of acromegaly. Their use in neuroendocrine tumours can lead to rapid symptom control (e.g. reducing diarrhoea), radically improving quality of life.

Actions Somatostatin inhibits cell proliferation (and thus tumour growth) and hormone production by acting on the somatostatin receptor, which is commonly expressed on neuroendocrine cells. Somatostatin analogues prevent release of vasoactive gastrointestinal and pancreatic peptides from normal tissue and neuroendocrine tumours. It also acts on G-protein-coupled receptors in the anterior pituitary gland to inhibit growth hormone, TSH and prolactin release.

Drugs The somatostatin analogues are:

- octreotide
- lanreotide
- pasireotide

Indications These drugs are used to treat:

- neuroendocrine tumours
- acromegaly
- thyrotropinoma (TSH-oma)

Routes Somatostatin analogues can be given as short-acting subcutaneous injections three times daily or as a deep subcutaneous depot injection (one to two monthly).

Adverse effects Because somatostatin analogues inhibit pancreatic and gastrointestinal function, many patients have intolerable diarrhoea. Antidiarrhoeal agents may help to control intractable cases.

Factors affecting choices Octreotide and lanreotide have similar efficacy and tolerability.

- In neuroendocrine tumours, they are used to relieve symptoms, for example flushing and diarrhoea in cases of carcinoid syndrome; they also stabilise tumour growth
- In pituitary tumours, they are either used to control hormone secretion before an operation or if an operation does not result in a cure

Cinacalcet

This drug binds to the calcium-sensing receptor of parathyroid cells. By mimicking calcium this way, cinacalcet signals to the cells that the calcium concentration in the blood is adequate, and thus inhibits parathyroid hormone production in patients with hyperparathyroidism.

Inhibition of hormone production

Some drugs reduce excessive production of a hormone by inhibiting its synthesis.

Antithyroid drugs

Antithyroid drugs are used to treat hyperthyroidism (overactive thyroid). They require careful monitoring to ensure patients are rendered euthyroid (normal levels) quickly, avoiding persistent hyperthyroidism or hypothyroidism.

Drugs Antithyroid drugs belong to the thioamide group:

- carbimazole or methimazole
- propylthiouracil

Methimazole is an active metabolite of carbimazole and has a similar mode of action.

Actions Antithyroid drugs decrease thyroid hormone synthesis primarily by inhibiting thyroid peroxidase enzyme. This action inhibits the organification of iodide (the incorporation of iodine into the thyroglobulin molecule), thus the coupling of iodothyronines is inhibited.

Propylthiouracil also inhibits the peripheral conversion of T_4 to the active hormone T_3.

Indication The one indication for antithyroid drugs is thyrotoxicosis.

Routes Only oral administration is used.

Adverse effects Adverse effects associated with antithyroid drugs (see page 201, Chapter 5)

Factors affecting choices Carbimazole (or methimazole) is preferred to propylthiouracil because they:

- have fewer adverse effects (propylthiouracil is rarely associated with severe liver injury)
- provide more rapid control of thyrotoxicosis
- have longer half-lives, so less frequent dosing is needed (carbimazole can be taken once daily, in contrast to propylthiouracil, which needs to be taken two or three times daily)
- are less expensive

One exception is in early pregnancy, when propylthiouracil is preferred. This is because treatment with carbimazole (or methimazole) in the first trimester is associated with rare congenital malformations in the fetus.

Metyrapone

A useful oral treatment for Cushing's syndrome, which is caused by cortisol excess, is metyrapone. Metyrapone inhibits the enzyme 11β-hydroxylase, which catalyses the final step in cortisol synthesis (see Figure 1.26). Thus this drug reduces serum cortisol. However, metyrapone also leads to a build-up of precursors of cortisol, such as adrenal androgens, and these accumulated hormones causes hirsutism in women over time.

This drug is short-acting and needs to be given three times a day to be effective.

Inhibition of the effects of the hormone

The effects of a hormone can be inhibited by:

- blocking binding of the hormone to its receptor
- increasing excretion of excessive substances, such as glucose

The physiological effects of excessive hormone production can be blocked by antagonists or partial agonists of the hormone receptor. Pegvisomant is an example of a receptor antagonist drug. It binds to the growth hormone receptor, thus blocking growth hormone binding, therefore it is used to treat acromegaly (overproduction of growth hormone). Other examples include the alpha-blockers.

Alpha-blockers

Alpha-blockers are usually second or third-line treatment for hypertension, but are the essential choice when a phaeochromocytoma is suspected.

Actions By blocking the α adrenergic receptor in blood vessel walls, these drugs prevent noradrenaline (norepinephrine) from causing vasoconstriction.

Drugs The alpha-blockers are:

- phenoxybenzamine
- doxazosin
- phentolamine
- labetolol (which provides alpha- and beta-blockade)

Indications These drugs are used to treat:

- phaeochromocytoma
- hypertension
- benign prostatic hyperplasia
- Raynaud's syndrome

Routes Alpha-blockers are administered orally or intravenously.

Adverse effects The most significant adverse effects are postural hypotension and tachycardia. These effects can be dramatic in patients with phaeochromocytoma, so they are told to take the first few tablets while sitting down and to rest for several hours afterwards.

Nasal congestion is associated with phenoxybenzamine use and makes this treatment intolerable to some patients. Doxazosin tends to be better tolerated.

Factors affecting choices Treatment of phaeochromocytoma starts with blockade of α adrenergic receptors with phenoxybenzamine or doxazosin to control peripheral vasoconstriction and hypertension. Only then is the use of a beta-blocker considered to control tachycardia.

Phenoxybenzamine offers the most complete alpha-blockade and can be used intravenously; however, it is not easily available. Phentolamine can be used as an alternative in patient with a phaeochromocytoma crisis.

Labetolol is often used on admission to hospital for patients with uncontrolled hypertension. It provides alpha- and beta-blockade.

Sodium-glucose transporter 2 inhibitors

These are also known as the gliflozins. They act by inhibiting glucose reabsorption in the kidney, thus increasing excretion of glucose and sodium and improving symptoms of hyperglycaemia and reducing blood pressure in patients with diabetes mellitus.

Sodium-glucose transporter 2 inhibitors produce weight loss and modest improvement in blood glucose control. However, these effects are at the expense of increased genital tract infections (e.g. *Candida*) and urinary tract infections, both of which are probably caused by glycosuria. Symptomatic hypotension also occurs due to the diuretic effects of sodium-glucose transporter 2 inhibitors.

Symptom control

Drugs to control symptoms are commonly used in combination with disease modifying drugs. This may augment the effect of treatments, such as codeine in addition to somatostatin analogues help control diarrhoea in patients with neuroendocrine tumours. Drugs for symptom control can be stopped when the underlying condition is treated, such as stopping beta-blockers when a patient with hyperthyroidism becomes euthyroid (normal function). Whilst there are many additional drugs that can be used for symptom control, the most common uses are discussed below.

Beta-blockers

Beta-blockers are a commonly prescribed group of drugs particularly for patients with angina. They have a broad range of uses outside of endocrinology, but are commonly used for a few weeks to control the sympathetic overdrive in thyrotoxicosis while medical management takes hold.

Actions Beta-blockers block β adrenergic receptors, which are present throughout the body, including in the heart, smooth muscle, bronchi, arteries and kidneys. These receptors are also present in the sympathetic nervous system; they are stimulated by adrenaline (epinephrine) to cause the 'fight or flight' response.

Drugs The most commonly used beta-blockers are:

- propranolol
- atenolol
- bisoprolol
- labetolol (mixed alpha and beta blocker)

Indications The endocrine uses of beta-blockers are:

- to treat tachycardia in cases of thyroid storm, thyrotoxicosis, thyroiditis, and phaeochromocytoma
- for symptomatic control, for example of tremor and anxiety in thyrotoxicosis

The non-endocrine indications for beta-blockers are cardiac arrhythmias; angina, myocardial infarction and cardiac failure; migraine prophylaxis; and glaucoma.

Routes Beta-blockers are given orally or intravenously.

Adverse effects They can cause bradycardia and hypotension. A few patients develop depression and insomnia. In men, beta-blocker use can cause loss of libido and erectile dysfunction.

Factors affecting choices In phaeochromocytoma, alpha-blockers are used to control blood pressure and beta-blockers to control heart rate.

Adequate alpha blockade must precede the start of beta-blocker therapy. If not, massive vasoconstriction may occur and a hypertensive crisis, with pulmonary oedema or intracranial haemorrhage, may develop. This can be life threatening.

Bisphosphonates

Bisphosphonates main role is to help to strengthen bones, but they are very slow to act with minimal changes seen before 6-12 months; therefore, they are often used over many years. In contrast, they rapidly act to reduce hypercalcaemia and are used acutely for that indication.

Actions Bisphosphonates attach to hydroxyapatite crystals in bone. This action reduces osteoclastic activity and thus inhibits bone turnover.

Drugs The bisphosphonates are:

- alendronic acid
- risedronate (risedronic acid)
- pamidronate (pamidronic acid)
- zoledronic acid

Indications These drugs are used to treat:

- osteoporosis
- hypercalcaemia not caused by excess
- acute hypercalcaemia in cases of hyperparathyroidism (less effective than in non parathyroid hormone related hypercalcaemia)
- malignant bone pain
- Paget's disease

Routes Alendronic acid can be taken orally once weekly. Pamidronic acid is used intravenously for acute treatment of hypercalcaemia. Zoledronic acid can be given once a year, but this is done intravenously.

Adverse effects Nausea and oesophageal reflux are common. Patients are told to swallow the tablets with plenty of water, on an empty stomach, while sitting or standing, and ≥ 30 min before eating or taking any other medication. Patients should stay upright for 30 min after each dose. This strict regimen is difficult for patients to tolerate, and because they do not see an immediate benefit, adherence to treatment is poor.

There have been reports of bisphosphonates causing osteonecrosis of the jaw and atypical femoral fractures.

Factors affecting choices Patients unable to tolerate oral treatment may be eligible for intravenous zoledronic acid, which is administered once yearly. Pamidronate is the most commonly used bisphosphonate for in patients with malignant hypercalcaemia.

Atypical analgesics

A number of atypical analgesics are used to treat painful diabetic neuropathy. These drugs are a mixture of antidepressant medication (e.g. amitriptyline) and anticonvulsants (e.g. gabapentin and pregabalin).

The atypical analgesics vary in their adverse effects and efficacy. Different patients have different responses to each medication. A long trial period is needed, because these drugs may take weeks to be effective, and the dose needs to be up-titrated. If a high dose of an atypical analgesic fails to control symptoms within 2–4 months then another of these drugs may be tried.

These medications control symptoms but do not reverse the pathology responsible for the neuropathic pain. The average effect is to reduce pain scores by less than half, so patients are warned that their pain will not resolve completely.

Antiandrogens

These are used to reduce hirsutism in conditions such as polycystic ovary syndrome. They are available as antiandrogens and eflornithine cream.

- Antiandrogens: cyproterone acetate (most commonly used), spironolactone, finasteride (which has limited use because of its liver toxicity) and flutamide (limited use because of liver toxicity)
- Eflornithine cream: this is applied topically and inhibits the L-orthinine decarboxylase enzyme which is essential for cell (and hair) growth.

Surgery

Surgical treatment of endocrine disease may:

- be curative
- reduce the symptoms of compression and help stabilise hormone release, when combined with pharmacological treatment and radiotherapy

Endocrine diseases (with the exception of diabetes mellitus) are rare, so surgeons with extensive experience yield better outcomes (improved cure rates and reduced complications). Close collaboration with the endocrinologist is essential to guide the appropriate type and timing of surgery.

The role of surgery is changing. Endocrine diseases may be detected incidentally, as patients undergo more blood tests and imaging studies for other reasons, and these conditions (e.g. mild hypercalcaemia due to primary hyperparathyroidism in the elderly) may require nothing more than occasional monitoring. In addition, pharmacological treatments, such as somatostatin analogues in acromegaly, are often available for patients for whom an operation would be high risk or offer no chance of a cure. However, most pharmacological treatments are expensive and not curative. Surgery is often the only way to achieve a cure, especially in cases of suspected malignancy.

Transplantation is a treatment option for some endocrine conditions. For example, whole pancreas or islet cell transplantation is carried out for some patients with type 1 diabetes mellitus.

Pharmacological treatment is sometimes used before surgery to help reduce the associated risks. For example, the use of somatostatin analogues in patients with acromegaly can normalise growth hormone concentration, thus reducing soft tissue swelling; consequently, the airway is easier to intubate when anaesthesia is induced. In addition, the use of somatostatin analogues is sometimes associated with tumour shrinkage, which may make the adenoma more accessible during the operation.

Surgery is used in endocrine diseases to:

- relieve obstructive or compressive symptoms
- stop hormone secretion
- remove cancer
- decrease morbidity and mortality
- treat complications of endocrine diseases

Large endocrine glands can cause symptoms of compression. For example, a retrosternal goitre can cause breathing difficulties by compressing the trachea, and a pituitary adenoma can cause visual loss by pressing on the optic chiasm. Surgery is often needed to relieve these compressive symptoms.

Surgery is also often necessary to address the oversecretion of a hormone, for example parathyroid hormone in hyperparathyroidism, and adrenaline (epinephrine) and noradrenaline (norepinephrine) in phaeochromocytoma and paragangliomas. Also, if the findings of imaging studies suggest malignancy, surgery is done to remove potential cancer from the gland. This is often the case with thyroid nodules, when the results of fine-needle aspiration and cytological investigation show cells suspected to be cancerous. In such cases, a thyroidectomy is done.

Bariatric surgery is done to induce weight loss and thus reduce the morbidity and mortality associated with obesity. The two most common operations for obesity are the laparoscopic adjustable gastric band insertion and the laparoscopic Roux-en-Y gastric bypass (**Figure 2.35**). Both reduce the effective volume of the stomach to reduce calorie intake. The gastric bypass also causes malabsorption by bypassing the duodenum and jejunum.

Corrective operations can help treat the complications of endocrine conditions, such as eye surgery for proptosis in Graves' disease ophthalmopathy.

Considerations for surgery

The following need to be considered by clinicians and patients when planning surgery.

- Will surgery be curative?
- Will the endocrine condition (e.g. phaeochromocytoma or thyrotoxicosis) affect the safety of surgery?
- What is the best surgical approach (e.g. a laparoscopic or an open approach for adrenal surgery)?
- What are the risks and expected benefits of surgery?
- What are the patients' expectations and understanding of the procedure?
- Who will carry out the operation? (Operations may be done in secondary or tertiary care, depending on the surgeon's degree of experience)

Surgical approaches

Three approaches are usually used in surgery for gland removal:

- enucleation
- partial resection of the gland
- total resection of the gland

Sometimes the lesion is easily visible to the surgeon. If it is likely to be benign, they can extract ('enucleate') it without having to remove any of the normal gland. This technique is often described as like popping a pea out of a pod. Enucleation is commonly used to remove neuroendocrine tumours of the pancreas, such as insulinomas, because pancreatic resection is associated with multiple complications.

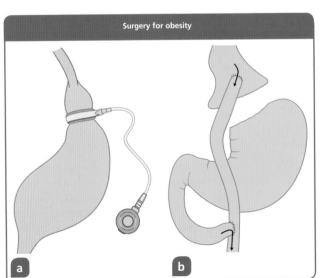

Figure 2.35 Surgery for obesity. (a) Adjustable gastric band. The band can be inflated to increase, or deflated to decrease, the size of the pouch at the proximal end of the stomach. (b) Roux-en-Y gastric bypass. The proximal transected stomach is connected directly to the jejunum, bypassing the stomach and duodenum. The distal end of the bypassed section is anastomosed to the ileum to allow drainage of gastric secretions.

Surgery for obesity

The common indications for partial or complete surgical resections are shown in **Table 2.27**. Surgeons may use different approaches to achieve the best chance of complete resection. Examples of different techniques and indications are shown in **Table 2.28**.

Patients with chronic endocrine disease often need special precautions for surgery, even if they are having an operation for a non-endocrine reason.

- Patients with hypoadrenalism require larger doses of steroid replacement and may need parenteral treatment if they are subject to a nil by mouth order in the perioperative period
- Patients receiving insulin may need intravenous insulin at the time of the operation, as well as adjustments to the dose (down if not eating, and up if they have a coexistent infection that would increase their blood glucose)

Endocrine gland resection and hormone replacement		
Surgery	Example indication(s)	Likely long-term hormone replacement
Parathyroidectomy		
Partial	Hyperparathyroidism	None
Total (all four glands removed)	Parathyroid hyperplasia	1,25-vitamin D (calcitriol) or 1α (OH) D3 (alfacalcidol)
Thyroidectomy		
Partial	Thyroid nodule or cyst	None
Total	Thyroid cancer	Levothyroxine
	Multinodular goitre	
	Graves' disease	
Adrenalectomy		
Unilateral	Adenoma	None (except temporary hydrocortisone deficiency if lesion was secreting cortisol)
	Carcinoma	
Bilateral	Uncured Cushing's disease	Hydrocortisone
		Fludrocortisone
Hypophysectomy		
Hemihypophysectomy	Pituitary adenoma	None
Total hypophysectomy	Failure of hemihypophysectomy to cure condition	Hydrocortisone
		Thyroxine
		Testosterone or oestrogen
		Growth hormone
		Desmopressin
Pancreatectomy		
Partial (resection of pancreatic tail or Whipple's procedure)	Neuroendocrine tumour	None
Total	Multiple neuroendocrine tumours	Insulin
		Pancreatic enzyme replacement (pancrelipase, e.g. Creon)

Table 2.27 Examples of indications for partial or complete endocrine gland resection and the associated need for hormone replacement

Endocrine gland surgical techniques			
Gland	Techniques	Indications	Reported benefits
Adrenal	Laparoscopic 'keyhole'	Small adenomas	Quicker recovery, shorter hospital stay and small scars
	Laparotomy (open procedure)	Large adrenal cancers	Easier to ensure complete resection without breaching the capsule and risking malignant spread
Pituitary	Direct visualisation (with microscope)	Pituitary adenomas	Reliable results with a traditional technique
	Endoscopic resection (camera on end of instruments)	Pituitary adenomas	Better for tumours extending into the cavernous sinus, and less postoperative scarring
	Craniotomy	Extensive macroadenomas, hypothalamic lesions (e.g. craniopharyngiomas) and cranial tumours (e.g. meningiomas)	Best technique tumours extending beyond the optic chiasm and pituitary fossa

Table 2.28 Different surgical techniques for operating on endocrine glands

Organ or tissue transplantation

Whole organ or cell transplantation is the surgical implantation of an endocrine organ or cells from a donor into a recipient. As the donor organ or cells are immunologically distinct from the patient's tissues, lifelong chemical immunosuppression is required to prevent rejection.

The commonest type of transplantation in patients with endocrine disease is a renal transplant for those with end-stage renal failure as a consequence of diabetes mellitus. To date, the only endocrine transplantations carried out in practice are in relation to the pancreas:

- pancreatic transplantation
- islet cell transplantation

Transplantation of other endocrine organs, such as the adrenal glands, has been done experimentally but is not considered in current clinical practice.

Pancreatic transplantation

Whole pancreas transplantation can 'cure' type 1 diabetes mellitus. It can restore normal insulin production and blood glucose control, and patients will no longer require insulin. However, whole organ pancreas transplantation is not commonly carried out, because the risks of major surgery and the adverse effects of immunosuppression outweigh the benefits of independence from insulin therapy. Transplantation is usually done in those who have had or who require renal transplantation for end-stage kidney disease associated with long-term diabetes, because these patients will already be using immunosuppressive drugs.

Islet cell transplantation

Transplantation of pancreatic beta cells also requires immunosuppression, but it does not result in long-term insulin independence. The main indication for beta-cell transplantation is severe recurrent hypoglycaemia.

Radiotherapy

In radiotherapy, ionising radiation is used to cause cell death in replicating cells by damaging their DNA. The ionising radiation is targeted to preferentially cause the death of cancerous or abnormal cells. However, it may also damage neighbouring healthy cells, such as normal optic nerve cells near abnormal pituitary cells. If the abnormal cells are replicating slowly, as in benign pituitary adenomas, cell death will be much slower than that in rapidly replicating malignant cells and therefore the treatment will take years to be effective.

Radiotherapy is usually an adjuvant to pharmacological and surgical treatments. It is used to treat:

- benign functional pituitary adenomas, such as Cushing's disease
- non-functioning lesions, such as non-functioning pituitary adenomas

Radiotherapy is also used as an adjuvant in the treatment of endocrine cancer, for example thyroid cancer. However, this option is usually reserved for patients for whom surgery has not achieved complete resection or cure. Occasionally, radiotherapy is a primary treatment for endocrine disease, when an operation is unlikely to produce a cure or if the patient is not well enough to be considered a candidate for surgery.

The age of the patient is also considered during treatment planning. Radiotherapy to the neck in childhood, which used to be part of treatment for leukaemia, can increase the risk of thyroid cancer in later life.

Modes of delivery of radiotherapy

Which method to use depends on the extent of the original disease and the proximity to surrounding organs, as well as the known effectiveness of treatment.

Internal radiotherapy

Radioactive molecules are administered systemically to treat certain endocrine disorders (**Table 2.29**). For example, radioactive iodine (iodine-131) is given by mouth to treat hyperthyroidism and thyroid cancer. Thyroid tissue takes up iodine avidly, so the radioactive isotope is incorporated by the thyroid tissue and destroys it from within.

After administration of systemic radiotherapy, the patient is radioactive. If treatment is given at a high dose, they must stay in hospital in a lead-lined room until discharge. Even after discharge, the patient will have a low level of radioactivity radiating to people nearby for several weeks. Patients can set off security alarms at airports for up to 12 weeks. It is essential for women to avoid pregnancy for up to 6 months, because of the potential risk of teratogenicity.

The treatments are slow to work and take effect over weeks or months, but they are well tolerated. Treatments can be repeated every few months if isotope uptake and tumour response continue. Evidence for a positive response to treatment is provided by the results of imaging studies and measurement of tumour markers showing stabilisation or reduction of the disease.

Systemic radiotherapy for endocrine diseases				
Condition	Radioisotope treatment	Preparation for treatment	Administration	Aim
Thyrotoxicosis	Low-dose radioiodine (^{131}I)	Stop antithyroid drugs (1 week before)	Oral (as an outpatient)	Cure
Thyroid cancer (papillary and follicular)	High-dose radioiodine (^{131}I)	Thyroidectomy Stop thyroid hormone replacement or use recombinant thyroid-stimulating hormone	Orally for 3–5 days (as an in patient)	Cure
Neuroendocrine tumours	Radiolabelled somatostatin receptor analogues	Stop somatostatin analogues	Intravenously (as an in patient)	Disease stabilisation
Neuroendocrine tumours	MIBG	Potassium iodide (to block thyroid uptake)	Intravenously for 3–5 days (as an in patient)	Disease stabilisation

MIBG, iodine-131 meta-iodobenzylguanidine, the commonest radioisotope used to treat neuroendocrine tumours.

Table 2.29 Systemic (internal) radiotherapy for endocrine diseases

External radiotherapy

In external radiotherapy, X-rays generated by a linear accelerator machine are targeted at a specific area of tissue. External radiotherapy is often required to treat endocrine conditions that cannot be cured by drug treatment or surgery, for example a non-functioning pituitary adenoma that has not been completely resected by surgery and that shows signs of regrowth. External radiotherapy is also used as an adjuvant to surgery for patients with malignant tumours such as anaplastic thyroid cancer.

The radiation beam passes through non-target tissues anterior and posterior to the target tissue. Damage to these structures must be minimised by carefully targeted treatment.

Conventional external beam radiotherapy

This is the commonest method of administering radiotherapy. It is used to treat:

- some inoperable malignant endocrine tumours (e.g. anaplastic thyroid cancer)
- some benign endocrine conditions (e.g. pituitary adenoma and active thyroid eye disease)

In cases of pituitary adenoma, multiple sessions may be required, during which the pituitary gland is targeted by radiation from a single beam (**Figure 2.36a**).

Stereotactic radiotherapy

In this type of radiotherapy, multiple narrow beams deliver highly focused and high-intensity radiation to a small target area. The use of multiple beams in this way minimises the exposure of other tissues to radiation (**Figure 2.36b**).

Gamma knife is a form of stereotactic radiotherapy that requires only a single session of treatment. In endocrinology, its use is limited to the treatment of a few types of pituitary tumour.

Adverse effects of radiotherapy

Radiotherapy has its drawbacks.

- External radiotherapy has adverse effects, including nausea, vomiting and fatigue
- External radiotherapy may damage adjacent structures, such as the optic chiasm, so there is a risk of visual loss when the pituitary gland is irradiated
- Functional endocrine structures may be damaged; hypopituitarism may develop over time, so hormone replacement is required after pituitary radiotherapy
- Pituitary radiotherapy is potentially damaging to surrounding brain tissue, resulting in reductions in mental function
- There is a small risk of the development of secondary tumours after radiotherapy
- There is a probable increased risk of cerebrovascular disease after pituitary radiotherapy

Radiotherapy is contraindicated in pregnant women.

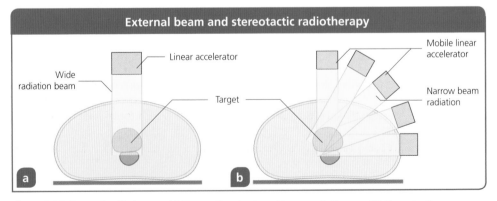

External beam and stereotactic radiotherapy

Linear accelerator

Wide radiation beam

Target

Mobile linear accelerator

Narrow beam radiation

a

b

Figure 2.36 Types of radiotherapy. (a) Conventional external beam radiotherapy. (b) Stereotactic radiotherapy.

Answers to starter questions

1. Many drug therapies alter investigation results, so it is important to know what drugs a patient has been taking, e.g. corticosteroids invalidate cortisol production tests. Other drugs, including alcohol, over-the-counter and internet-sourced medicine, affect hormone metabolism and alter biochemistry results.

2. Most endocrine conditions are a constellation of non-specific symptoms. Initially, patients may put these symptoms down to stress (e.g. at work) or relationship difficulties, and therefore will not present to a doctor. If there are no obvious 'trigger points' in the history (such as a change in relationship or job) this points to a potential pathological cause.

3. Symptoms such as erectile problems can be hard to admit to and discussing them with patients can be difficult. Asking a direct question when they are not expecting it often leads to patients denying there is a problem. Explaining that a condition is often associated with symptoms, such as erectile dysfunction, can allow them to open up. If the patient attends with someone else, ask during an examination rather than when taking a history, as this can be more private and patient won't have to talk about it in front of someone else.

4. Careers that involve machinery can be restricted (e.g. HGV driving) or prohibited (e.g. armed forces, airline pilot) if a patient takes insulin. Patients given radioactive iodine must also avoid close contact with children for weeks after treatment. Smoking worsens the prognosis of thyroid eye disease and hugely increases the risk of cardiovascular disease in diabetes mellitus, while alcohol use alters the metabolism of some hormone treatments lowering their effectiveness.

5. Old photographs can show very gradual changes in facial appearance over time which may not have been noticed by the patient, or their friends and family. Cushing's syndrome and acromegaly are two conditions that are accompanied by very slow changes in appearance.

6. Acromegaly can often be diagnosed 'on sight' because it causes a stereotypical appearance of large hands and feet, prognathism (protruding jaw), macroglossia (large tongue) and interdental separation (widened spaces between the teeth). Cushing's syndrome is also fairly characteristic with central adiposity, a round flushed face and thin arms and legs. Other conditions that the trained eye can often quickly recognise are Turner's syndrome (short stature and webbed necks), Klinefelter's syndrome (tall with long arm span) and Graves' disease (large goitre and thyroid eye disease).

7. Short stature is a frequent presentation in children and adolescents. Knowing the height of the parents can help predict the expected normal height range for the adolescent. The final predicted height is based on the mid parental height minus 7 cm for girls and plus 7 cm for boys. In addition, conditions run in families and spotting a condition in a parent, such as neurofibromatosis, can help with the diagnosis of the child's problem.

Answers *continued*

8. Hormone concentrations in the blood vary, often from minute to minute, so it is difficult to interpret levels in blood drawn at a single time point. However, most hormones have a corresponding stimulatory hormone: administration of the stimulatory hormone tests whether the gland responds normally. Conversely, pathological hypersecretion of a hormone is frequently independent of the usual suppressive feedback mechanisms: if administration of a suppressor fails to suppress hormone production in the normal manner, this confirms hypersecretion.

9. No. Whilst a positive test is diagnostic in the majority of cases, the sensitivity and specificity of tests mean that some patients will have a 'positive' result and not have the disease (false positive) and others will have a 'negative' result and still have the condition (false negative).Therefore clinical suspicion is vital. In conditions such as Cushing's syndrome, often multiple tests are required to reach a diagnosis.

10. An incidentaloma is a mass in an endocrine gland, discovered when using imaging to look for something else. These are common in the adrenal, pituitary and thyroid glands. Once identified the significance of the mass is determined by clinical assessment and biochemical and imaging tests, to see if the mass is functional (hormone-secreting) or if it changes over time (growth of a benign or malignant tumour).

11. The investigation of many endocrine diseases is very complicated requiring a multitude of tests to make a diagnosis. Without protocols it would be easy for practice to vary between clinicians to the detriment of patients. Investigation protocols standardise what constitutes a normal or abnormal test result, ensuring that patients receive consistent quality care.

12. Pancreas transplantation results in insulin independence and normal blood glucose. However, it carries the significant risks of major surgery, lifelong immunosuppression, graft failure and rejection. There is also a shortage of organs to transplant. Pancreatic transplants are usually restricted to patients who will already have to have lifelong immunosuppressive therapy because of planned or previous renal transplantation.

13. With almost all management options there is a balance of risks and benefits to consider before offering potentially curative treatment, and management can do more harm than good if the risks are not properly considered. For example, transsphenoidal surgery for a pituitary mass will cure acromegaly but will leave the patient with hypopituitarism. Weighing up pros and cons, and discussing these with patients, is a fundamental part of ensuring that patients receive an appropriate treatment that will benefit them with as few risks as possible.

14. A management plan should be agreed on that is acceptable to both the patient and their healthcare professionals. Communicating this often takes time and repetition. After delivering an important message such as the need for an operation, it is necessary to pause, to allow the patient time to reflect and ask questions. Encouraging the patient to bring a friend or relative can help them to recall the conversation. Often providing written information (a letter or information sheet) or scheduling follow-up appointments is helpful to the patient as repeating the information can help them to understand.

15. Continuity of care helps manage chronic endocrine conditions more effectively. It allows the patient to develop trust and understanding with their doctor and allows the doctor to have a better understanding of the patient's personality, health beliefs and social situation. The downside is that dependence can develop, and if the relationship has to end, e.g. the doctor relocates, it can be hard for the patient to place trust in a new doctor.

Chapter 3
Diabetes mellitus, obesity and lipid disorders

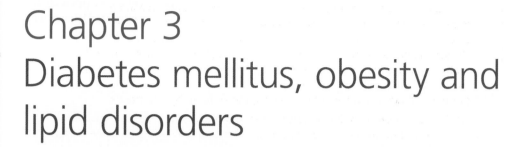

Starter questions

Answers to the following questions are on page 171.

1. Do all obese patients develop diabetes?
2. Can surgery cure diabetes?
3. Why do some women develop diabetes in pregnancy?
4. Why do some ethnic groups have a higher incidence of diabetes than others?
5. Should all patients with type 2 diabetes be treated the same way?
6. Are all new diabetes patients symptomatic?

Introduction

Certain diseases, such as diabetes, obesity and hyperlipidaemia, are grouped together as they share long-term metabolic consequences. They all increase the risk of ischaemic heart disease, peripheral vascular disease and stroke. The conditions often overlap and it is not uncommon for patients to simultaneously suffer from all three, with one contributing to the cause of the other. These conditions are occasionally caused by single gene defects, but in the vast majority of patients the conditions develop because of a combination of genetic factors and lifestyle decisions. Treatment of type 2 diabetes, obesity and hyperlipidaemia often share common goals of maintaining a healthy lifestyle and optimal weight.

Diabetes mellitus is a condition of chronically elevated blood glucose concentrations usually caused by:

- total or relative deficiency of insulin or,
- failure to of the tissues respond appropriately to the insulin produced (insulin resistance).

Diabetes mellitus is common; 4.5% of the UK population currently have it and its incidence is rising globally because of changes in dietary habits, increase in obesity, sedentary lifestyles and aging of the population. Although the search for a cure continues for diabetes mellitus, particularly type 1, the main focus is on preventing the epidemic of type 2 diabetes mellitus brought on by obesity.

Case 1 Weight loss, thirst and excessive amounts of urine

Presentation

Tom is 24 years old. He presents to his general practitioner (GP) with a weight loss of 4kg over the past month. He has also been feeling thirstier and has been waking more frequently to pass urine.

Initial interpretation

Unintentional weight loss of 4kg in 1 month, without change in lifestyle, is significant. Weight is lost for numerous reasons (see page 70), but common endocrine causes, such as thyrotoxicosis and type 1 diabetes mellitus, should always be considered.

Excessive thirst (polydipsia) and passing excessive amounts of urine (polyuria) suggest the presence of excessive solute, such as glucose, in urine forming in the kidneys. During filtration, transport proteins in the renal tubules become saturated with the solute; the filtered load of solute exceeds the reabsorption capacity.

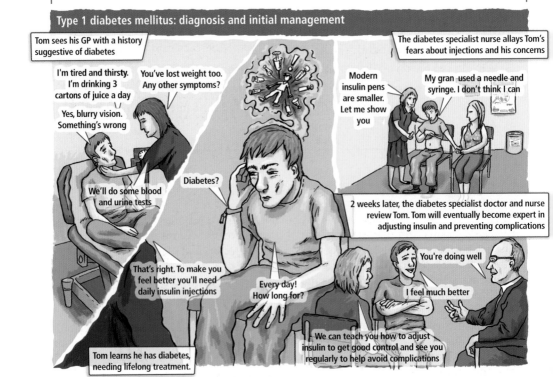

Case 1 *continued*

The solute remaining in the urine then draws water into the urine by osmosis.

History

Tom has noticed that his clothes have become ill fitting and loose. He always feels thirsty and is drinking up to 4 L of water and fruit juice daily.

He plays football regularly, but he has to take a break in the game to pass urine. Furthermore, he feels exhausted at the end. He also wakes up to four times at night to pass large amounts of urine.

Interpretation of history

Urgent investigation is needed, because Tom's symptoms have developed quickly and are progressively worsening. Diabetes mellitus should always be excluded.

> Patients presenting with diabetes mellitus are often drinking lots of sweet drinks to quench their thirst. However, these drinks only make the problem worse because of their sugar content (10% for fruit juice). Switching to water or unsweetened drinks often significantly reduces blood glucose, with the patient's symptoms improving within a couple of days.

Further history

On further questioning, Tom says that he has been feeling very tired for a few weeks. He has been experiencing blurred vision for the past week.

At the age of 18 years, Tom learned that he had autoimmune hypothyroidism when his GP diagnosed the condition, so he takes levothyroxine. He does not smoke, and he drinks up to 20 units of alcohol every week. There is no family history of diabetes mellitus in his parents, but his mother has primary hypothyroidism.

Tom works shifts as a heavy goods vehicle driver for a supermarket chain. He has no fixed mealtimes.

Examination

On examination, Tom is thin, with a body mass index (BMI) of 20 kg/m². He has a resting heart rate of 80 beats/min, and his blood pressure is 110/66 mmHg. The rest of the examination is normal.

Interpretation of findings

Significant weight loss with polydipsia, polyuria, blurred vision and lethargy suggests diabetes mellitus. Tom is thin, young and has autoimmune hypothyroidism, which is associated with type 1 diabetes (**Table 3.1**). The severity of his symptoms, his weight loss and his young age make a diagnosis of type 1 diabetes mellitus likely.

Tom's thyroid function should be checked to ensure that his dose of levothyroxine, used for thyroxine replacement

Autoimmune conditions associated with type 1 diabetes mellitus	
Condition	Description
Autoimmune thyroid disease	Hashimoto's thyroiditis (autoimmune hypothyroidism) and Graves' disease (autoimmune thyrotoxicosis)
Pernicious anaemia	Loss of intrinsic factor leading to B12 deficiency
Coeliac disease	Hypersensitivity to gluten
Vitiligo	Loss of skin pigmentation leading to white patches
Addison's disease	Primary adrenal insufficiency
Premature ovarian failure	Early menopause and menstruation stops

Table 3.1 Autoimmune conditions associated with type 1 diabetes mellitus

Case 1 *continued*

therapy, is appropriate. Weight loss usually results if the dose is too high.

Investigations

Urinalysis shows glycosuria and an excessive concentration of ketones. Capillary blood glucose is high, at 22.8 mmol/L, and this finding is confirmed by measurement of venous glucose. Haemoglobin A1c (glycated haemoglobin; haemoglobin with glucose permanently bound to it) is increased at 70 mmol/mol. Glutamic acid decarboxylase and islet cell antibody tests are positive.

Tom's thyroid function tests showed appropriate replacement dose of levothyroxine.

Diagnosis

Tom has type 1 diabetes mellitus, given positive glutamic acid decarboxylase and islet cell antibody results, the short history and his young age. The family history of autoimmune disease is also suggestive.

He is started on insulin therapy the same day. He receives basic dietary education, including the advice to stop consuming fruit juice and to drink water instead. Tom is also taught about testing capillary blood glucose and how to recognise hypoglycaemia.

Tom is initially upset with the diagnosis of diabetes mellitus and the prospect of insulin injections. He must inform the appropriate authority of his diagnosis. In the UK, to continue with his heavy goods vehicle license, Tom needs to provide 3 months' worth of frequent capillary blood glucose measurements. Therefore his employer will have to find him an alternative job while he gathers this information.

> **In the UK, patients need to inform the Driver and Vehicle Licensing Agency that they have started insulin treatment.** Commercial transport drivers can continue driving, but only after providing sufficient evidence over time that their blood glucose is stable. Certain occupations, such as being a pilot or being on the front line in the armed forces, are currently prohibited to those taking insulin. The requirements differ in other countries.

Case 2 Recurrent thrush

Presentation

Mrs Evans, aged 55 years, presents to her GP with white vaginal discharge and severe pruritus (itching) of 1 week's duration.

Initial interpretation

When considering the cause of vaginal discharge, sexually transmitted diseases should be considered. However, in a woman over 50 years old the most common cause is *Candida albicans* (thrush).

Further history

Mrs Evans has had two episodes of thrush in the past 6 months, which she treated with cotrimazole pessaries (medicine-containing devices that are inserted into the vagina) from the pharmacy. Her symptoms improved but then recurred a few weeks later. She finds the itching troublesome and seeks an explanation for these recurrent episodes.

Her partner has no symptoms, and she has had no new sexual contacts in the past 30 years. She feels tired most of the time

Case 2 *continued*

and has put on 10 kg of weight over the past year. She has osteoarthritis in her right knee, which limits her mobility.

Mrs Evans takes ramipril for high blood pressure, which was diagnosed 3 years ago. She smokes 20 cigarettes a day. Type 2 diabetes mellitus has recently been diagnosed in her older sister. Her mother had diabetes mellitus and died at 64 years of age after a stroke.

Examination

On examination, Mrs Evans is obese, with a BMI of 34.2 kg/m^2. She does not have acanthosis nigricans (dark, thickened skin) or abdominal striae (stretch marks). Her blood pressure is increased, at 150/92 mmHg.

Her vagina has a thick, white curdy discharge, a sample of which is sent for smear and culture.

Interpretation of findings

Mrs Evans is an obese woman of 55 years with recurrent candidiasis and a strong family history of diabetes mellitus. High blood glucose allows yeasts such as *Candida* to flourish.

Obesity is likely to be contributing to her osteoarthritis. The tiredness is a consequence of hyperglycaemia or other obesity-related complications, such as sleep apnoea. Type 2 diabetes mellitus must be suspected.

Investigations

Urinalysis shows glycosuria. Random venous blood glucose is increased, at 12 mmol/L. Haemoglobin A1c is also high, at 69 mmol/mol. The diagnostic criteria for diabetes mellitus are shown in **Table 3.2**.

Diagnosis

Type 2 diabetes mellitus has predisposed Mrs Evans to recurrent candidiasis. She also has a high risk of cardiovascular disease, because she is obese, smokes, has hyperlipidaemia, is hypertensive and has a family history of vascular disease. She is given diet and lifestyle advice to treat her diabetes and will be reassessed after 3 months to see how effective this has been. Her risk of further episodes of candidiasis will improve as her glucose is controlled but this episode is treated with a further vaginal clotrimazole pessary.

> Many people fear a diagnosis of diabetes, because they have seen a relative develop complications such as a leg amputation or severe hypoglycaemic episode on insulin. Early education usually helps allay the fear associated with the diagnosis and engage patients in the necessity of good control.

Diagnosis of diabetes mellitus			
Measurement	Result in diabetes	Result in impaired glucose tolerance or prediabetes	Normal result
Haemoglobin A1c (mmol/mol)	≥48*	42–47	≤41
Fasting glucose (mmol/L)	≥7	6.1–6.9 (impaired fasting glucose)	≤6
Random plasma glucose (mmol/L)	≥11.1		
2-h glucose in oral glucose tolerance test (mmol/L)	≥11.1	7.8–11 (impaired glucose tolerance)	≤7.7
*A repeat confirmatory test is required in most cases.			

Table 3.2 Diagnosis of diabetes mellitus

Type 1 diabetes mellitus

Type 1 diabetes mellitus results from insulin deficiency. The deficiency is caused by decreased or absent insulin production as a consequence of destruction of pancreatic beta cells. This is an autoimmune process: the immune system attacks 'self' proteins.

Rising levels of obesity has made diagnosis of the type of diabetes more challenging. Diabetes in an obese child may be type 2 (rather than the typical picture of type 1 diabetes in childhood). Conversely, type 1 diabetes can still develop in an overweight adult.

Epidemiology

Type 1 diabetes mellitus accounts for 5–10% of cases of diabetes mellitus in the UK. After asthma, it is the second most common chronic disease of childhood. It presents at any age, but the peak age of presentation is 11–13 years.

The incidence of type 1 diabetes is rising worldwide. Between 1990-1999 the global incidence of type 1 diabetes increased by 3% per year.

The risk of having the condition shows wide geographical variation, increasing with increasing distance from the equator. Furthermore, relocating to an area of higher risk increases the risk of developing type 1 diabetes. These phenomena support a role for environmental factors in its pathogenesis.

Aetiology

The incidence of type 1 diabetes is increasing, however the cause of this increase is not firmly established. Genetic and environmental factors each have an influence, and may explain the wide geographical variation seen.

Autoimmunity

In type 1 diabetes mellitus, an autoimmune reaction destroys pancreatic beta cells. Postmortem studies have also shown insulitis (inflammation of the islet cells of Langerhans). The common autoantibodies detected in serum are:

- glutamic acid decarboxylase antibody
- anti–tyrosine phosphate antibody
- islet cell antibody

If all three autoantibodies are present, the patient has about a 90% risk of developing type 1 diabetes mellitus over 10 years.

Genetic factors

Genetic susceptibility for type 1 diabetes mellitus is polygenic; several genetic factors contribute to its susceptibility. The greatest contribution is from the human leukocyte antigen (*HLA*) region on the short arm of chromosome 6. These are genes that encode for cell surface proteins that regulate the immune system and common variations in *HLA* are linked to autoimmune diseases such as type 1 diabetes. *HLA DR3* and *HLA DR4* alleles are present in 90% of patients with type 1 diabetes mellitus in the UK.

The Greek physician Aretaeus first described diabetes mellitus in the first century. The name diabetes comes from a word for 'siphon' or 'passing through', referring to polyuria, and mellitus is derived from the Latin word meaning 'sweetened like honey'.

Environmental factors

The recent increase in the incidence of type 1 diabetes suggests that environmental factors are involved in its pathogenesis. Early exposure to viral agents, such as rubella, and the early introduction of cows' milk have been proposed as environmental factors that start the autoimmune process in genetically susceptible people.

Prevention

There is no way to prevent type 1 diabetes mellitus. However, research suggests that it is possible to synthesise monoclonal antibodies that prevent further beta-cell destruction.

Vaccines to prevent the immune system from destroying these pancreatic cells have been developed in mice, and it is hoped that this research may yield a vaccine for use in humans.

Pathogenesis

Type 1 diabetes mellitus is a chronic, organ-specific autoimmune disease that is induced by an environmental event, or events, in a genetically susceptible person. The activation of immune cells and autoantibodies leads to selective destruction of pancreatic beta cells over a variable period of time.

Clinical features

Patients with type 1 diabetes mellitus usually present with symptoms of hyperglycaemia. The classical triad of symptoms of insulin deficiency is as follows.

- Polyuria: the result of osmotic diuresis caused by the presence of glucose in urine in the kidneys
- Polydipsia: thirst as the result of loss of fluid
- Weight loss: insulin deficiency leads to accelerated breakdown of fat and muscle

Others symptoms include:

- hyperphagia (excessive hunger)
- blurred vision, the consequence of high glucose levels causing fluid influx (by osmosis) and lens swelling causing a refractive error
- fatigue and lassitude
- muscle cramps
- fungal or bacterial infection
- features of diabetic ketoacidosis (see page 307)

> Glycosuria (glucose in the urine) occurs in diabetes because the blood contains too much glucose for the renal tubules to reabsorb from the filtrate. It represents a loss of pure chemical energy, hence the weight loss that occurs in type 1 diabetes mellitus.

Most signs of diabetes come from developing complications. However, a rare inflammato-

ry skin condition called necrobiosis lipoidica occasionally occurs in type 1 and type 2 diabetes (**Figure 3.1**). It causes shiny red-brown or yellowish patches on the skin, usually on the shin, and rarely precedes the diagnosis of diabetes.

Between 5 and 10% of patients with type 1 diabetes mellitus present with diabetic keto-acidosis. They can have rapid metabolic decompensation because of intercurrent illness such as sepsis. Mortality in patients with diabetic ketoacidosis has decreased significantly over the past 10 years because of early recognition and standardised treatment pathways; it is now < 2%.

Diagnostic approach

The general approach in establishing a diagnosis of type 1 diabetes mellitus is based on:

- confirmation of diabetes mellitus
- classification of the type of diabetes mellitus

Confirmation of diabetes mellitus

The diagnosis of diabetes mellitus is based on the finding of increased blood glucose or haemoglobin A1c (**Table 3.2**). The World Health Organisation has advocated haemoglobin A1c measurement for the diagnosis of diabetes mellitus; its value represents the average blood glucose concentration over the previous 8–12 weeks (the normal lifespan of red blood cells). Therefore if patients present with a very short history of symptoms,

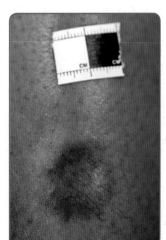

Figure 3.1
Necrobiosis lipoidica presents as an irregular shaped lesion with reddish-brown pigmentation, most commonly seen on the pre-tibial area.

haemoglobin A1c does not always reflect blood glucose concentration in the preceding days.

Table 3.3 lists the occasions when haemoglobin A1c is unreliable for use in diagnosing or monitoring diabetes mellitus. The threshold for making a diagnosis of diabetes with haemoglobin A1c is based on the risk of micro- and macrovascular complications above that value. However, this is an arbitrary threshold, and the real risk is a continuum: the higher the risk, the higher the haemoglobin A1c.

> The glucose concentration at which glucose enters the urine is the renal threshold. It is reduced in renal disease and pregnancy, and urinalysis cannot be used solely as a diagnostic test.

Classification of diabetes mellitus

The type of diabetes mellitus is determined based on additional information. A young patient with a normal BMI who presents with weight loss is likely to have type 1 diabetes mellitus. These patients often have significant ketosis, with ketones detected on urinalysis or in capillary blood tests. Table 3.4 shows the differences between type 1 and type 2 diabetes mellitus.

Investigations

Having established an elevated blood glucose (diabetes), attention is then given to the cause of the diabetes. As with all endocrine conditions, the cause is often clear from the history and examination, and urine and blood tests are performed to confirm this. Imaging and cytology is rarely useful in the diagnosis of diabetes unless a secondary cause of pancreatic

Diagnosis of diabetes mellitus: when not to use haemoglobin A1c	
Condition(s)	Details
Rapid onset of diabetes mellitus	Suspected type 1 diabetes mellitus
	Use of steroids and antipsychotics
	After pancreatitis or pancreatic surgery
	Gestational diabetes
Conditions with reduced red cell survival (lower haemoglobin A1c)	Haemoglobinopathy (sickle cell anaemia or thalassemia)
	Renal dialysis for patients on erythropoietin
	Splenomegaly
	Haemolytic anaemia
	Severe blood loss or transfusion
	Use of antiretroviral drugs
Conditions with increased red cell survival (high haemoglobin A1c)	Splenectomy
Iron and vitamin B12 deficiency	Decreased erythropoiesis

Table 3.3 Conditions in which haemoglobin A1c is unreliable for the diagnosis of diabetes mellitus

Differentiating type 1 and type 2 diabetes mellitus	
Type 1	Type 2
Sudden onset with short history	Gradual onset
Patients usually <25 years old	Patients often older
Severe symptoms; some present acutely with diabetic ketoacidosis	May be asymptomatic, but can present with severe dehydration and hyperglycaemia (hyperosmolar hyperglycaemic state)
Severe ketosis possible	Ketosis usually mild, if present
Patients usually lean	Patients typically overweight or obese
Recent weight loss	Weight loss rarely develops
C-peptide usually low	Increased C-peptide
Positive autoantibodies (glutamic acid decarboxylase and tyrosine phosphatage-related islet antigen 2 (IA$_2$)) in 80% of patients)	Autoantibodies rarely positive

Table 3.4 Differences between type 1 and type 2 diabetes mellitus

failure, such as cancer, is suspected from the history and examination.

Antibody tests

After confirming a diagnosis of diabetes mellitus, glutamic acid decarboxylase, anti–tyrosine phosphate antibody and islet cell antibodies are checked if a diagnosis of type 1 diabetes is suspected. A small percentage of patients with type 1 diabetes mellitus are antibody-negative, in which case the diagnosis is made on clinical suspicion and the presence of ketosis.

C-peptide concentration

C-peptide is a cleavage product (molecule derived from splitting of a complex molecule into two or more simpler molecules) in the production of insulin from proinsulin, and its concentration in urine or plasma is measured to help differentiate type 1 diabetes from type 2 diabetes. Low C-peptide indicates insulin deficiency and supports a diagnosis of type 1 diabetes mellitus. However, this result does not confirm the diagnosis, for the following reasons.

- Many patients with type 1 diabetes still have some endogenous insulin production, and therefore C-peptide, at diagnosis; this means that a detectable amount of C-peptide does not exclude type 1 diabetes
- Type 2 diabetes mellitus occasionally progresses to insulin deficiency, therefore low C-peptide does not exclude type 2 diabetes

The honeymoon phase is the period shortly after diagnosis of type 1 diabetes mellitus, when the pancreas is still able to produce insulin. This period lasts for weeks, months, or in some cases years, during which patients usually require small insulin doses to control their blood glucose.

Other tests

During the process of diagnosing the type of diabetes mellitus, various other tests are carried out (**Table 3.5**) to ensure no other

Tests associated with diagnosis of type 1 diabetes mellitus	
Condition	Investigation
Associated risk factors	
Hyperlipidaemia	Blood test for fasting lipid profile (includes cholesterol, triglycerides, high-density and low-density lipoproteins)
Complications	
Diabetic nephropathy	Early morning albumin: creatinine ratio spot urine test Serum creatinine
Retinopathy	Retinal photographs
Associated autoimmune conditions	
Autoimmune thyroid disease	Blood test for thyroid stimulating hormone (TSH)
Coeliac disease	Blood test for anti-transglutaminase (TTG) antibodies

Table 3.5 Tests for associated risk factors, complications and other autoimmune disorders in type 1 diabetes

associated autoimmune conditions are present and that there are no complications at diagnosis (although this is rare for type 1 diabetes as complications take time to develop).

Management

The diagnosis of type 1 diabetes necessitates many changes to a patient's life. They are required to inject insulin every day for the rest of their life, and the condition has implications for their work, social life, participation in sports and insurance arrangements. Patients also have to follow legal requirements for driving, and travel plans may be more complicated. Care should be provided by a specialist diabetes mellitus team, including a diabetes specialist nurse, an endocrinologist, a dietician, a podiatrist and a psychologist. Patients are always reviewed annually, but this can be more frequent if a patient is experiencing difficulty with their control or experiencing complications.

The goals of therapy are to:

- lower blood glucose concentration to as near normal range as possible
- avoid hypoglycaemia
- maintain a healthy body weight
- prevent or delay the onset of complications
- avoid episodes of diabetic ketoacidosis and the need for hospital admission
- engage patients in self-management of their condition

Structured education

Patients with type 1 diabetes mellitus are offered individual or a structured group programme of education covering:

- the aims of insulin therapy
- delivery of insulin
- self-monitoring of blood glucose
- the effects of diet, physical activity and intercurrent illness on glycaemic control
- the detection and management of hypoglycaemia

> **Any illness, including a cold, flu or a urinary tract infection, usually upsets glycaemic control.** Insulin requirement increases during periods of illness, because of the increased level of stress hormones such as cortisol. Therefore frequent blood glucose monitoring (hourly if necessary) and urinary or blood ketone testing are required at these times, and extra doses of insulin are needed.

Dietary advice

Patients should follow a healthy balanced diet (**Figure 3.2**). They should have frequent small meals and aim to make the following dietary changes:

- reduce refined sugars
- increase complex carbohydrates with a low glycaemic index (such as porridge and wholegrain bread). Complex carbohyrates are polysaccharides which take longer to be broken down, leading to a lower delayed peak of glucose (or lower glycaemic index).
- limit saturated fats to < 10% of calorie intake

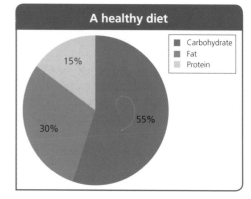

Figure 3.2 A healthy diet. Healthy carbohydrates include unprocessed whole grains, vegetables, fruits and beans, as opposed to refined choices such as white bread and chips. Monounsaturated and polyunsaturated fats such as olive oil, nuts and fatty fish are healthier choices than saturated fats from processed food, fatty meat and cheese. Healthier protein options tend to be those which are low in saturated fat such as eggs, pulses, lean meat and fish.

- reduce alcohol intake to < 21 units/week for men and < 14 units/week for women
- reduce salt intake

Carbohydrate rapidly increases blood glucose concentration. Therefore patients with type 1 diabetes practise 'carbohydrate counting' to enable them to adjust their insulin dose according to the carbohydrate content of their food. The aim is to maintain tight glycaemic control while allowing flexibility in mealtimes and meal content.

Patients with type 1 diabetes often refer to their carbohydrate ratios. For example, 1 unit of insulin for 10 g of carbohydrate is considered a 1:1 ratio. Patients whose condition is more insulin-resistant may need 2 units of insulin for every 10 g of carbohydrate (a 2:1 ratio) to achieve the same reduction in blood glucose.

Exercise

This maintains general well-being and reduces the risk of cardiovascular complications. It also improves insulin sensitivity and lowers blood glucose. The effects of exercise depend on its duration and intensity, but prolonged exercise frequently leads to increased insulin sensitivity for at least 16 h after the activity. During this time, there is an increased risk of hypoglycaemia if the insulin dose or carbohydrate intake is not adjusted.

The type and duration of exercise determine any changes in insulin doses or food intake. Hypoglycaemia is avoided by:

- taking extra carbohydrate during and after exercise
- reducing the insulin dose before prolonged exercise
- monitoring blood glucose closely after exercise

Capillary blood glucose monitoring

Patients normally use electronic devices to monitor their blood glucose (**Figure 3.3**). These blood glucose meters often have inbuilt memories to store previous readings. Some also calculate the insulin dose needed and are used to measure ketones if the patient is feeling unwell, which is an important early sign of metabolic deterioration and acidosis.

Most meters require the patient to draw blood by pricking one of their fingers. However, some devices provide continuous monitoring by measuring the patient's blood glucose, through an electrode just below the skin, at frequent intervals. The optimal frequency of self-monitoring varies between patients, but it is usually done before meals or when a high or low reading is suspected.

Insulin therapy

The aims of insulin therapy are to maintain euglycaemia (normal blood glucose level) by trying to reproduce the physiological pattern of insulin production through the regular administration of animal, analogue or biosynthetic human insulin. Insulin is given through subcutaneous injections unless the patient is acutely unwell, in which case it is given intravenously. Other methods of delivery, such as inhaled insulin, have been developed but are not yet used in everyday practice. A wide variety of insulins are available with different durations of action and insulin release profiles (**Figure 3.4**). Most patients deliver insulin by using a pen device (**Figure 3.5**).

- Rapid-acting insulins usually have a peak action within minutes; they are used to counteract the rapid increase in blood glucose at mealtimes and usually last up to 6 h
- Isophane insulins are intermediate-acting, with an onset of action typically over 2 hours and a typical duration of action of 14–20 h; they are usually given once or twice daily to provide a 'background' insulin
- Long-acting analogue insulins have a slow onset and long duration of action (> 18 h); they are associated with fewer peaks and troughs of insulin delivery and therefore reduce the likelihood of hypoglycaemia in patients with tight glycaemic control
- Animal insulin, the first insulin to be used, is extracted from the pancreas of pigs (porcine insulin) and cows (bovine insulin); however, these insulins are used less frequently now

Insulin regimens are tailored to meet the patient's needs. Patients choose to use mixed insulin (with rapid-acting and intermediate-acting insulin premixed in the same injection) or a basal bolus regimen (longer-acting insulin once or twice daily with shorter-acting insulin at mealtimes). The latter option allows much greater flexibility and is there-

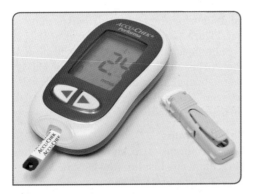

Figure 3.3 A glucose meter with glucose test strip inserted and lancet (for drawing blood). A small drop of blood is placed on the test strip and a rapid glucose measurement is made within a couple of seconds. The meters can store multiple readings and newer meters can be downloaded.

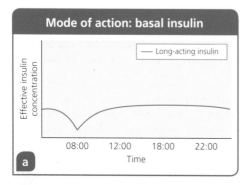

Mode of action: basal insulin

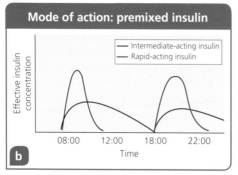

Mode of action: premixed insulin

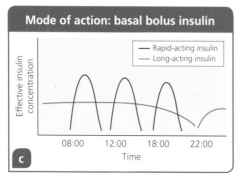

Mode of action: basal bolus insulin

Figure 3.4 Modes of action of different insulins. (a) Basal insulin: twice-daily intermediate-acting and once-daily long-acting insulin. (b) Twice-daily premixed insulin. (c) Basal bolus insulin regimen.

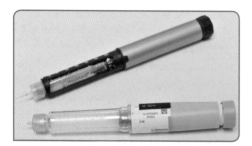

Figure 3.5 Insulin pen delivery device with dial-up dose control, changeable needle and prefilled insulin cartridge.

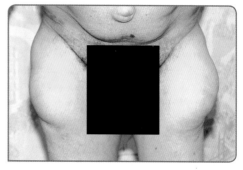

Figure 3.6 Lipohypertrophy.

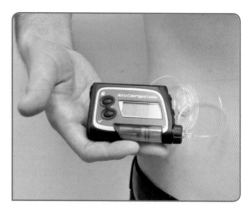

Figure 3.7 Insulin pump with plastic-giving set and subcutaneous needle to allow delivery of the insulin

fore particularly suitable for patients with less predictable lifestyles, including variable mealtimes.

Lipoatrophy (thinning of subcutaneous fat) and lipohypertrophy (excessive deposition of fat, **Figure 3.6**) occasionally occurs at sites of insulin injection and changes the absorption time of insulin. Therefore patients are advised to rotate their injection sites. The main patient concerns with insulin are weight gain and fear of hypoglycaemia.

Insulin pumps

Insulin pumps, also known as continuous subcutaneous insulin infusions, deliver frequent tiny pulses of subcutaneous insulin through a plastic infusion tube and a subcutaneous needle that remains in situ (**Figure 3.7**). The device allows a variable 'basal' insulin infusion in addition to boluses at mealtimes or to correct high blood glucose. Insulin pumps are used by patients with total insulin deficiency. However, patients need to be motivated for optimal control to be achieved.

These devices are more expensive than insulin injections. However, when used by motivated patients, insulin pumps help improve hyperglycaemia and reduce the frequency and severity of hypoglycaemia.

Pumps that monitor information from continuous glucose measurement are being introduced. It is hoped that they will act as a 'closed loop', automatically adjusting insulin delivery according to blood glucose concentration. This system is called the 'artificial pancreas'.

> **Long-distance travel can be challenging for patients with type 1 diabetes.**
>
> - Insurance can be more expensive
> - Airlines often require a letter from a physician before allowing patients to carry insulin and blood glucose meters in the cabin
> - Travel eastwards results in a shorter day and requires patients to inject less insulin or have an extra snack
> - Travelling west prolongs the day, so patients may require an extra insulin dose

Surgery

Pancreatic transplantation is usually considered in combination with renal transplantation. The morbidity and mortality from pancreatic transplantation alone usually outweighs the benefit of the chance of insulin independence and 'cure' of type 1 diabetes.

Donor islet cell transplantation is occasionally considered, particularly in patients with signficant problems with unrecognised hypoglycaemia, but they need lifelong immunosuppression after the procedure (see page 140). Stem cell research is ongoing and holds tremendous promise for the future treatment of many diseases, including type 1 diabetes.

Complications

Type 1 diabetes leads to short-term and long-term complications which have an impact on quality of life, hospital admissions and life expectancy. In the short term, hyperglycaemia and diabetic ketoacidosis (see Chapter 11) or hypoglycaemia can occur. In chronic cases, macrovascular and microvascular complications are screened for (see Chapter 4).

Hypoglycaemia

For most people with type 1 diabetes, hypoglycaemia occurs when blood glucose is < 4 mmol/L. At this concentration, treatment is needed to prevent any further reduction. As glucose concentration decreases, the hypoglycaemic episode (a 'hypo') is typically recognised by the patients as:

- hunger
- sweating
- dizziness
- fatigue
- blurred vision
- tremor
- pallor
- palpitations
- difficulty concentrating
- confusion and irritability
- tingling lips

Hypoglycaemia usually results from:

- misjudging the dose of insulin
- an increase in physical activity
- changes in other hormones (e.g. during the menstrual cycle)
- changes in carbohydrate absorption (e.g. with delayed gastric emptying or coeliac disease)
- failure of action of counter-regulatory hormones (e.g. glucagon)

The glucose concentration at which symptoms are detected varies from person to person. However, a few patients lose the ability to recognise or control their hypoglycaemic episodes. In such cases, tertiary referral is necessary. Management of hypoglycaemia is detailed in Chapter 11.

> **Worsening serial episodes of hypoglycaemia or decreasing insulin requirement in a patient with type 1 diabetes can indicate other conditions.** These include adrenal insufficiency, coeliac disease and renal or hepatic failure.

Vascular complications

Vascular complications, which are associated with diabetes, are covered in Chapter 4.

Prognosis

Without insulin replacement patients with type 1 diabetes will die within days or weeks of developing the disease. Even with treatment, type 1 diabetes is associated with lower life expectancy. However, the difference in life expectancy between people with and without the condition is narrowing.

Poor glycaemic control increases the risk of the development and progression of diabetes complications, which increase morbidity and mortality (see Chapter 4).

Type 2 diabetes mellitus

Type 2 diabetes mellitus is characterised by insulin resistance and relative insulin deficiency, which result in hyperglycaemia. In contrast to type 1 diabetes mellitus, it tends to have an insidious onset and is often diagnosed through screening of high-risk populations.

The increasing incidence of type 2 diabetes worldwide is attributed to rising obesity levels and population ageing. A healthy diet, exercise and weight loss are the cornerstones of prevention and treatment.

Epidemiology

Type 2 diabetes mellitus accounts for 85-95% of cases of diabetes mellitus in adults globally. Its prevalence increases with age. However, its incidence in childhood is increasing, because of a reduction in physical activity and an increase in obesity. Asian, Hispanic and African ethnic groups are at increased risk of developing the disease which is, in part, due to increased obesity and lack of physical exercise in these groups. The incidence of type 2 diabetes is also higher in urban populations; lack of exercise and easy access to high-calorie convenience foods are contributory factors.

Aetiology

The aetiology of type 2 diabetes mellitus is multifactorial, involving multiple genetic and environmental factors.

Genetics

Type 2 diabetes is a polygenic disorder. There is no *HLA* predilection, as there is in type 1 diabetes. However, in monozygotic twins the concordance rate of type 2 diabetes or impaired glucose tolerance approaches 100%, underlining a strong genetic component. Furthermore, 10% of patients with type 2 diabetes have an affected sibling, and 40% have at least one affected parent. However, most families are exposed to similar environments, so this concordance is not necessarily the result of genetic factors alone.

Environmental risk factors

People with obesity are at increased risk of developing type 2 diabetes and are usually insulin-resistant. Over 10 years, an obese person (BMI $>30\,kg/m^2$) is 10 times more likely to develop type 2 diabetes. Certain foods that are high in sugar and high in saturated fats are independent risk factors for the development of diabetes mellitus. In addition, people living in affluent countries are much less active and life expectancy is rising, which contributes to the surge in its prevalence.

Pathogenesis

Type 2 diabetes mellitus is characterised by insulin resistance in the peripheral tissues and relative insulin deficiency. Insulin resistance increases as fat mass increases. The more obese and insulin-resistant a person becomes, the more insulin secretion is necessary to maintain euglycaemia. The beta-cell function of the pancreas becomes unable to cope with the demand for insulin. Eventually, the pancreas atrophies (waste away), which leads to relative insulin deficiency.

Insulin resistance

Adipose tissue is metabolically active. Adipocytes (fat cells) release adipokines (hormones such as leptin, as well as other cytokines). Adipocytes also store free fatty acids as triglyceride. Excessive release of hormones and cytokines from adipose tissue is responsible for insulin resistance by impairing glucose uptake in skeletal muscle. This leads to increased glucose in the blood which is used to make free fatty acids that increase serum triglyceride concentration.

Pancreatic beta-cell failure

Patients also have significantly reduced beta-cell function at diagnosis. The toxic effects of free fatty acids and hyperglycaemia on beta cells further impair insulin secretion. A progressive loss of beta-cell function occurs over time.

Clinical features

Patients with type 2 diabetes mellitus typically present in four ways:

- with incidental diagnosis on screening or routine blood glucose testing (e.g. when admitted to hospital)
- with osmotic symptoms (e.g. dry mouth, thirst and polyuria) usually developing over weeks or months
- with complications of diabetes mellitus (e.g. neuropathic foot ulcer or macrovascular event such as myocardial infarction)
- as an acute presentation with a hyperosmolar hyperglycaemic state (blood glucose > 30 mmol/L, hypovolaemia and raised serum osmolality)

A minority of patients present with a short history. However, most cases of type 2 diabetes have a more prolonged course, with patients reporting malaise, thirst, nocturia and blurred vision over many months before presentation. Hyperosmolar hyperglycaemic state usually occurs with extremely high blood glucose (which may be precipitated by an underlying infection) combined with dehydration; this state develops more frequently in the elderly (see Chapter 11). Ketonuria is occasionally present in patients with type 2 diabetes mellitus at low levels, particularly when they are unwell.

Acanthosis nigricans (blackish patches on the skin of the axillae or neck) are frequently found on examination of patients with severe insulin resistance (see page 84).

Diagnostic approach

In patients who have symptoms of type 2 diabetes, a single positive test result suffices for diagnosis. Asymptomatic patients whose screening test results are just at the threshold for diagnosis, for example a haemoglobin A1c value of 48 mmol/mol, require repeated tests; if the results are positive, type 2 diabetes is confirmed. Patients presenting with precursory symptoms of type 2 diabetes receive advice on healthy living to try to prevent the development of diabetes mellitus.

As well as differentiating type 1 from type 2 diabetes (see page 152), secondary causes of diabetes mellitus must be considered. These include Cushing's syndrome and acromegaly (**Table 3.6**).

Investigations

Diagnosis is usually made with a haemoglobin A1c or random blood glucose test, in the context of a supportive clinical history (e.g. obesity, family history, prolonged symptoms). Investigations are then focused on:

- assessing blood glucose control
- looking for complications

A haemoglobin A1c test is usually sufficient for assessing control on treatment, but if patients are taking agents that cause fluctuations in blood glucose (such as insulin) then glucometers are used by patients to measure their own glucose at home. These readings can be downloaded or recalled from the meter to assess patterns, and fine tune current dosing if necessary.

Investigations for complications are discussed further in Chapter 4.

Management

Medical treatments for diabetes mellitus should be used in conjunction with lifestyle

Classification of diabetes mellitus

Category	Causes
Type 1 diabetes mellitus	Autoimmune disease
Type 2 diabetes mellitus	Genetic and environmental causes (e.g. obesity)
Monogenic diabetes mellitus	Single gene mutations
Exocrine pancreatic deficiency plus diabetes mellitus	Trauma
	Pancreatitis
	Pancreatectomy
	Haemochromatosis
	Cystic fibrosis
Secondary diabetes mellitus	Endocrine (e.g.Cushing's syndrome and acromegaly)
	Drug-induced (e.g. through use of corticosteroids, nicotinic acid, thiazides and β-adrenergic agonists)
Infections	Congenital rubella
	Cytomegalovirus
Diabetes mellitus associated with other genetic syndromes	Down's syndrome
	Klinefelter's syndrome
	Turner's syndrome
	Wolfram's syndrome
	Friedreich's ataxia
	Laurence-Moon syndrome
	Prader–Willi syndrome
Gestational diabetes mellitus	Genetic predisposition and obesity

Table 3.6 Aetiological classification of diabetes mellitus

changes to reduce blood glucose to concentrations that are as near normal as possible, without risking hypoglycaemia. All patients require regular review, at least annually. The purpose of these reviews is to assess glycaemic control and detect and treat diabetes complications; attention should also be given to other risk factors, including control of serum lipids and hypertension.

> Elderly patients are more at risk of the adverse effects of hypoglycaemia, including impaired consciousness, which may cause falls. Maintenance of adequate glycaemic control still needs to be considered, but targets are often relaxed to avoid hypoglycaemic episodes, which usually present with episodes of confusion or recurrent falls.

Figure 3.8 shows the management algorithm for type 2 diabetes mellitus. The cornerstone of diabetes mellitus management is sustained lifestyle modification: a healthy diet, exercise, weight loss and smoking cessation.

Diet

Dietary education is delivered as part of group education or at an individual or family appointment. Dietary advice often focuses on the following.

- Weight loss:
  - limiting calorie-rich convenience food
  - reducing portion sizes
- Healthy eating:
  - choosing options that are low in saturated fat and low in sugar
  - eating fibre-rich, wholegrain alternatives
  - including at least five portions of fruit and vegetables daily
- Low alcohol intake and avoidance of binge drinking

Carbohydrates should comprise 55% of the diet; proteins, 15%; and saturated fats, 30% (**Figure 3.2**).

If obesity is the main precipitant in the development of diabetes mellitus, patients should be considered candidates for bariatric surgery (see page 138). Bariatric surgery frequently allows years of 'remission' of diabetes mellitus after weight loss.

Exercise

Regular exercise improves insulin sensitivity. It also helps lower blood pressure and

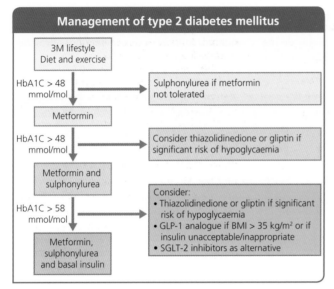

Management of type 2 diabetes mellitus

3M lifestyle
Diet and exercise

HbA1C > 48
mmol/mol → Sulphonylurea if metformin not tolerated

Metformin

HbA1C > 48
mmol/mol → Consider thiazolidinedione or gliptin if significant risk of hypoglycaemia

Metformin and sulphonylurea

HbA1C > 58
mmol/mol →

Consider:
- Thiazolidinedione or gliptin if significant risk of hypoglycaemia
- GLP-1 analogue if BMI > 35 kg/m² or if insulin unacceptable/inappropriate
- SGLT-2 inhibitors as alternative

Metformin, sulphonylurea and basal insulin

Figure 3.8 Stepwise management of type 2 diabetes mellitus. HbA1c, haemoglobin A1c. GLP-1, glucagon-like peptide-1.

cholesterol. Sometimes 'exercise on prescription' group classes or gym memberships are available in primary care in the UK.

Smoking cessation

Smoking increases the risk of vascular complications in patients with diabetes mellitus. For smokers with type 2 diabetes, a meta-analysis of cardiovascular risk reduction trials has shown that smoking cessation has a greater overall survival benefit than any other intervention (page 118).

Structured education

All patients with diabetes mellitus should be offered structured education, which includes:

- education about their condition
- healthy diet and exercise advice
- information on daily self-management, including monitoring, driving, sick day rules (how to manage blood glucose and medications on days of illness) and hypoglycaemia
- explanation of the importance of screening and the prevention of long-term complications

Patients often also benefit from written information and an opportunity to join patient groups.

Not all patients with type 2 diabetes mellitus need to monitor their blood glucose regularly. However, they should do this if receiving insulin or if hypoglycaemia is suspected. Particular circumstances put patients at risk of altered blood glucose concentration, such as a short course of steroid treatment.

Patients with a diagnosis of diabetes are ideally offered the opportunity to take part in clinical trials to evaluate the effectiveness of established and new treatments and interventions. Trials of treatments for chronic conditions such as diabetes have to be done over many years and recruit thousands patients to be able to show any significant benefit in morbidity and mortality.

Oral medications

Tablets are usually recommended if glycaemic control remains suboptimal despite lifestyle and dietary changes. Early intensive glycaemic control reduces the risk of cardiovascular and cerebrovascular morbidity, as well as continuing to reduce the risk of microvascular complications.

Most agents, except insulin, reduce haemoglobin A1c by a modest amount (often <11 mmol/mol). Therefore patients with very poor control of blood glucose often need more than one agent, unless they have made significant lifestyle changes. Some people do not respond to certain tablets. Therefore if there is no reduction in haemoglobin A1c after 6 months, a change of therapy should be considered. A list of oral medications is provided in **Table 3.7.**

Oral treatment for type 2 diabetes mellitus			
Type	When used	Drug action(s)	Adverse effects and benefits
Biguanides (e.g. metformin)	First-line treatment for most patients with type 2 diabetes mellitus	Decrease hepatic gluconeogenesis	Gastrointestinal adverse effects (e.g. diarrhoea and bloating)
		Increase glucose uptake	Epigastric discomfort occurs in 50% of patients but is often transient
		Increase muscle metabolism	Risk of lactic acidosis in patients with renal, hepatic or cardiac failure, in whom these drugs are contraindicated
			Reduce cardiovascular risk, independent of blood glucose
			Weight neutral
Sulfonylureas (e.g. tolbutamide, gliclazide and glibenclamide)	Used in addition to metformin or if metformin is not tolerated	Bind to ATP-dependent potassium channels on the surface of beta cells to stimulate insulin release	Weight gain

Hypoglycaemia |
| Thiazoledinediones | Third-line treatment | Increase insulin sensitivity by interacting with peroxisome proliferator-activated receptor-γ (a nuclear receptor that regulates many genes, reducing hepatic glucose production and improving peripheral glucose uptake) | Modest reduction of blood glucose

Associated with bladder cancer

Increased risk of fractures |
| Acarbose | Third-line treatment (rarely used) | Inhibits α-glucosidase

Inhibits carbohydrate absorption in the gut | Poorly tolerated gastrointestinal adverse effects |
Meglitinides	Third-line treatment	Promote insulin secretion in beta cells in response to meals	Adverse effects of weight gain and hypoglycaemia
		Short-acting (so taken before meals)	Reduction in post-prandial blood glucose concentration.
Dipeptidyl peptidase-4 inhibitors (e.g. gliptins such as sitagliptin and saxagliptin)	Third-line treatment (safe to use in renal failure) although some gliptins need dose reduction	Block action of the enzyme dipeptidyl peptidase-4	Weight neutral
		Prevent breakdown of glucagon-like peptide-1	Modest reduction of blood glucose
Sodium–glucose transport protein-2 inhibitors (e.g. gliflozins such as dapagliflozin or canagliflozin)	Third-line treatment (newest on the market)	Inhibit glucose reabsorption in the kidney	Weight loss

Modest improvement in glycaemic control

Increased urinary tract infections because of glycosuria |

Table 3.7 Oral treatments for type 2 diabetes mellitus

Injectable medications

Injectable treatment is the next step after oral medication has failed to control the blood glucose. Patients commonly have a fear of injections, particularly insulin. This is partly the fear of injecting themselves, but also because they may know friends who have had diabetes complications while on insulin and therefore associate the two (rather than focussing on how insulin works towards preventing the complications associated with poor control). As insulin delivery systems such as pens have become easier to administer and more people are on injectable treatment, patients are more amenable to trying it.

Glucagon-like peptide-1 analogues (incretin mimetics)

These drugs are similar to the incretin hormone glucagon-like peptide-1, which is usually broken down by dipeptidyl peptidase-4 (see page 131). They:

- increase insulin secretion
- inhibit glucagon secretion
- delay gastric emptying, thus slowing glucose absorption and producing early satiety

These actions result in patients reducing their portion sizes, because they feel full and often nauseous if they continue eating. This reduction in dietary intake improves glycaemic control and aids weight loss.

Glucagon-like peptide-1 analogues are given by injection twice daily, daily or weekly, depending on the drug. Because of their association with weight loss, they are frequently used in overweight patients. However, these drugs are expensive, so their effectiveness should be proven for their use to continue beyond 6 months.

Concerns have arisen that glucagon-like peptide-1 analogues increase the risk of pancreatitis and pancreatic cancer. Therefore this potential adverse effect is under surveillance.

Insulin therapy

The indications for insulin therapy in patients with type 2 diabetes mellitus are:

- suboptimal glycaemic control on treatment with first-line agents
- failure to tolerate, or contraindications to, oral agents
- signs of insulin deficiency (weight loss, ketonuria and low C-peptide concentration)
- acute illness, sepsis or treatment that increases blood glucose (such as prednisolone)
- perioperative management

Metformin, sulfonylureas and some glucagon-like peptide-1 analogues are licensed for use with insulin in the European Union and USA. Patients with type 2 diabetes often need only one daily injection of intermediate-acting insulin, because their body is still providing some of its own insulin, which reduces high postprandial blood glucose concentration.

> **Vitamin D** has been shown in some studies to reduce insulin resistance, aid weight loss and improve appetite control.

Prognosis

In type 2 diabetes, the prognosis depends on glycaemic control and the development of complications (see Chapter 4). The main cause of death is cardiovascular disease.

The degree of insulin deficiency tends to progress over time. Therefore many patients with type 2 diabetes mellitus eventually require insulin treatment.

Monogenic diabetes mellitus

Monogenic diabetes mellitus is a group of rare, usually autosomal dominant causes of diabetes mellitus resulting from a single gene defect. The condition is also called maturity-onset diabetes of the young (MODY). It affects 1–2% of people with diabetes mellitus and the type often goes unrecognised with patients assumed to have type 1.

The main features of monogenic diabetes mellitus are:

- diabetes mellitus, which usually develops before the age of 25 years
- continued production of insulin
- a family history of diabetes mellitus over several generations, with the condition developing in childhood or early adulthood (in an autosomal dominant inheritance pattern)

The correct identification of monogenic diabetes is important, because some forms of the condition are treated effectively with sulfonylureas. However, monogenic diabetes mellitus is often misclassified as type 1 diabetes mellitus, and patients are consequently treated with insulin unnecessarily.

Clinical features

The two commonest types of monogenic diabetes are caused by mutations in the human nuclear transcription factor-1α and glucokinase genes.

The diagnosis should be considered in children or young adults with a strong family history of the disease and presenting in the absence of ketosis or autoantibodies. Monogenic diabetes mellitus should always be suspected in cases of neonatal diabetes mellitus. Patients with neonatal diabetes do not produce enough insulin (but this deficiency is sometimes transient), and the condition is not autoimmune in nature (unlike type 1 diabetes mellitus).

Patients with monogenic diabetes are not normally obese. The presence of C-peptide suggests this is not type 1 diabetes. However, C-peptide concentration is not excessive, which is associated with insulin resistance and type 2 diabetes mellitus. Patients with glucokinase mutations often have impaired fasting glucose but a normal response to glucose. Diagnosis is confirmed by genetic testing.

Management

Diabetes mellitus caused by human nuclear transcription factor-1α mutations is very sensitive to treatment with sulfonylureas as these drugs bind to a receptor that bypasses the beta cell defect present, thus directly stimulating insulin secretion. The initial response to these drugs is better than that to insulin therapy. Diabetes mellitus resulting from a glucokinase mutation rarely needs treatment as it doesn't cause symptoms or complications.

Family members of patients with a diagnosis of monogenic diabetes are offered genetic testing to determine their risk of developing diabetes mellitus.

Prognosis

The type of monogenic diabetes determines prognosis. Diabetes mellitus caused by human nuclear transcription factor-1α mutations carries a risk of microvascular and macrovascular complications if the hyperglycaemia is not controlled. Diabetes mellitus resulting from a glucokinase mutation has a benign course, and the hyperglycaemia does not normally result in complications.

Gestational diabetes

Gestational diabetes mellitus is diabetes mellitus that develops during pregnancy. The condition occurs because of an increase in insulin resistance caused by increases in the concentrations of:

- growth hormone
- placental lactogen
- progesterone
- cortisol

Between 2 and 3% of pregnant women develop gestational diabetes. Its incidence is increasing because of rising incidence of overweight mothers.

Clinical features

Most patients are asymptomatic, so the condition is usually diagnosed after screening with an oral glucose tolerance test in the 2nd trimester. Risk factors for gestational diabetes mellitus are:

- BMI $> 30 \, \text{kg/m}^2$
- previous macrosomic (large) baby weighing $> 4.5 \, \text{kg}$
- previous gestational diabetes mellitus
- first-degree relative with type 2 diabetes mellitus
- ethnic origin with a high prevalence of diabetes mellitus

> **Gestational diabetes mellitus usually develops in the 2nd or 3rd trimester.** Patients with hyperglycaemia in early pregnancy are likely to have previously undetected type 2 diabetes mellitus, or more rarely early type 1 diabetes mellitus.

Management

Mothers should be informed that untreated gestational diabetes mellitus increases the risk of:

- a large (macrosomic) baby
- instrumental birth
- neonatal hypoglycaemia

Reducing blood glucose concentration reduces these risks. Most patients respond to dietary advice, with only 10–20% requiring metformin or insulin. Fetal size is usually monitored monthly in the 3rd trimester, and birth is often induced before term.

Post-delivery treatment is rarely required, except in cases of pre-existing diabetes mellitus. Blood glucose concentration is measured 6 weeks after the birth to exclude type 2 diabetes.

Prognosis

Uncontrolled gestational diabetes carries an increased risk of perinatal morbidity. Forty per cent of patients with gestational diabetes will develop type 2 diabetes within 10 years. However, this risk is reduced by lifestyle modification and weight loss.

The risks of gestational diabetes (described above) are minimised by careful blood glucose control.

Diabetes mellitus in pregnancy

Established diabetes mellitus before pregnancy confers a much higher risk of fetal and maternal complications. The purposes of preconception care are to optimise control of blood glucose, stop fetotoxic medications and start high-dose folic acid to reduce the risk of congenital malformations. Regular review in pregnancy, tight glycaemic control and fetal monitoring are essential to reduce the risk of the complications shown in **Table 3.8.**

Complications of pre-existing diabetes mellitus in pregnancy	
Fetal	Maternal
Fetal macrosomia	Induction of labour or caesarean section
Congenital malformations	Miscarriage
Stillbirth, neonatal death and birth trauma (shoulder dystocia)	Birth trauma, and increased risk of instrumentation and caesarean delivery
Transient neonatal morbidity (hypoglycaemia)	Progression of microvascular complications (e.g. retinopathy and nephropathy)
Obesity, diabetes mellitus or both developing in later life	Increased risk of pre-eclampsia

Table 3.8 Fetal and maternal complications of pre-existing diabetes mellitus in pregnancy

Obesity

Obesity is defined by the World Health Organization as a BMI of $> 30 \, \text{kg/m}^2$. The condition is associated with increased mortality, not only from cardiovascular disease and diabetes mellitus but also from cancer. Obesity also significantly increases morbidity from many associated conditions, such as arthritis and sleep apnoea (**Table 3.9**).

Consequences of obesity	
Category	Consequence
Metabolic	Hypertension
	Type 2 diabetes mellitus and insulin resistance
	Dyslipidaemia
Vascular	Ischaemic heart disease
	Cerebrovascular disease
Reproductive	Polycystic ovary syndrome and reduced fertility
	Increased obstetric complications
Cancer	Endometrial cancer
	Post-menopausal breast cancer
	Renal cell cancer
	Colorectal cancer
	Oesophageal cancer
Gastrointestinal	Non-alcoholic fatty liver disease
	Gallstones
Respiratory	Obesity hypoventilation syndrome
	Sleep apnoea
Musculoskeletal	Osteoarthritis
Psychiatric	Depression
	Anxiety and stress
Increased operative complications	Cardiac ischaemia, infection, venous thromboembolism, anaesthetic complications, increased length of stay

Table 3.9 Health consequences of obesity

Epidemiology

Obesity is becoming a global epidemic. In the UK, a quarter of adults are obese and more than half are overweight (or obese). In the USA this increases to 39% obese and 69% overweight (or obese). This places a huge burden on medical resources.

> **The public perception of 'normal' weight has increased in recent years.** This is a consequence of changes in their 'normality' as the average weight of the people they see in their daily lives has increased. Explaining body mass index to patients, and offering evidence on the adverse impact being overweight has on their health, is an important first step in making a lifestyle change.

Aetiology

Lifestyle factors are key to the rise in obesity and include:

- excessive food intake
- consumption of high-calorie, high-sugar foods
- increased portion sizes
- sedentary lifestyle

A limited number of cases arise from a monogenic mutation, an endocrine cause or the use of certain medications.

Clinical features

Patients who are obese have certain clinical features:

- 'Apple' body shape with increased abdominal girth, or a 'pear' body shape, which has increased deposition of fat around the gluteal region and upper leg girth
- Signs of insulin resistance: skin tags, acanthosis nigricans, hirsutism (in women)
- Signs of organ failure: cardiomegaly, respiratory compromise, tender hepatomegaly from nonalcoholic steatohepatitis (NASH)
- Signs of complications: candida infections, pressure ulceration, osteoarthritis

Diagnostic approach

Body mass index is generally used to define obesity. However, BMI is less accurate in certain groups, such as highly muscular people or those with a leg amputation.

People in some ethnic groups, such as South Asian adults, are at higher risk of cardiovascular disease at a lower BMI, which may be due to the increased accumulation of abdominal fat. Waist: hip ratio also confers risk; people with an 'apple' body shape (central obesity) are more at risk than those with a 'pear' shape and are more likely to develop the metabolic syndrome.

Examination of a patient presenting with obesity should cover both physical and psychological evaluation (**Table 3.10**).

History of patients with obesity	
Evaluation	Details
Clinical	History of weight gain (including its duration) and weight loss attempts
	Family history of obesity
	Current diet and level of physical activity
Underlying psychiatric disease	Depression
	Eating disorders (e.g. bulimia nervosa)
	Abnormal food behaviours (e.g. secretive eating)
	Consideration of secondary causes of obesity
	Assessment of other vascular risk factors and the presence of other comorbidities

Table 3.10 History of patients presenting with obesity

Management

The aims of management are to:

- reduce and maintain weight loss
- address any precipitants of weight gain (e.g. depression and bulimia nervosa)
- reduce morbidity and mortality associated with obesity

Multidisciplinary teams including dieticians, psychologists, physicians, physiotherapists and specialist nurses usually run obesity services. The purpose of these services is to ensure that lifestyle changes are maintained in the long term.

Behavioural interventions

Psychologists try to support goal setting and self-monitoring, slowing the rate of eating and addressing strategies for dealing with relapse. It is also essential to tackle eating disorders. These disorders are frequently associated with previous physical, emotional and sexual abuse.

Dietary modification

Weight loss is ensured when calorie intake is reduced to below daily requirements. The normal daily calorie intake is 2500 kcal for a man and 2000 kcal for a woman. An initial target weight loss of 5–10% of body weight over 6 months is realistic, with no more than 0.5–1 kg of weight loss per week.

> **Unduly restrictive and nutritionally unbalanced diets are ineffective for weight loss in the long term.** They can also be harmful (resulting in loss of muscle mass and vitamin deficiencies) and lead to rebound weight gain as the patient resumes a normal diet. There may be a role for these diets when rapid weight loss is essential, e.g. ahead of a joint replacement.

Medication

Oral medications are frequently used to supplement weight loss efforts. However, the effects are modest and difficult to maintain over time.

Orlistat works by inhibiting pancreatic lipases and increasing faecal excretion of fat. In the UK and USA, it can be bought over the counter. Adverse effects include flatus, faecal incontinence and intestinal cramps. Orlistat has a modest short-term benefit.

Glucagon-like peptide-1 analogues (see page 131) are also commonly used to aid weight loss if the patient has type 2 diabetes mellitus.

Surgery

Bariatric surgery is considered for patients for whom previous methods of non-surgical weight loss have failed and who meet one of the following criteria.

- BMI $> 40\,kg/m^2$
- BMI $> 35\,kg/m^2$ and obesity-related comorbidities, including hypertension, diabetes mellitus, sleep apnoea, dyslipidaemia and joint disease
- Previous treatment from a specialist obesity service and the patient's commitment to long-term follow-up

Surgery is considered as first-line treatment if the patient's BMI is $> 50\,kg/m^2$ and can be considered in patients diagnosed with type 2 diabetes within 10 years, and who have a BMI of $30-34.9\,kg/m^2$.

The two commonest operations to treat obesity are:

- insertion of an adjustable gastric band
- gastric bypass, such as a Roux-en-Y gastric bypass (see page 135 and Figure 2.35)

Long-term follow-up is needed to prevent complications such as nutritional deficiencies and hypoglycaemia. Insertion of a gastric band is a potentially reversible procedure and has a lower complication rate than that of other operations to treat obesity, such as gastric bypass but usually with less impressive weight loss results.

Prognosis

Successful bariatric surgery leads to an improvement in diabetes mellitus, hypertension and sleep apnoea.

A 10-kg weight loss usually results in:

- a 30% decrease in deaths related to diabetes mellitus and a 50% reduction in fasting blood glucose (in patients with newly diagnosed diabetes mellitus)
- a reduction of 10 mmHg in systolic blood pressure and 20 mmHg in diastolic blood pressure
- a 10% reduction in total cholesterol concentration and a 30% reduction in triglyceride concentration

Lipid disorders

Hyperlipidaemia is a heterogeneous group of disorders characterised by an excess of lipids in the bloodstream.

Types

The different types of hyperlipidaemia are:

- hypercholesterolaemia (predominantly cholesterol is increased)
- hypertriglyceridaemia (predominantly triglycerides are increased)
- mixed hyperlipidaemia (both cholesterol and triglycerides are increased)

These disorders are inherited or acquired. Hyperlipidaemia is a modifiable risk factor for cardiovascular disease.

Epidemiology

Genetically inherited heterozygous familial hypercholesterolaemia has an prevalence of 1 in 500, and the prevalence for homozygous familial hypercholesterolaemia is 1 in 1,000,000. Polygenic hypercholesterolaemia is common.

Aetiology

Hyperlipidaemia is caused by a combination of genetic and lifestyle factors. Patients have primary or secondary (acquired) hyperlipidaemia (**Table 3.11**).

Triglyceride concentration increases with a high-fat diet and excessive alcohol intake.

Causes of hyperlipidaemia	
Type of hyperlipidaemia	Causes
Familial primary hypercholesterolaemia	Homozygous familial hypercholesterolaemia: both pairs of low-density lipoprotein receptor genes are mutated
	Heterozygous familial hypercholesterolaemia: one pair of low-density lipoprotein receptor genes is mutated
Secondary or acquired hyperlipidaemia	Diabetes mellitus
	Hypothyroidism
	Renal failure and nephrotic syndrome
	Certain drugs (e.g. diuretics, beta-blockers, oestrogen and antiretrovirals)
	Obesity
	Excessive alcohol intake

Table 3.11 Causes of primary and secondary hyperlipidaemia

Pathogenesis

Lipoproteins, which include chylomicrons, very-low-density lipoprotein (VLDL), low-density lipoprotein (LDL) and high-density lipoprotein (HDL), allow cholesterol and triglycerides to be transported in the bloodstream. Triglycerides are carried by chylomicrons and VLDL. Cholesterol is carried mainly by LDL and HDL, and to a small extent by VLDL. HDL helps remove fat from cells and atheromas, so HDL cholesterol is labelled 'good cholesterol'.

Most familial hypercholesterolaemia is an autosomal dominant condition caused by a mutation in the LDL receptor gene. The excessive circulating LDL cholesterol in this condition is responsible for premature atherosclerosis and cardiovascular disease.

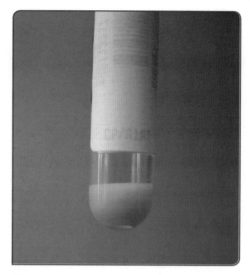

Figure 3.9 Lipaemic serum.

Clinical features

Tendon xanthomas (accumulations of lipid-laden macrophages in the tendons) are frequently present in patients with familial hypercholesterolaemia. Some patients also have xanthelasma.

Hypertriglyceridaemia is associated with eruptive xanthomas (xanthomas manifesting as papules all over the body), lipaemia retinalis (milky white appearance of retinal veins and arteries) lipaemic serum (milky white appearance of serum, **Figure 3.9**) and increased risk of pancreatitis.

Diagnostic approach

Patients are considered to have a clinical diagnosis of familial hypercholesterolaemia if they have serum cholesterol concentration > 7.5 mmol/L and any of the following:

- tendon xanthomata
- a first- or second-degree relative with cholesterol concentration > 7.5 mmol/L
- a family history of myocardial infarction before the age of 50 years in a second-degree relative (or before the age of 60 years in a first-degree relative)

Other considerations are other modifiable risk factors for premature cardiovascular disease (e.g. smoking), conditions associated with increased lipid concentration (e.g. hypothyroidism and diabetes mellitus) and a previous history of cardiovascular events.

> **'Fat-free' usually means high in sugar, refined carbohydrate and calories instead of fat.**

Investigations

A fasting lipid profile usually includes total cholesterol, LDL, HDL and triglycerides. Total cholesterol is mainly a sum of the lipoprotein components (particularly HDL and LDL).

Genetic testing is offered for familial hypercholesterolaemia if the patient fits the clinical criteria.

Management

Dietary advice on lipid-lowering and weight management is necessary, as well as optimal treatment of any conditions that predispose the patient to hyperlipidaemia. Drug treatment, usually with a statin, is added if also needed.

Not all dietary fats are the same.
'Good fats' include monounsaturated fats (e.g. those in vegetable oils and nuts) and polyunsaturated fats (e.g. in fatty fish and seeds), which help lower cholesterol. 'Bad fats', which increase cholesterol, include trans-fats (in commercially produced cakes, fried foods, etc.) and saturated fats (in animal fats and dairy products).

Primary prevention

Patients with familial hypercholesterolaemia are offered 3-hydroxy-3-methylglutaryl-coenzyme A reductase inhibitors (statin therapy). Treatment should be instituted to achieve a > 50% reduction in LDL cholesterol.

Patients with homozygous familial hypercholesterolaemia whose condition fails to respond to medical treatment or who develop severe adverse effects are referred for LDL apheresis. In this procedure, blood is dialysed to remove lipid; access to the blood is usually through a surgically created fistula.

In the absence of familial hypercholesterolaemia, a decision guiding whom to treat for hypercholesterolaemia is based on other associated risk factors, as well as cost-effectiveness. A patient's 10-year risk of having a vascular event is determined by using a 'risk engine' (**Table 3.12**), which is based on findings from large clinical trials. Statins are usually recommended as primary prevention if the 10-year risk of developing cardiovascular disease is > 10%.

Secondary prevention: lipid-lowering medications

Lipid-lowering treatment provides secondary prevention. It is started in all patients with a history of cardiovascular, cerebrovascular or peripheral vascular disease to help prevent further episodes.

A statin is the first-line treatment for most patients, unless hypertriglyceridaemia is the predominant feature, in which case a fibrate is preferable. Statin therapy carries a risk of

Factors used to calculate 10-year cardiovascular risk	
Risk factor	Fixed or modifiable
Age	Fixed
Sex	Fixed
Blood pressure	Modifiable
Total cholesterol, high-density lipoprotein cholesterol and triglyceride concentration	Modifiable
Smoking	Modifiable
Diabetes mellitus, duration of diabetes mellitus and degree of glycaemic control	Modifiable
Left ventricular hypertrophy and atrial fibrillation	Modifiable
Central obesity	Modifiable
Ethnic origin (particularly South Asian)	Fixed
First-degree family history of a cardiovascular event	Fixed

Table 3.12 Risk factors commonly used to calculate 10-year risk of a cardiovascular event when considering statin treatment for primary prevention

transaminitis (increased liver transaminase). Patients should be warned to report muscle aches or weakness, because of the risk of myositis and rhabdomyolysis.

If treatment is not tolerated or the target is not reached, consideration could be given to adding or replacing the statin with:

- fibrate (effective for hypertriglyceridaemia)
- ezetimibe (reduces cholesterol absorption)
- nicotinamide
- anion exchange resin such as colestyramine (which prevents bile reabsorption)

Prognosis

Patients with untreated heterozygous familial hypercholesterolaemia commonly develop cardiovascular disease in their thirties or forties. The increase in cardiovascular disease correlates most closely to the concentration of LDL cholesterol.

Answers to starter questions

1. Obesity is a major risk factor for diabetes but other risk factors such as family history, ethnicity and age are also important in contributing to its onset. Obesity alone does not make developing diabetes inevitable.

2. Pancreatic transplantation has been able to cure patients with type 1 diabetes mellitus by replacing destroyed pancreatic cells and some complications, such as autonomic neuropathy, have been shown to improve afterwards, although the diabetes recurs if the transplant is rejected. Bariatric surgery is effective for patients with type 2 diabetes mellitus, although as they age or if they regain weight the diabetes mellitus may still return.

3. A combination of change in hormone levels, genetic risk, the mother's age and weight gain can all lead to diabetes developing during pregnancy. Pre-existing diabetes mellitus is often diagnosed in pregnancy as it is usually the first time the patient has sought medical attention.

4. Many researchers believe that some African, South Asian and Latin American groups selectively inherited a 'thrifty gene' which helped their ancestors store food when it was plentiful to survive during times when it was scarce. These previously helpful genes now put these groups at a higher risk for type 2 diabetes.

5. There are many guidelines suggesting a standard model of care for people with type 2 diabetes. However, there is emerging evidence that some patients don't respond to certain drugs and that treatment should be individually tailored using the guidelines as a framework. Elderly or pregnant patients, or those not requiring tight blood glucose control, are often placed on different treatment regimes.

6. Type 2 diabetes frequently does not show symptoms and is only picked up on screening, for example, measuring for hypertension. Some patients, especially men, ignore symptoms such as fatigue until it is significantly disrupting their life.

Chapter 4
Complications of diabetes

Starter questions

Answers to the following questions are on page 192.

1. Why is tight blood glucose control not always the safest management in patients with complications of diabetes?
2. What makes diabetic foot infections particularly difficult to treat?
3. Are the complications of diabetes inevitable?
4. Will diabetes patients have improved life expectancies in the future?

Introduction

Diabetes mellitus results in increased blood glucose. Blood glucose concentration may become sufficiently high to cause short-term emergencies (e.g. diabetic ketoacidosis and hyperosmolar hyperglycaemic state; see Chapter 11) or chronic damage to body tissues. Long-term complications of diabetes mellitus are divided into two categories:

- macrovascular (large blood vessel) complications
- microvascular (small blood vessel) complications

Large-scale trials have provided evidence that maintaining blood glucose below a certain threshold prevents or delays the onset of these complications. Prevention of complications also involves modifying other vascular risk factors, such as:

- hypertension
- hyperlipidaemia
- smoking

Case 3 Red swollen foot

Presentation

Mr Baker is a 58-year-old patient with long-standing type 2 diabetes mellitus. He presents to his general practitioner (GP) with a 5-day history of a red, swollen right foot. He does not remember any trauma to the foot, but it is throbbing. He feels generally well in himself, with no fevers or sweats.

Initial interpretation

There are many causes for a red swollen foot in a patient with diabetes mellitus (**Table 4.1**). It is a potentially serious problem and requires urgent investigation and treatment.

Causes of a red, swollen foot in a patient with diabetes	
Infective	Cellulitis
	Infected ulcer
	Osteomyelitis
Trauma	Fracture
	Soft tissue injuries
Vascular	Ischaemia
	Deep vein thrombosis
Inflammatory	Charcot's arthropathy
	Gout
	Other inflammatory arthritis

Table 4.1 Causes of a red, swollen foot in a patient with diabetes mellitus

History

Mr Baker has had diabetes for 15 years. He admits that he does not pay much atten- tion to his health. He has complained over the past 12 months of a nagging,

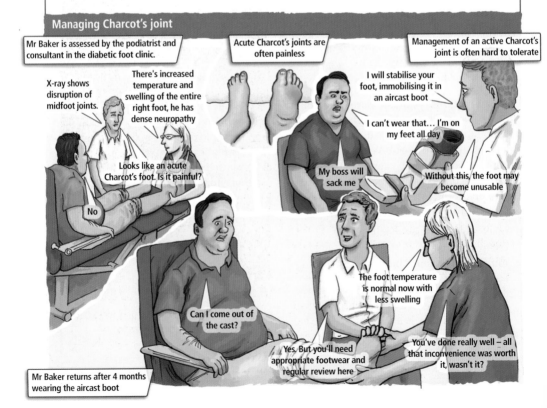

Managing Charcot's joint

Mr Baker is assessed by the podiatrist and consultant in the diabetic foot clinic.

X-ray shows disruption of midfoot joints.

There's increased temperature and swelling of the entire right foot, he has dense neuropathy

Looks like an acute Charcot's foot. Is it painful?

No

Acute Charcot's joints are often painful

I will stabilise your foot, immobilising it in an aircast boot

I can't wear that... I'm on my feet all day

My boss will sack me

Management of an active Charcot's joint is often hard to tolerate

Without this, the foot may become unusable

Can I come out of the cast?

The foot temperature is normal now with less swelling

Yes. But you'll need appropriate footwear and regular review here

You've done really well – all that inconvenience was worth it, wasn't it?

Mr Baker returns after 4 months wearing the aircast boot

Case 3 *continued*

aching pain in both feet. His feet also feel numb, 'like walking on cotton wool'. He works long hours as a hospital porter and spends all day on his feet.

He noticed the redness and swelling in his foot 5 days ago but did not seek attention at that point. He only occasionally checks his capillary blood glucose, and it is usually about 9–14 mmol/L.

Interpretation of history

The numbness and pain in Mr Baker's feet are typical of diabetic peripheral sensory neuropathy. The lack of feeling means that a fracture could go unnoticed, and the foot is at risk of Charcot's arthropathy.

Infection or gout are also possibilities. Infection would usually be associated with fever and an entry wound, and gout is often recurrent so there might be a previous history.

Further history

Mr Baker has been working with his practice nurse to try to reduce his blood glucose. His GP had wanted him to go on to insulin 2 years ago. However, Mr Baker was keen to avoid this, preferring to try to lose weight and improve his diet. As well as diabetes, he has hypertension and increased cholesterol.

Examination

Mr Baker's right foot is red and swollen compared with the left, but neither is deformed. The right foot is warm to the touch. The skin is intact, but the toenails are in poor condition.

The posterior tibial and dorsalis pedis pulses are easily palpated bilaterally, and capillary refill time is <2 s. There is dense neuropathy in the feet; Mr Baker is unable to detect the 10 g monofilament on either foot. He is apyrexial.

Interpretation of findings

Mr Baker has dense peripheral neuropathy and a red, hot, swollen foot with no vascular compromise or ulceration. The

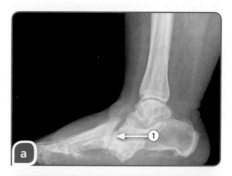
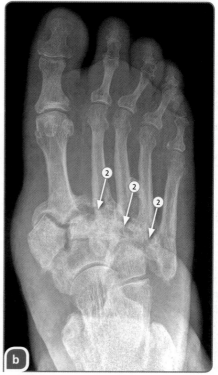

Figure 4.1 X-rays of the right foot, showing bony destruction ① and subluxation of the midfoot ② joints. (a) Lateral view. (b) Anteroposterior view.

lack of signs of infection and dense neuropathy mean that a Charcot's arthropathy is the most likely diagnosis. Gout is still possible.

Investigations

The GP arranges urgent assessment in the local diabetic foot clinic. Mr Baker has blood tests that show a normal white cell count and normal urate and C-reactive protein (CRP) concentrations. Haemoglobin A1c value is increased at 98 mmol/mol. X-ray of the right foot shows bony destruction and subluxation of the midfoot joints (**Figure 4.1**).

Diagnosis

In the absence of ulceration or biochemical evidence of infection (normal CRP and white cell count), acute Charcot's arthropathy is the likely diagnosis. Once the diagnosis of acute Charcot's arthropathy is made the foot must be immobilised as soon as possible in either an aircast boot or total contact cast. This must be worn continuously for 2–6 months until the inflammatory process has ceased.

Macrovascular complications

Macrovascular complications of diabetes are:

- ischaemic heart disease
- cerebrovascular disease
- peripheral vascular disease

Macrovascular complications are a common cause of morbidity. They are also the leading cause of mortality in patients with both type 1 and type 2 diabetes mellitus. Treating vascular risk factors (hypertension, hyperlipidaemia, obesity and smoking) and having good diabetic control reduce the risk of developing these complications.

If achieving tight glycaemic control (aiming for near normal blood glucose levels) increases the risk of hypoglycaemia, this may conversely expose the patient to a higher risk of cardiovascular events.

Epidemiology

Macrovascular disease of all types is more common in patients with diabetes mellitus (**Table 4.2**).

- 65% will die of heart disease or cerebrovascular disease.
- Myocardial infarction and stroke are two to four times more common in patients

Increased macrovascular risk in patients with diabetes	
Complication*	Increased risk
Ischaemic heart disease	Eight-fold in women
	Five-fold in men
Stroke	Three-fold
Transient ischaemic attack	Six-fold

*Not including peripheral vascular disease, which is often asymptomatic, so the true risk is difficult to estimate.

Table 4.2 Increased macrovascular risk in patients with diabetes mellitus

with diabetes than in matched populations without diabetes
- About one in three patients with diabetes in the UK over the age of 50 years have peripheral vascular disease

Aetiology

Atherosclerosis is the process by which diabetes mellitus causes an increased risk of macrovascular disease. The exact process by which hyperglycaemia causes atherosclerosis is unclear, but elevated blood glucose levels are thought to cause an increase in reactive oxygen species that contribute to damage of the arterial wall.

Pathogenesis

Diabetes mellitus increases the risk of macrovascular disease by accelerating atherosclerosis. However, the mechanism by which hyperglycaemia promotes atherosclerosis is unclear. Atherosclerotic plaques develop in the arterial wall through a process of inflammation and narrowing of the arterial lumen (**Figure 4.2**). Rupture of these plaques exposes the blood to a thrombogenic surface. The subsequent platelet aggregation occludes the artery. Furthermore, in addition to being at risk of atherosclerosis, patients with diabetes are in a hypercoagulable state, with impaired fibrinolysis.

Arterial atherosclerosis restricts blood flow, thus causing tissue ischaemia. Acute occlusion of the arterial lumen results in critical ischaemia and infarction of the target tissue.

Prevention

National and international guidelines help direct the care of patients with type 1 and type 2 diabetes mellitus. Guidance provides treatment targets that are applicable to most patients.

Glycaemic control

In the United Kingdom Prospective Diabetes Study (UKPDS), patients with type 2 diabetes mellitus and tight glycaemic control had a significant reduction in the risk of cardiovascular disease compared with those with less tight glycaemic control.

In the Diabetes Control and Complications Trial (DCCT), patients with type 1 diabetes mellitus were randomised to intensive therapy or usual therapy. Intensive therapy consisted of:

- the use of at least three insulin injections daily or insulin pumps
- adjustment of insulin dose to food intake and exercise
- testing of capillary blood glucose concentration at least four times daily
- following a diet and exercise plan
- monthly visits to diabetes healthcare providers

The intensely treated group achieved a significantly reduced mean haemoglobin A1c value over a mean of 6.5 years during the study. Patients in the intensive therapy group had a 42% lower risk of cardiovascular events over the 17 years of follow-up.

Blood pressure control

Hypertension is twice as likely in patients with type 1 and 2 diabetes mellitus than in

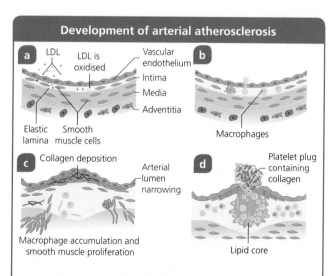

Development of arterial atherosclerosis

a. LDL / LDL is oxidised / Vascular endothelium / Intima / Media / Adventitia / Elastic lamina / Smooth muscle cells

b. Macrophages

c. Collagen deposition / Arterial lumen narrowing / Macrophage accumulation and smooth muscle proliferation

d. Platelet plug containing collagen / Lipid core

Figure 4.2 The development of arterial atherosclerosis. (a) LDL is taken up into the arterial wall. (b) Macrophages migrate into the arterial wall and ingest the LDL developing into foam cells. (c) Macrophages and collagen accumulate and smooth muscle cells proliferate in the intimal layer causing lumen narrowing. (d) The endothelial layer above the lipid core of the atherosclerotic plaque fissures resulting in platelet accumulation, thrombus formation and arterial occlusion.

comparable populations without diabetes. The UKPDS confirmed that tight blood pressure control in patients with type 2 diabetes reduces the risk of diabetes complications. In patients in the tight blood pressure group, whose mean blood pressure was 144/82 mmHg (standard care group, 154/87 mmHg), there were significant reductions in:

- the risk of stroke (decreased by one third)
- the risk of death from macrovascular complications (decreased by one third)

Lipid control

Patients with type 2 diabetes mellitus usually have an adverse lipid profile. This puts them at increased risk of macrovascular complications.

Reducing low-density lipoprotein and total cholesterol decreases the risk of macrovascular end points (by 22% in primary prevention) and death (18% in secondary prevention). Therefore tight lipid control is desirable, particularly in patients with type 2 diabetes mellitus, who are at high risk of macrovascular disease due to the presence of other features of the metabolic syndrome such as obesity and hypertension.

> It is difficult to reduce serum cholesterol to a target concentration through exercise and diet manipulation alone. Patients often want to avoid taking tablets to reduce their cholesterol. However, evidence from clinical trials strongly supports the use of statins in patients with diabetes who are at risk of cardiovascular events.

Smoking cessation

Smokers with diabetes have twice the risk of premature death as that of non-smokers with diabetes. Smoking cessation is probably the most important therapeutic step in patients with diabetes mellitus in terms of preventing macrovascular complications and death. The risk of serious complications in former smokers returns to that of never smokers within about 10–20 years of quitting.

Clinical features

The clinical features depend on the type of macrovascular complication.

Ischaemic heart disease

This condition causes chest pain resulting from myocardial tissue ischaemia. In patients whose coronary plaques are stable, myocardial ischaemia causes predictable angina or breathlessness on exertion. Acute plaque rupture and arterial occlusion causes acute myocardial infarction when the pain occurs at rest. Cardiac chest pain may also be associated with sweating and nausea.

> **Some patients with diabetes mellitus have silent ischaemic heart disease.** This is the occurrence of angina or myocardial infarction without chest pain. They also may not experience chest pain because of neuropathic destruction of the cardiac sensory fibres.

Cerebrovascular disease

This presents as stroke or transient ischaemic attacks. Patients have unilateral weakness of the face, the limbs, or both, as well as visual loss, speech disturbance and sensory and balance disturbances. Most events are embolic, but 20% of strokes are haemorrhagic.

Peripheral vascular disease

The chronic ischaemia associated with peripheral vascular disease contributes to the development of diabetic foot disease. When combined with poor microvascular circulation and sensory or motor neuropathies, serious, limb-threatening abnormalities often occur. The primary problems in peripheral vascular disease are:

- intermittent claudication (pain in the muscles of the leg due to tissue ischaemia that occurs with exercise and is relieved by rest)
- pain at rest, signifying critical ischaemia
- ulceration (usually of the distal limbs especially the feet)
- necrosis and autoamputation (**Figure 4.3**)

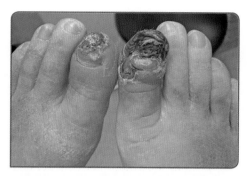

Figure 4.3 Necrosis of the toes in a patient with diabetes mellitus and peripheral vascular disease.

The ischaemic diabetic foot is also at high risk of infection due to ulceration and poor tissue perfusion by blood resulting in a deficiency of immune cells to fight infection. Once infection occurs, treatment is more challenging because of poor blood supply to the tissues and consequent impaired antibiotic penetration.

Diagnostic approach

For the diagnosis of macrovascular disease, the arteries supplying the organ of interest need to be assessed. This is done directly or indirectly.

Direct assessment is through imaging studies:

- Doppler ultrasound
- angiography, done percutaneously or non-invasively with computerised tomography or magnetic resonance imaging (MRI)
- perfusion scanning

Indirect assessment is done by:

- examining electrocardiograms
- blood tests, such as measurement of cardiac enzymes

Investigations

Table 4.3 summarises investigations for macrovascular disease.

Investigations for macrovascular complications of diabetes		
Complication	Investigation(s)	Reason for investigation
Ischaemic heart disease	ECG and exercise ECG	ECG changes at rest and during exercise highlight underlying acute and chronic IHD
	Myocardial perfusion scan	Demonstrates extent and location of cardiac hypoperfusion
	CT coronary angiogram	Demonstrates location and extent of coronary artery stenosis and coronary arterial calcification
	Percutaneous coronary angiogram*	Demonstrates location and extent of coronary artery stenosis, provides an option for revascularisation
Cerebrovascular disease	CT or MRI of the head	Demonstrates acute and chronic cerebral ischaemia and haaemorrhage
	Doppler ultrasound carotid arteries	Identifies carotid artery stenosis that predisposes to stroke
	Percutaneous angiogram*	Demonstrates location and extent of carotid artery stenosis, provides an option for revascularisation
Peripheral vascular disease	Doppler arterial ultrasound scan	Identifies peripheral artery stenosis
	CT or magnetic resonance angiogram	Demonstrates location and extent of peripheral artery stenosis
	Percutaneous angiogram*	Demonstrates location and extent of peripheral artery stenosis, provides an option for revascularisation

CT, computerised tomography; ECG, electrocardiography; IHD, ischaemic heart disease; MRI, magnetic resonance imaging.

*Invasive percutaneous angiogram has the advantage of providing an option for revascularisation.

Table 4.3 Investigations for macrovascular complications of diabetes

Management

Management of macrovascular diseases is considered in terms of:

- primary prevention
- secondary prevention
- specific treatment of the complication itself

Prevention is a combination of lifestyle adjustment and medication. Complications frequently require a combination of medical and surgical treatments.

Medication

The specific treatment of diabetes mellitus and treatment of risk factors is detailed in Chapter 3. Patients at high risk of macrovascular disease, and those with existing macrovascular disease, should adhere to strict targets for blood pressure control and lipid-lowering. A number of medications have proved efficacious in reducing the risk of macrovascular complications:

- angiotensin-converting enzyme (ACE) inhibitors to treat hypertension
- statins to reduce cholesterol
- beta-blockers to treat ischaemic heart disease
- aspirin and other antiplatelet drugs used in the secondary prevention of ischaemic heart disease, peripheral vascular disease and stroke

Rapid treatment of embolic strokes with thrombolytic therapy reduces disability and improve prognosis.

> **The commonest adverse effect of ACE inhibitors is a dry cough.** It invariably resolves after discontinuation of the drug, although this can take some weeks. If the cough is intolerable for the patient, an angiotensin II receptor blocker can be prescribed as an alternative.

Surgery

Vascular disease of the heart, brain and larger peripheral arteries may be treated with percutaneous transluminal angioplasty and stenting of narrowed vessels. Another therapeutic option is open surgical procedures. These include endarterectomy (plaque removal) and bypass grafting with native blood vessels or synthetic grafts.

In patients with non-disabling strokes and transient ischaemic attacks, secondary prevention is vital. Carotid artery stenosis > 70% on the ipsilateral side of the stroke is treated successfully by carotid endarterectomy to reduce the risk of future strokes.

Prognosis

Patients with diabetes mellitus who have a myocardial infarction, have a death rate or reinfarction rate of 18% at 6 months (compared to 11% in non-diabetics). Mortality due to stroke is 25% in patients with diabetes (compared to 17% in non-diabetics).

Survival and prognosis for macrovascular disease has greatly improved over the years. This is largely attributable to the advent of medications such as statins and ACE inhibitors. The advent of percutaneous angioplasty for acute myocardial infarction has also dramatically improved the prognosis for acute myocardial infarction.

Management of patients after ischaemic cardiac and cerebral events has been enhanced by the advent of cardiac rehabilitation and the establishment of dedicated stroke units.

Microvascular disease

Microvascular disease refers to a group of common complications that occur in patients with type 1 and 2 diabetes mellitus. Microvascular disease is comprised of:

- retinopathy
- nephropathy
- neuropathy

There is a common pathophysiology to all forms of microvascular complications. Damage occurs to small arterioles resulting in tissue ischaemia, causing fibrosis, cell death and proliferation of collateral blood vessels (**Figure 4.4**). Microvascular disease takes many years to develop and progress.

Diabetic retinopathy

Diabetic retinopathy is the leading cause of new blindness in adults of working age in the UK. Internationally, cataracts are the leading cause of blindness.

The development and progression of diabetic retinopathy can be prevented by good glycaemic and blood pressure control.

Epidemiology

Almost all patients with type 1 diabetes mellitus, and 60% of those with type 2 diabetes mellitus, have some degree of retinopathy 20 years after diagnosis. About a fifth of patients with type 1 diabetes would be expected to have proliferative diabetic retinopathy 20 years after diagnosis.

Prevention

The DCCT showed that tight glycaemic control is effective for both primary prevention of retinopathy and reducing progression of established retinopathy (secondary prevention). Hypertension is an independent risk factor for the development of diabetic retinopathy in patients with either type 1 or type 2 diabetes.

Table 4.4 outlines targets for blood pressure and glycaemic control in primary and secondary prevention of microvascular disease. Glycaemic control is achieved by titrating anti-diabetic medication and insulin (see Chapter 3). Blood pressure control is achieved by use of multiple anti-hypertensive drugs but the angiotensin-converting enzyme inhibitors (ACEi) are the most effective at preventing microvascular disease. Tight control of serum lipids is also required for the prevention of diabetic retinopathy.

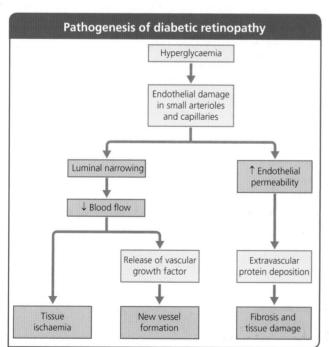

Pathogenesis of diabetic retinopathy

Figure 4.4 The pathogenesis of diabetic retinopathy. Hyperglycaemia causes endothelial damage to small arterioles and capillaries. This results in a reduction in blood flow and abnormalities in the endothelial permeability. Poor blood flow results in tissue ischaemia, vascular growth factor release and new vessel formation (e.g. neovascularisation in proliferative diabetic retinopathy). Tissue damage also occur through fibrosis from protein deposition due to increased vascular permeability.

Targets for prevention of microvascular disease		
Patient group	Blood pressure (mmHg)	Haemoglobin A1c (mmol/mol)
Primary prevention	140/80	<58 (type 1)
		<48 (type 2)
Established diabetic retinopathy	130/80	<48*
Established diabetic nephropathy	130/80	<48*

*Glycaemic targets are individualised.

Table 4.4 Targets for prevention of microvascular disease

Pregnant women with pre-existing diabetes mellitus are at particular risk for the development and progression of diabetic retinopathy. Retinal screening before and during pregnancy, and treatment of retinopathy with laser photocoagulation, helps to slow the progression of established proliferative retinopathy.

Pathogenesis

In most patients, diabetic retinopathy develops asymptomatically. In others, noticeable visual symptoms develop because of the following.

- Retinopathy at the macula: the high concentration of light-detecting cells at the macula means that oedema here decreases visual acuity
- Haemorrhage: large retinal or vitreous haemorrhages cause sudden and devastating loss of vision
- Retinal detachment: this causes sudden unilateral loss of vision

Diabetes also increases the risk of cataracts.
The precise cause of diabetic retinopathy is uncertain. However, several pathological processes progress to cause retinal damage and visual loss.

Dysfunction of capillary beds

Increased blood glucose causes anatomical and functional disruption of the retinal capillary bed. This permits protein and fluid to leak into the retina. Capillary fluid leakage at the macula causes macular oedema.

Hyperviscosity

The diabetic state leads to increased blood coagulability and platelet activation. This results in micro-occlusion and weakening of capillary walls, culminating in retinal ischaemia, capillary aneurysms and haemorrhage.

Retinal hypoxia

This causes necrosis of retinal light-detecting cells. Ischaemia also stimulates the release of vascular endothelial growth factors, which encourages the formation of new vessels (neovascularisation).

Neovascularisation

New blood vessels form on the retina but are fragile and may bleed. Neovascularisation also causes fibrosis of the retina and traction, which leads to retinal tears and detachment.

Clinical features

The early features of retinopathy are often asymptomatic. Later features include:

- floaters
- visual distortion
- blurred vision
- reduction in vision

The retina is examined either by using digital retinal photography or by an ophthalmologist with the use of a slit lamp. Visual acuity is reduced in advanced diabetic retinopathy.

Diagnostic approach

The findings of retinal screening are graded in a retinopathy classification (**Table 4.5**).

Management

General management of diabetic retinopathy comprises tight control of blood glucose,

Grading of diabetic retinopathy			
Grade	Findings	Symptoms	Action
R0 (**Figure 4.5**)	No diabetic retinopathy	None	Annual screening
R1 (mild non-proliferative retinopathy; **Figure 4.6**)	Dot-and-blot haemorrhages and microaneurysms	None	Inform the diabetes team to tighten diabetes and blood pressure control
R2 (severe non-proliferative retinopathy; **Figure 4.7**)	Hard exudates, venous bleeding and cotton wool spots (ischaemia)	None	Referral to an ophthalmologist
R3 (proliferative retinopathy; **Figure 4.8**)	New blood vessel formation (the macula is spared), vitreous or preretinal haemorrhage and fibrovascular changes leading to retinal detachment	Floaters or sudden visual loss (central in preretinal haemorrhage or retinal detachment)	Urgent referral to an ophthalmologist for consideration of laser treatment
M1 (maculopathy)	Signs of retinopathy (e.g. microaneurysms or haemorrhages) present at the macula	Floaters or loss of central vision	Urgent referral to an ophthalmologist for consideration of laser treatment
P (treated with photocoagulation; **Figure 4.9**)	Evidence of scarring from laser photocoagulation	Reduced night vision	Follow up depends on current activity of retinopathy as graded above

Table 4.5 Grading of diabetic retinopathy

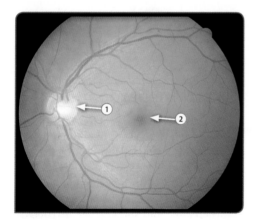

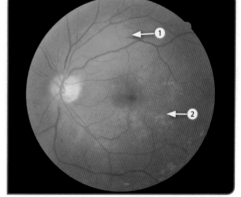

Figure 4.5 Grade R0 diabetic retinopathy: the absence of retinopathy. ① Optic disc. ② Macula.

Figure 4.6 Grade R1 diabetic retinopathy: mild and non-proliferative. ① Dot haemorrhages. ② Hard exudates.

hypertension and hyperlipidaemia. This is the primary therapeutic strategy for the early stages of retinopathy (R1 and R2).

Specific treatments for established retinopathy include laser photocoagulation, vitrectomy and intravitreal injections of anti–vascular endothelial growth factor (VEGF).

Laser photocoagulation

This is a non-invasive treatment in which a laser is used to burn the retina. This reduces retinal ischaemia by destroying peripheral parts of the retina that are less important for maintenance of detailed vision (and therefore

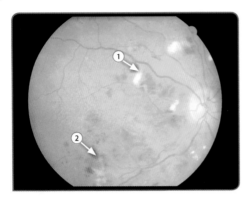

Figure 4.7 Grade R2 diabetic retinopathy: severe and non-proliferative. ① Cotton wool spot. ② Blot haemorrhage.

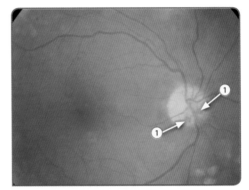

Figure 4.8 Grade R3 diabetic retinopathy: proliferative. Note the multiple new vessels at the disc ①.

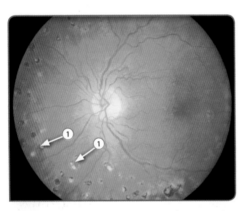

Figure 4.9 Grade P diabetic retinopathy: treated with photocoagulation. Laser scarring ①.

reducing the oxygen demand), which decreases the production of vascular growth factors, thereby reducing new vessel formation.

Two major strategies are used in laser photocoagulation.

- Panretinal photocoagulation: the ischaemic retina is burned with multiple applications of laser; this technique is used to treat proliferative retinopathy and macula oedema
- Focal or grid photocoagulation: small areas are burned to treat macula oedema

Vitrectomy

Surgical removal of vitreous humour is used to treat cases of vitreous haemorrhage and retinal detachment caused by scarring.

Intra-vitreal injections of anti-VEGF

These injections reduce the proliferative effect of VEGF. They are used as adjunct treatment for proliferative diabetic retinopathy.

Prognosis

Pan-retinal photocoagulation slows progression of proliferative retinopathy. With early detection and optimal treatment of diabetic retinopathy, blindness can be prevented in 90% of cases.

Diabetic nephropathy

Diabetic nephropathy is damage done to the kidneys by the effects of chronic hyperglycaemia. Diabetes mellitus is the leading cause of chronic kidney disease in the UK. Diabetic nephropathy is asymptomatic until progression occurs to end-stage renal failure and therefore close surveillance is required for patients with diabetes mellitus.

Epidemiology

Diabetic nephropathy is rare in patients with type 1 diabetes mellitus of < 10 years' duration. After 30 years duration of type 1 diabetes 40% will develop microalbuminuria. The worldwide prevalence of diabetic nephropathy is increasing in line with the increase in the overall prevalence of type 1 and 2 diabetes.

Aetiology

The exact aetiological mechanism of diabetic nephropathy remains unclear. However, it has been postulated that a combination of inflammation, vascular growth factor release, glycosylation of proteins and excess collagen synthesis occur as a result of hyperglycaemia. The effects of hyperglycaemia are exacerbated if there is coexisting hypertension.

It is likely that genetic factors determine the development of diabetic nephropathy. Evidence for this comes from the differing rate of nephropathy in various ethnic groups, and the fact that some patients with poor diabetic control progress more slowly than others to diabetic nephropathy.

Prevention

Reducing blood pressure significantly decreases the risk of the occurrence and progression of diabetic nephropathy. Certain antihypertensive drugs (e.g. ACE inhibitors) have a particular role in the management of complications.

Patients with diabetic nephropathy should avoid potentially nephrotoxic drugs where an alternative exists. For example choosing opiate analgesia as opposed to non-steroidal anti-inflammatory drugs.

Pathogenesis

Three major histological phenomena are seen in diabetic nephropathy:

- thickening of the capillary basement membrane
- excessive production of extracellular matrix
- scarring of the glomeruli (glomerulosclerosis)

These histological changes result in microalbuminuria (small amounts of protein in the urine), and this progresses to overt proteinuria. A decline in renal excretory and synthetic function occurs later in the disease. Progressive diabetic nephropathy both causes and exacerbates hypertension.

Clinical features

Like diabetic retinopathy, early diabetic nephropathy is asymptomatic until it has progressed to an end stage and irreversible degree. Microalbuminuria is the early hallmark of diabetic nephropathy. Clinical features of end-stage renal failure include:

- fatigue and breathlessness (caused by anaemia resulting from deficiency of erythropoietin, which is produced by the kidneys and occasionally by pulmonary oedema)
- osteoporosis secondary to the inability to activate vitamin D
- accelerated cardiovascular disease
- electrolyte abnormalities (e.g. hyperkalaemia)
- uraemia (causing itching, nausea and skin discoloration)
- fluid retention
- hypertension

Diagnostic approach

Simple urine dipstick tests, using the first-pass urine of the day, have been superseded by quantitative laboratory measures of albuminuria and proteinuria by calculating the urine albumin:creatinine ratio (ACR). Microalbuminuria detected on urine ACR identifies the early stages of nephropathy, when the condition is potentially reversible.

Serum creatinine is also measured but does not increase in a linear manner alongside progression of renal disease. Therefore estimated glomerular filtration rate (eGFR) is calculated.

All patients with diabetes require at least annual determination of urine ACR, creatinine and eGFR.

Classification of diabetic nephropathy

This is based on urine ACR and the severity of impaired kidney function. A urine ACR test will show:

- Microalbuminuria: urine ACR > 2.5 mg/mmol in men and > 3.5 mg/mmol in women

- Proteinuria: urine ACR > 30 mg/mmol (or positive protein on urine dipstick)

Microalbuminuria is albumin excretion at a rate of 30–300 mg/24 h. This degree of albuminuria is not detectable through urine dipstick testing. Renal function can be normal at early stages of diabetic nephropathy with microalbuminuria and proteinuria.

> **Microalbuminuria is the first sign of diabetic nephropathy**. However, it also develops in patients with hypertension, those with a family history of microalbuminuria, smokers and patients who are overweight.

As diabetic nephropathy progresses, renal function deteriorates. **Table 4.6** shows the classification of chronic kidney disease used internationally.

Management

Intensive anti-diabetic therapy with the aim of tight glycaemic control and optimal blood pressure control may reverse early nephropathy and delays its progression. Establishing ACE inhibitor treatment in patients with microalbuminuria slows the progression of diabetic nephropathy.

Patients approaching end-stage renal failure require specific dietary advice to maintain a low-sodium, potassium and phosphate diet and to maintain correct fluid and electrolyte balance.

Specific therapies that may be required in advanced renal failure include:

- activated vitamin D (alfacalcidol)
- intravenous iron replacement (because renal failure results in poor intestinal absorption of iron)
- erythropoietin
- phosphate binders
- diuretics for fluid overload

When end-stage renal failure is established, the options for renal replacement therapy are:

- peritoneal dialysis
- haemodialysis
- renal transplantation (which may be from cadaveric or live donors)
- conservative management in those too elderly, too unfit for or unwilling to accept renal replacement therapy

Prognosis

Microalbuminuria is an independent risk factor for cardiovascular disease in patients with diabetes mellitus, and it increases all-cause mortality. End-stage renal failure is more common in patients with type 2 diabetes, reflecting its overall higher prevalence. End-stage renal failure accounts for 21% of deaths in people with type 1 diabetes, and for 11% in those with type 2 diabetes.

Classification of chronic kidney disease		
Stage	Estimated glomerular filtration rate (mL/min/1.73m²)	Description
1	> 90	Normal kidney function but detection of microalbuminuria points to early kidney damage
2	60–89	Mildly reduced kidney function
3A	45–59	Moderately reduced kidney function
3B	30–44	
4	15–29	Severely reduced kidney function
5	< 15	Established renal failure (end-stage renal failure)

The suffix p is used to denote significant proteinuria when classifying patients with chronic kidney disease (e.g. chronic kidney disease stage 3Ap)

Table 4.6 Classification of chronic kidney disease

Diabetic neuropathy

Chronic diabetes mellitus damages peripheral and autonomic nerves; this is termed diabetic neuropathy. Diabetic neuropathy tends to present as a symmetrical polyneuropathy that is predominantly sensory but may also affect motor nerves.

Epidemiology

The prevalence of neuropathy depends on the duration of type 1 or 2 diabetes and the degree of blood glucose control. Clinically detectable sensory neuropathy affects about half of patients after two decades of diabetes. In the same period, about 35% develop symptoms of painful diabetic neuropathy.

Aetiology

The aetiology of diabetic neuropathy is multifactorial. Factors include duration of diabetes, degree of glycaemic control, hypertension, hyperlipidaemia, smoking, alcohol use and genetic susceptibility.

Prevention

Prevention of diabetic neuropathy focuses on good glycaemic control. A quarter of patients with type 2 diabetes mellitus have evidence of diabetic neuropathy at the time of diagnosis.

Pathogenesis

Diabetic neuropathy probably develops through a combination of pathological processes including the following.

- Increased intraneuronal glucose leads to metabolic effects, including reduced axonal transport of proteins, abnormal cell protein transport and axonal breakdown
- Increased oxidative stress causes microvascular damage, resulting in damage to neurons
- Increased glucose leads to an increase in glycation end products, which may disrupt neuronal structure and metabolism

Clinical features, investigations and management

Diabetes mellitus can affect 3 major types of nerves resulting in:

- Sensory neuropathy
- Autonomic neuropathy
- Motor neuropathy

The clinical features of diabetic retinopathy are summarised in **Table 4.7**.

Sensory neuropathy

Diabetic sensory neuropathy first affects the longest nerves, i.e. those supplying the periphery. This results in symmetrical sensory neuropathy, which tends to affect the feet and lower limbs first and may progress to affect the hands and arms. Common symptoms include:

- numbness
- paraesthesia (tingling)
- pain (often described as shooting, burning or aching)
- hyperaesthesia or allodynia: the sensation of pain resulting from a stimulus that does not usually cause pain (often the bedclothes brushing against the feet at night)

Clinical features of diabetic neuropathy		
Type of neuropathy	Symptoms	Signs
Sensory	Numbness	Reduced sensation in glove-and-stocking distribution
	Hyperaesthesia	Evidence of recurrent trauma to hands and feet
	Pain (shooting, burning and gnawing) in glove-and-stocking distribution	
Motor	Muscle weakness	Reduced power
		Abnormal limb posture
Autonomic	Palpitations	Tachycardia
	Dizziness	Postural hypotension
	Sweating	Loss of diurnal variation in blood pressure
	Hypo- or hyperthermia	Delayed gastric emptying
	Erectile dysfunction	
	Nausea, vomiting, constipation and diarrhoea	

Table 4.7 Clinical features of diabetic neuropathy

Sensory neuropathy can be diagnosed by clinical examination with soft touch, use of a monofilament and vibration testing (e.g. by using a neuroaesthesiometer). Sensory loss occurs in a glove and stocking distribution.

Investigations
Formal nerve conduction studies are rarely required to make the diagnosis of diabetic sensory neuropathy.

Management
Various atypical analgesics are used to treat painful diabetic neuropathy. The atypical drugs are a heterogeneous group of of anti-depressant medications (amitriptyline and duloxetine) and anticonvulsants (gabapentin and pregabalin).

These medications control symptoms but do not reverse the pathology that originally caused the neuropathic pain.

Other analgesia, such as local anaesthetic applied to a painful region, or acupuncture, are sometimes effective if pain remains uncontrolled.

> **Pain from diabetic neuropathy can be distressing for patients and is difficult to control.** Specialist pain teams provide non-medical therapies, such as acupuncture and spinal nerve stimulators, as well as psychological support.

Autonomic neuropathy

Diabetic autonomic neuropathy is damage to the involuntary nervous system, by diabetes mellitus, which controls heart rate, blood pressure, sweating and digestion.

Autonomic neuropathy can cause various symptoms:
- palpitations (as a result of effects on vagal tone in the heart)
- dizziness (caused by postural hypotension)
- sweating (which can be excessive or in response to eating, i.e. gustatory sweating)
- vomiting, diarrhoea, constipation and other gastrointestinal symptoms caused by gut dysmotility
- erectile dysfunction
- urinary incontinence or retention

Signs of autonomic dysfunction include postural hypotension and sinus tachycardia.

Investigations
Autonomic neuropathy may be detected by autonomic function tests. Investigation of gut dysmotility (gastroparesis) is by way of gastric-emptying studies.

Management
Prokinetic agents such as metaclopramide (for short durations <5 days) and low-dose erythromycin can be used to treat autonomic neuropathy causing gastroparesis.

Motor neuropathy

Motor neuropathy causes weakness that tends to be mild and symmetrical. Symptoms affect distal or proximal muscle groups. Common symptoms are proximal muscle weakness of the hips (difficulty climbing stairs) or the shoulder girdle (unable to lift the arms above the head).

> **Diabetic amyotrophy is a distinct form of diabetic neuropathy.** In this condition, lower motor neuron weakness is associated with pain in the same distribution.

Motor neuropathies are detected by lower motor neurone weakness and muscle wasting.

Management
As with all microvascular complications, control of blood glucose and risk factor modification are helpful to slow the progression of established neuropathy. Physiotherapy helps in rehabilitation.

Mononeuritis multiplex
This syndrome is characterised by painful sensory and motor neuropathy that may affect multiple nerves. A common presentation would be of a unilateral, incomplete 3rd cranial nerve palsy. Patients present with unilateral eye pain, drooping of the eyelid and double vision. Clinically, there is a ptosis, with 'down and out' gaze palsy but pupillary sparing.

Mononeuritis multiplex is often acute in onset when caused by diabetes. However, other causes include vasculitis and inflammatory joint diseases. Mononeuritis multiplex is a disabling condition that usually resolves with good diabetes control over 3-6 months. Occasionally, mononeuritis multiplex may be permanent.

Prognosis

Diabetic neuropathy increases both morbidity and mortality. Peripheral sensory neuropathy increases the risk of trauma, ulceration and amputation. Medical treatments for painful neuropathy rarely fully control symptoms.

Diabetic foot disease

Diabetic foot disease encompasses a range of pathological processes that combine to cause limb-threatening disease. Diabetic neuropathy combined with damage to the macro- and microvascular peripheral circulation cause ulceration and superadded infection.

> **All hospital patients with diabetes should have their feet examined on admission.** Simple visual and peripheral neurological examination identifies those at high risk of developing complications such as ulceration. Measures to reduce the risk of complications, such as the use of pressure-relieving mattresses and protective boots, are required for these patients.

Epidemiology

People with diabetes are 30 times more likely to have a limb amputation than those without diabetes. In the UK there are 2.6 major limb amputations (amputation above the ankle joint) per 1000 patients with diabetes per year.

Aetiology

Diabetic neuropathy predisposes the foot to unrecognised trauma. The trauma is either acute (e.g. from treading on a sharp, penetrating object) or chronic (e.g. rubbing from ill-fitting shoes).

Trauma may lead to skin abrasions and ulceration. Impaired blood-flow to the foot from the large arteries and small capillaries results in tissue ischaemia and slow wound healing. These factors combine to allow infection to occur. Furthermore, poor blood supply impairs the immune response and the penetration of antibiotics from the circulation to the tissues. Poor glycaemic control also increases the risk of infection by providing a favourable environment for bacterial growth.

Charcot's arthropathy is a complex inflammatory joint reaction that occurs in patients with neuropathic feet. The precipitant of an acute Charcot's joint may be trauma but is usually not identifiable.

Ulceration of diabetic feet can result in bacterial ingress into deep tissues (such as bone) resulting in osteomyelitis (infection and destruction of the bone).

Clinical features

The following clinical features are hallmarks of diabetic foot disease.

- Ulceration: if ulcers probe deeply (i.e. to bone), suspect osteomyelitis (**Figure 4.10**)
- Ischaemia: cool foot, delayed capillary refill time and weak or impalpable pulses
- Deformity: caused by neuropathy (**Figure 4.11**) or after amputation
- Erythema: the result of inflammation from infection or in active Charcot's arthropathy (**Figure 4.12**)
- Temperature: infection and Charcot's arthropathy cause a hot foot, whereas ischaemia causes a cool foot
- Malodour: this arises from necrotic, infected tissue

Diagnostic approach

The key to diagnosis is assessment of the impact of the various factors contributing to

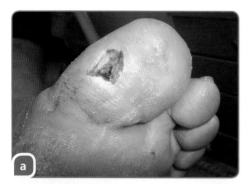

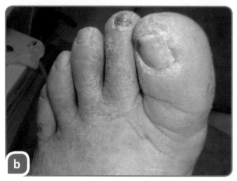

Figure 4.10 Ulceration in diabetic foot disease (note the red, swollen great toe).

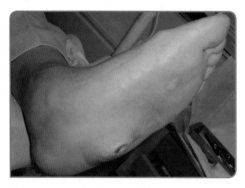

Figure 4.11 Deformity caused by neuropathy in diabetic foot disease resulting in a neuropathic ulcer on the plantar aspect of the foot.

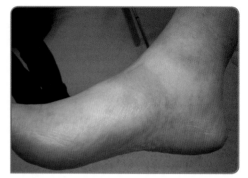

Figure 4.12 Erythema in a patient with active Charcot's arthropathy.

Investigations

Wound swabs and tissue samples are cultured, and the findings used to guide antibiotic therapy. Superficial skin and wound swabs grow bacteria that may colonise the wound or skin but do not necessarily cause infection. More clinically useful results are yielded from cultures of tissue samples or deep swabs done after sterile debridement.

Arterial blood supply is assessed by using Doppler ultrasound and percutaneous, CT or MR angiography.

Plain radiographs of the foot may show pathology:

- fractures
- osteomyelitis (lucencies in bone; **Figure 4.13**)
- Charcot's arthropathy (joint subluxation and inflammatory joint destruction)

Magnetic resonance imaging is sometimes used to try to distinguish Charcot's arthropathy from infection. However, pathological features seen on MRI such as tissue oedema are seen in both Charcot's and infection, and this can make it difficult to differentiate between the two.

Management

Rapid assessment and treatment by an expert multidisciplinary team are essential in cases of an acute diabetic foot problem such as ulceration and infection. The diabetic foot team includes a diabetologist, a podiatrist,

diabetic foot disease, such as vascular and nervous supply and foot deformity. Accurate assessment of the degree of ischaemia, neuropathy and infection guides management. Certain conditions, such as osteomyelitis and Charcot's arthropathy, require specific treatments (see page 191).

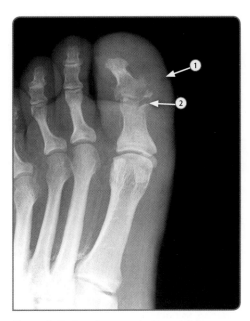

Figure 4.13 Anterior-posterior X-ray (of the same patient as in Figure 4.10) showing lucencies in the bones of the great toe in osteomyelitis. ① Gas in soft tissue. ② Bone resorption.

vascular and orthopaedic surgeons, a diabetic specialist nurse and an orthotist (footwear specialist).

Basic foot care

Wound care consists of regular debridement of hard, necrotic or infected tissue and the application of clean dressings.

Charcot's arthropathy is managed by immobilisation of the foot in an air cast or total contact cast for 2–6 months.

Footwear must be assessed. Ill-fitting footwear exacerbates ulceration, especially in deformed neuropathic limbs. Orthotists construct specific footwear that fits well, provides support and relieves pressure on vulnerable areas.

Medication

Aggressive treatment of diabetic foot infections with broad-spectrum antibiotics is essential. The choice of antibiotics is guided by the results of cultures of microbiological samples from the wound, tissue and blood.

The infecting organisms tend to be streptococci and staphylococci. However, atypical infections may be detected in patients with diabetes; they include infection by gut or anaerobic organisms. Diabetic patients are susceptible to atypical infections, because of their high tissue glucose, immunosuppression and poor blood supply (resulting in anaerobic conditions). Courses of antibiotics for infections of the feet of diabetic patients are generally prolonged, because the tissue is slow to heal.

Indications for intravenous antibiotics are:

- cellulitis extending widely around an area of ulceration
- systemic illness (fever and deteriorating diabetes control)
- inability to tolerate oral antibiotics (vomiting)
- failure to respond despite treatment with oral antibiotics

Surgery

Vascular surgeons perform a huge variety of operations, from revascularisation of the ischaemic foot to debridement and amputation of necrotic tissue and limbs. Limb preservation is generally attempted to maintain an optimally functioning limb after the operation.

Orthopaedic surgeons perform reshaping surgery to deformed feet to improve their function and to minimise the risk of ulceration secondary to deformities.

Orthotists design footwear for patients with diabetes. The aim is to spread the load across the foot and thus offload particularly vulnerable areas and prevent ulceration caused by friction to the skin.

Vascular supply must be assessed in patients with diabetic foot ulcers before they undergo surgery (e.g. wound debridement and amputation). If blood supply is poor, the wounds are unlikely to heal.

Prognosis

The condition of feet at high risk of diabetic foot disease should be closely and regularly monitored by specialist podiatrists. If infection, ischaemia or ulceration develop, a good outcome depends on swift, aggressive treatment. Delays in optimal treatment can lead to limb loss and, rarely, death.

Major amputation, i.e. above the ankle, results in a lower rate of postoperative independent mobility than a minor amputation. The mortality rate is 50–80% at 5 years.

Answers to starter questions

1. Although controlling blood glucose reduces the risk of complications in diabetes, there are risks associated with achieving this (e.g. hypoglycaemia and adverse effects of medications). Individual blood glucose targets should be agreed with each patient to avoid adverse effects of medication, reduced quality of life from frequent blood glucose monitoring and hypoglycaemia and the potential loss of consciousness or cardiovascular events.

2. Patients with diabetes are at increased risk of peripheral nerve and blood vessel disease. This predisposes patients to ulcers which provide entry points for bacteria. Damaged arteries mean that there is reduced access to the foot for immune cells and antibiotics. This makes infections harder to fight and allows microbes that are not usually pathogenic to cause infection.

3. The development and progression of diabetic complications can be prevented or dramatically delayed with good blood glucose control and the reduction of other cardiovascular risk factors such as high blood pressure, high cholesterol and smoking. Genetics factors are highly influential in who develops complications, particularly nephropathy, which has led to a search for the specific mutations responsible.

4. New technological and pharmaceutical developments, such as insulin pumps, 'closed loop systems' (integrated continuous blood glucose monitors and insulin pumps), islet cell transplantation,pancreas transplantation and new drugs ,will help improve blood glucose control and reduce complications leading to longer life expectancies.

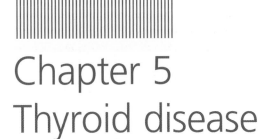

Chapter 5
Thyroid disease

Starter questions

Answers to the following questions are on page 213.

1. Does stress cause thyroid disease?
2. Why is thyroid disease more common in women?
3. What is a thyroid storm?
4. What might lead you to suspect a thyroid lump is 'sinister'?

Introduction

Thyroid diseases are the most common endocrine disorders in the general population, and affect all ages. Patients present with diverse clinical features, including weight gain or loss, tremor, anxiety and depression. Because many of these symptoms are non-specific, patients initially present to a wide range of healthcare professionals. Thyroid diseases result from several different mechanisms, including:

- excessive or inadequate amounts of thyroid hormones
- inflammation or infection of the thyroid gland
- benign or malignant growth

Case 4 Tremor and irritability

Presentation

Samantha, who is 26 years old, is referred to the endocrinology clinic with tremor in her hands. Her husband remarks that she has been uncharacteristically irritable in recent weeks. Her general practitioner noticed a small diffuse swelling in her neck.

Initial interpretation

The characteristics of tremor usually provide a clue to the diagnosis (**Table 5.1**).

In a young woman such as Samantha, who also has a goitre, thyrotoxicosis is the most likely cause.

Further history

Samantha first noticed the tremor about 6 weeks ago, when she was working as a waitress. She first thought that it was related to stress at work, but it persisted on her days off. She also started to have palpitations, sweating and frequent loose bowel motions. At her GP appointment,

Causes of tremor	
Cause	Description of tremor
Physiological (severe anxiety or fear)	High frequency and low amplitude, often not apparent unless amplified by outstretching the hands
Chronic alcoholism and alcohol withdrawal	Low amplitude, postural tremor
	Flapping tremor (jerking movement of the hand outstretched) in severe alcoholic liver disease causing encephalopathy
Hypoglycaemia	Fine and rapid
	Associated with hunger, sweating and palpitations
	Common in patients with diabetes and taking hypoglycaemic agents (e.g. insulin and sulfonylureas)
Thyrotoxicosis	Fine and rapid
	Pronounced when the hands are outstretched
Essential tremor	Typically occurs in people aged > 40 years
	Coarse and irregular
	Present both at rest and during movement
Parkinsonism	'Pill rolling' tremor
	Often with other extrapyramidal signs (e.g. cogwheel rigidity, hypokinesia and short-shuffling gait)
Dystonia	Involuntary writhing movements
	Irregular in amplitude and frequency
Cerebellar diseases	Cerebellar (intention) tremor during movement
	Associated with cerebellar signs (e.g. nystagmus, ataxia, past-pointing and dysdiadochokinesia)
Psychogenic	Often starts abruptly
	Variable frequency and amplitude
	Increased frequency and amplitude at the time of stress

Table 5.1 Causes of tremor

Case 4 *continued*

she was surprised to learn she had lost 5 kg of weight.

She has no personal history of serious illness, and reports no recent short-term viral illnesses before the appearance of her symptoms. She is not on regular medications, and she denies taking any unprescribed over-the-counter drugs.

Samantha goes out once a week with her friends, when she drinks about 5 units of alcohol. She smokes 10 cigarettes daily. Her menstrual periods are regular. She has no intention of becoming pregnant in the near future and uses barrier contraception.

Interestingly, Samantha's mother suffers from hypothyroidism, and one of her cousins had a thyroidectomy for hyperthyroidism.

Examination

Samantha looks anxious and has a fine tremor of her outstretched hands. Her palms are warm and clammy. She has tachycardia, with a regular heart rate of 105 beats/min. Her blood pressure is 142/66 mmHg.

She has a small, smooth and non-tender swelling in the neck, which moves with swallowing. Her eyes are prominent, with bilateral lid retraction. However, there is no eyelid swelling, conjunctival redness or chemosis (oedema of the conjunctiva), exophthalmos, limitation of eye movement or decreased visual acuity. No skin changes are visible on her legs and feet. She has no signs of cardiac failure.

Interpretation of findings

Tremor of the hands, together with unintentional weight loss, palpitations, sweating, loose bowel motions and irritability in a young woman strongly suggest thyrotoxicosis (**Figure 5.1**). The findings of warm sweaty palms, tachycardia and

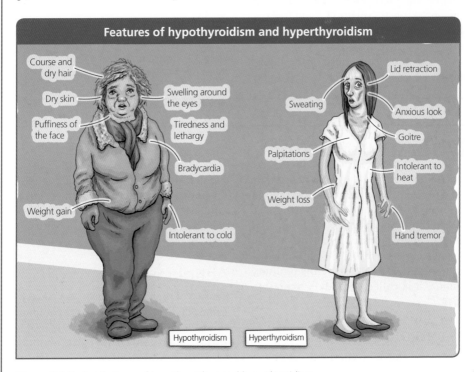

Features of hypothyroidism and hyperthyroidism

Course and dry hair

Dry skin

Puffiness of the face

Bradycardia

Weight gain

Intolerant to cold

Swelling around the eyes

Tiredness and lethargy

Lid retraction

Sweating

Anxious look

Goitre

Palpitations

Intolerant to heat

Weight loss

Hand tremor

Hypothyroidism   Hyperthyroidism

Figure 5.1 Typical features of hypothyroidism and hyperthyroidism.

Case 4 *continued*

eyelid retraction also support this diagnosis.

History and physical examination are vital in elucidating the cause of thyrotoxicosis. In Samantha's case, the family history of autoimmune thyroid diseases suggests Graves' disease. The goitre in Graves' disease is typically diffuse, smooth and bilaterally symmetrical.

Thyroid eye disease and pretibial myxoedema occur only in thyrotoxicosis resulting from Graves' disease. However, lid retraction without other signs of thyroid eye disease, as in Samantha's case, can occur in all cases of thyrotoxicosis.

Investigations

In view of the symptoms and signs of thyrotoxicosis, Samantha's GP sends her blood sample to the laboratory to test thyroid function. The test results are shown in **Table 5.2**. The fully suppressed thyroid-stimulating hormone (TSH) with increased free thyroxine (T_4) and free tri-iodothyronine (T_3) are consistent with the diagnosis of thyrotoxicosis.

To determine the cause of the thyrotoxicosis, a blood test for TSH receptor antibodies is carried out and shows high titres of these antibodies. Tests for TSH receptor antibodies are positive in > 95% of cases of Graves' disease.

Diagnosis

The diagnosis of thyrotoxicosis caused by Graves' disease is confirmed. The GP prescribes Samantha propranolol for symptom relief and an antithyroid drug, carbimazole, to reduce the thyroid hormone level. She is referred to an endocrinologist.

Test results from a patient with thyrotoxicosis		
Measurement	Result	Normal reference range
Thyroid-stimulating hormone (mIU/L)	<0.01	0.35–4.5
Free thyroxine (pmol/L)	36.5	12–24
Free tri-iodothyronine (pmol/L)	9.5	4.0–6.8

Table 5.2 Thyroid function test results from a patient with thyrotoxicosis

Hyperthyroidism

Hyperthyroidism (or thyrotoxicosis) is caused by excessive amounts of thyroid hormones in the circulation. Hyperthyroidism resulting from disorders of the thyroid gland is called primary hyperthyroidism. When it occurs as a result of a pituitary disease, for example a TSH-secreting pituitary adenoma, it is called secondary hyperthyroidism.

Epidemiology

Hyperthyroidism is a common condition, with a prevalence rate of about 2% in women and 0.2% in men in the general population. The annual incidence of hyperthyroidism in women is about 1 in 1000 in the general population. The incidence increases with age in both sexes.

Aetiology

Causes of hyperthyroidism are shown in **Table 5.3**. Graves' disease is the commonest cause, accounting for about 75% of all cases. Toxic nodular goitre, either toxic multinodular goitre or a single toxic nodule, is the next most common.

Causes and pathogenesis of thyrotoxicosis	
Cause	Pathogenesis
Graves' disease	Stimulation of thyroid follicular cells by TSH receptor antibodies
Toxic multinodular goitre	Multiple autonomous nodules secreting excess thyroid hormone
Toxic nodule	Single autonomous nodule secreting excess thyroid hormone
Thyroiditis (including subacute or de Quervain's thyroiditis, silent thyroiditis and post-partum thyroiditis)	Release of preformed thyroid hormone following inflammatory destruction of thyroid follicles
Certain drugs (e.g. amiodarone, excessive intake of thyroxine, iodine, lithium or interferon α)	Different mechanisms including excess thyroid hormones or iodine, autoimmunity and thyroiditis
Gestational hyperthyroidism	β-chorionic gonadotrophin stimulating thyroid follicular cells
Hydatidiform mole and choriocarcinoma	β-chorionic gonadotrophin stimulating thyroid follicular cells
Struma ovarii (a teratoma of the ovary, containing thyroid tissue)	Excess thyroid hormone secretion from thyroid tissues within the ovarian tumour
Thyroid-stimulating hormone–secreting pituitary adenoma	Excess TSH from pituitary adenoma stimulating secretion of thyroid hormones

Table 5.3 Causes and pathogenesis of thyrotoxicosis

Pathogenesis

Pathogenesis of hyperthyroidism is variable and depends upon the aetiology.

Graves' disease In this autoimmune disorder, TSH receptor antibodies bind and activate TSH receptors on thyroid follicular cells. This stimulates thyroid hormone secretion, resulting in hyperthyroidism, and cell division, resulting in goitre.

Toxic nodular goitre Hyperthyroidism caused by toxic nodular goitre results from oversecretion of thyroid hormones by one or more autonomous thyroid nodules.

Thyroiditis In subacute thyroiditis (also called de Quervain's thyroiditis), silent thyroiditis and post-partum thyroiditis, a destructive inflammation causes release of stored thyroid hormones. This, in turn, results in transient thyrotoxicosis (see page 207).

Drug-induced hyperthyroidism Drugs cause hyperthyroidism in several different ways. For example, iodine (or iodine-containing drugs such as amiodarone) can cause uncontrolled oversecretion of thyroid hormones in a process known as the Jod-Basedow phenomenon. Amiodarone can also cause thyrotoxicosis as a result of thyroiditis.

> **Be cautious when using iodine-containing contrast medium** for computerised tomography (CT) scans in patients with multinodular goitre. This can precipitate thyrotoxicosis in these patients due to exposure to supraphysiological levels of iodine (the Jod-Basedow phenomenon).

Gestational hyperthyroidism This condition is caused by increased production of thyroid hormones by thyroid follicular cells in response to excess placental β-human chorionic gonadotrophin secretion in some pregnant women in the first trimester. The phenomenon occurs because β-human chorionic gonadotrophin is structurally and functionally similar to TSH.

Gestational hyperthyroidism improves spontaneously as the secretion of β-human chorionic gonadotrophin decreases in the second trimester.

Hydatidiform mole and choriocarcinoma
Hyperthyroidism in hydatidiform mole and choriocarcinoma is also mediated through β-human chorionic gonadotrophin.

Struma ovarii This is a rare tumour of the ovary containing thyroid tissue, which secretes excess thyroid hormone.

Thyroid-secreting pituitary adenoma This is a rare condition in which hyperthyroidism results from stimulation of thyroid follicular cells by excessive TSH secreted by a pituitary adenoma.

Clinical features

The most common symptoms and signs of hyperthyroidism are shown in **Table 5.4** and **Figure 5.1**. These clinical features may be present in thyrotoxicosis of any cause.

In thyrotoxicosis with a specific cause, several clinical features are apparent. For example, subacute thyroiditis is usually associated with a tender thyroid gland. Thyroid eye disease, pretibial myxoedema (also called thyroid associated dermopathy) and thyroid acropachy (finger clubbing) are hallmarks of Graves' disease (**Figure 5.2**).

- About a quarter of patients with Graves' disease have some degree of thyroid eye disease
- Pretibial myxoedema is less common, and patients with this sign typically have concomitant thyroid eye disease
- Thyroid acropachy is very rare

Patients with Graves' disease usually have diffuse, bilaterally symmetrical and smooth goitre. In contrast, a nodular goitre or a single nodule may be palpable in hyperthyroidism caused by toxic multinodular goitre or toxic nodule, respectively.

Clinical features of hyperthyroidism	
Symptoms	Signs
Weight loss	Weight loss
Tremor	Tremor
Palpitations	Tachycardia
Tiredness	Atrial fibrillation
Heat intolerance	Systolic hypertension and wide pulse pressure
Sweating	
Muscle weakness	Warm, clammy hands
Loose bowel motions	Proximal myopathy
Anxiety	Prominent eyes, lid retraction and lid lag
Breathlessness and decreased exercise tolerance	Thyroid bruit
	Signs of high-output cardiac failure
Menstrual irregularities	
	Hyper-reflexia

Table 5.4 Clinical features of hyperthyroidism

> An elderly patient with hyperthyroidism will not always present with classical symptoms of thyrotoxicosis. Consider the diagnosis in an elderly patient presenting with unexplained weight loss despite the absence of other symptoms and signs of thyrotoxicosis.

Diagnostic approach

Thyroid function tests (including TSH, free T_4 and T_3) are required to confirm hyperthyroidism. Following that, further investigations, such as measurement of TSH receptor

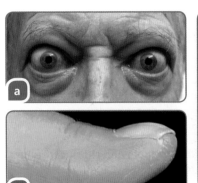
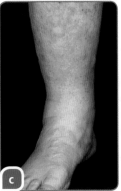

Figure 5.2 Extrathyroidal manifestations of Graves' disease. (a) Thyroid eye disease: proptosis and eyelid retraction. Also note upper and lower eyelid swelling and mild conjunctival redness. (b) Thyroid acropachy: a convexly curved nail. (c) Pretibial myxoedema (thyroid-associated dermopathy): thickened waxy skin on the lower leg.

antibodies and radionuclide thyroid uptake scan, may be necessary to define the aetiology of hyperthyroidism.

Investigations

A range of blood tests and radionuclide scans are useful.

Thyroid function tests

Thyroid function tests include measurement of TSH, free T_4 and free T_3 concentration levels in the serum. In primary hyperthyroidism, serum free T_4 and/or serum free T_3 concentrations are elevated with suppression of serum TSH concentration due to negative feedback (**Table 5.2**). In secondary hyperthyroidism (e.g. hyperthyroidism resulting from TSH secreting pituitary adenoma), serum free T_4 and serum free T_3, as well as serum TSH concentrations are elevated.

Primary hyperthyroidism is confirmed by suppressed serum TSH, together with increased serum free T_4, free T_3, or both. If serum TSH is suppressed but serum free T_4 and free T_3 are normal, the condition is subclinical hyperthyroidism.

> If the results of thyroid function tests show suppressed serum TSH but normal serum free T_4, serum free T_3 must be measured to exclude T_3 toxicosis. T_3 toxicosis is a type of thyrotoxicosis in which only free T_3 is increased. The condition is common in toxic multinodular goitre and toxic nodule, and it can also occur in early Graves' disease.

Inflammatory marker tests

Measurement of inflammatory markers is sometimes useful if clinical history and physical examination (for example, a recent history of viral illness with neck pain or tenderness) raise the suspicion of subacute thyroiditis. These markers include erythrocyte sedimentation rate, plasma viscosity and C-reactive protein, which are usually increased in subacute thyroiditis.

TSH receptor and thyroid peroxidase antibodies

Graves' disease can be confirmed by a blood test for TSH receptor antibodies, which are present in >95% of patients with the condition. Tests for thyroid peroxidase antibodies are less sensitive and specific, because these antibodies are present in about 75% of patients with Graves' disease and up to 10% of the general healthy population.

Radionuclide uptake scan

These scans, using radioactive iodine or technetium, are helpful, particularly if tests for TSH receptor antibodies are negative (**Figure 5.3**). Radionuclide scans show:

- diffuse increased uptake in Graves' disease
- a single area of uptake in cases of toxic nodule
- patchy uptake in cases of toxic multinodular goitre
- absent or markedly decreased uptake in thyroiditis

Radionuclide uptake scan is the investigation of choice if thyroiditis is suspected.

Generally, thyroid ultrasound is not a useful investigation for identifying the cause of hyperthyroidism because many patients with Graves' disease have small nodules on ultrasound making the distinction between Graves' disease and toxic nodular goitre difficult. In addition, if a nodule is seen on ultrasound, it is not possible to determine whether the nodule is the cause of excess thyroid hormone secretion or a non-secretory incidental lesion.

Management

The management of hyperthyroidism depends on the cause. However, a beta-blocker can be used to relieve the symptoms of thyrotoxicosis of any cause.

Graves' disease Management options for Graves' disease are antithyroid drug therapy, radioiodine treatment and thyroidectomy (see page 201).

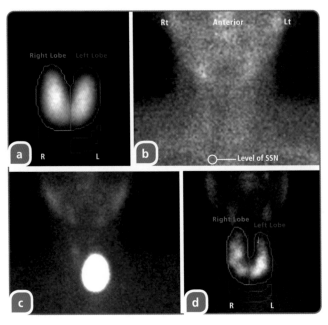

Figure 5.3 Thyroid uptake scans in thyrotoxicosis. (a) Graves' disease: increased bilaterally symmetrical diffuse uptake. (b) Thyroiditis: absence of radionuclide uptake in the thyroid. (c) Toxic nodule: increased uptake by a single autonomous nodule. Note the decreased radionuclide uptake in other parts of the thyroid. (d) Toxic multinodular goitre: patchy uptake by several autonomous nodules. L, left; R, right.

> **Patients in a thyrotoxic state find it difficult to concentrate and to retain information.** It is helpful if a family member is present to ask questions and note answers. A repeat discussion may be necessary when the thyrotoxicosis has improved.

Toxic nodular goitre Both toxic multinodular goitre and toxic nodules can be treated with antithyroid drugs, radioiodine or surgery. All cases of toxic nodular goitre relapse once antithyroid drug therapy is stopped, therefore radioiodine is the treatment of choice.

Thyroiditis Thyrotoxicosis caused by thyroiditis is a transient condition and resolves spontaneously. Antithyroid drugs are not indicated, but beta-blockers may be used to control symptoms.

Drug-induced hyperthyroidism The treatment of drug-induced thyrotoxicosis depends on the mechanisms causing thyrotoxicosis. For example, type 1 amiodarone-induced thyrotoxicosis is associated with hyper-secretion of thyroid hormone in response to excess iodine in amiodarone and is treated with antithyroid drugs. In contrast, type 2 amiodarone induced thyrotoxicosis is caused by inflammation of the thyroid (thyroiditis) with release of pre-formed thyroid hormones and is best treated with corticosteroids.

Gestational hyperthyroidism Gestational hyperthyroidism improves spontaneously in the second trimester. Most cases of gestational hyperthyroidism do not require treatment with antithyroid drugs.

Struma ovarii This is treated with surgical resection of the affected ovary. Some patients also need ablation with radioactive iodine (performed after total thyroidectomy to prevent accumulation of radioactive iodine in the thyroid rather than in the ovarian tumour) to control thyrotoxicosis.

Thyroid-secreting pituitary adenoma The treatment of choice for hyperthyroidism due to TSH-secreting pituitary adenoma is trans-sphenoidal resection of the adenoma. Somatostatin analogues are useful in controlling hyperthyroidism before the surgery or when surgery is not feasible.

Medication

The drugs used to treat hyperthyroidism belong to the thionamide group and include carbimazole, methimazole and propylthiouracil. Methimazole is an active metabolite of carbimazole; the two drugs have a similar mode of action.

All three antithyroid drugs (carbimazole, methimazole and propylthiouracil) decrease thyroid hormone synthesis primarily by inhibiting thyroid peroxidase enzyme. This action inhibits both the organification of iodide (the incorporation of iodine into thyroglobulin molecules) and the coupling of iodothyronines (see page 12).

Propylthiouracil also inhibits the peripheral conversion of T_4 to active hormone (T_3). However, carbimazole (or methimazole) is preferred to propylthiouracil. This is because carbimazole and methimazole:

- have fewer adverse effects (propylthiouracil is rarely associated with severe liver injury)
- provide more rapid control of thyrotoxicosis
- have longer half-lives, allowing less frequent dosing (carbimazole can be taken once daily, whereas propylthiouracil needs to be taken two or three times a day)
- are less expensive

The exception is for antithyroid drug therapy in early pregnancy. Propylthiouracil is preferred, because carbimazole (or methimazole) treatment in the first trimester is associated with rare congenital malformations in the fetus, including aplasia cutis (loss of skin on the scalp), dysmorphic facial features and gastrointestinal and respiratory abnormalities.

Serious adverse effects associated with antithyroid drugs are shown in **Table 5.5**. The most significant of these are as follows.

- Carbimazole or propylthiouracil: agranulocytosis (a reduction in white blood cells); a full blood count is indicated if the patient develops a sore throat, mouth ulcers or a high fever
- Propylthiouracil: fulminant hepatitis with features including jaundice, nausea and vomiting, dark-coloured urine and pale stool

Patients must be given written warnings of the serious potential adverse effects of antithyroid drugs.

Adverse effects of antithyroid drugs	
Carbimazole (or methimazole)	Propylthiouracil
Skin rash and itchiness	Skin rash and itchiness
Nausea, vomiting and change in taste sensation	Nausea, vomiting and change in taste sensation
Joint pain	Joint pain
Agranulocytosis, thrombocytopenia and aplastic anaemia	Agranulocytosis, thrombocytopenia and aplastic anaemia
Cholestatic liver disease*	Fulminant hepatic failure*
Congenital malformations*	Antineutrophil cytoplasmic antibody-positive vasculitis*

*These adverse effect profiles are different in the two groups of antithyroid drugs.

Table 5.5 Adverse effects of antithyroid drugs

Antithyroid drugs are used in two regimens.

- Titration regimen: the dose of carbimazole or propylthiouracil is titrated based on the results of thyroid function tests, to partially block T_4 secretion
- Block-and-replace regimen: an antithyroid drug is started at a high dose, and the high dose is kept constant throughout the treatment period to block T_4 secretion completely; then, when serum free T_4 and free T_3 concentrations are normal, levothyroxine is added for thyroid hormone replacement

In general, patients with a new diagnosis of Graves' disease are treated with antithyroid drugs. Patients unable to tolerate antithyroid drugs due to side-effects or those who relapse following a course of antithyroid drugs are treated with radioactive iodine therapy or total thyroidectomy.

In the treatment of Graves' disease, the use of either of these two regimens for 12–18 months is associated with an about 50% chance of long-term remission. Male sex, smoking, large goitre and very high free T_4 concentration at presentation are risk factors for relapse of Graves' disease after stopping antithyroid drug therapy.

Radioiodine treatment

Radioiodine (iodine-131) is generally used as second-line treatment if a patient is unable to tolerate, develops adverse effects from or has a recurrence of thyrotoxicosis while receiving antithyroid drug therapy. It is the treatment of choice for thyrotoxicosis due to toxic multinodular goitre and toxic nodule. Radioiodine is given orally in the form of capsule or liquid drink.

Radioiodine is contraindicated in pregnant women and breastfeeding mothers. Furthermore, patients should follow several precautions during and after radioiodine treatment.

> **Precautions for during and after radioiodine treatment include:** avoiding close and prolonged physical contact with children and pregnant women for several days, depending on the dose. For a woman of reproductive age undergoing radioiodine treatment, a pregnancy test is performed to ensure that she is not pregnant at the time of the treatment and is advised to avoid pregnancy for at least 6 months.

Hypothyroidism is a common adverse effect of radioiodine treatment. Therefore close monitoring with thyroid function tests is necessary to detect this condition before symptoms develop. Radioiodine can also worsen thyroid eye disease, particularly in patients who smoke and whose hypothyroidism is inadequately treated after radioiodine treatment.

Surgery

Total thyroidectomy is an effective treatment for Graves' disease and is increasingly preferred to subtotal thyroidectomy, because the latter is usually associated with persistent or recurrent thyrotoxicosis.

Total thyroidectomy is indicated in the following groups of patients:

- Patients who have developed adverse effects from antithyroid drugs and who decline radioiodine treatment
- Those whose thyrotoxicosis is inadequately controlled by antithyroid drug therapy, or who have recurrent disease and decline radioiodine treatment
- Patients who have a large goitre that is causing obstructive symptoms or is considered a cosmetic problem
- Patients with active thyroid eye disease, in whom radioiodine should be avoided because radioiodine treatment can worsen the eye disease

Before surgery, the patient must be euthyroid. A euthyroid state is achieved through antithyroid drug therapy and/or potassium iodide or Lugol's iodine. This is done to prevent excessive bleeding and thyrotoxic crisis during the operation.

Other potential complications of total thyroidectomy are transient or permanent hypoparathyroidism and vocal cord paralysis caused by damage to the recurrent laryngeal nerve. Patients develop hypothyroidism following total thyroidectomy and require long-term levothyroxine replacement.

> **Patients with Graves' disease must be advised to stop smoking.** Smoking:
>
> - makes thyroid eye disease six times more likely
> - delays the action of antithyroid drugs
> - increases the risk of thyroid eye disease after radioiodine treatment

Prognosis

Hyperthyroidism is associated with increased mortality as a result of cardiovascular disease. Poorly treated hyperthyroidism increases the risk of cardiac arrhythmias and osteoporosis.

Thyroid eye disease

Thyroid eye disease is an autoimmune disorder affecting the tissues around the eyes. The condition is usually associated with Graves' disease, but it can also be associated with autoimmune hypothyroidism or develop in patients with normal thyroid function. In

Graves' disease, eye symptoms can occur before, concurrently or after thyrotoxicosis.

Epidemiology

Thyroid eye disease affects up to 25% of patients with Graves' disease. A majority of these patients have mild disease, with only about 3% developing severe or sight-threatening disease.

Aetiology and pathogenesis

Thyroid eye disease is caused by an autoimmune reaction to an antigen shared by the thyroid and retro-orbital tissues. The reaction produces inflammatory swelling of the extraocular muscles and retro-orbital tissues.

Smoking is associated with a greater than sixfold increase in the risk of thyroid eye disease. This thought to be due to immune modulation associated with smoking. Radioiodine treatment and poorly controlled thyroid dysfunction (both thyrotoxicosis and hypothyroidism) are other risk factors.

Clinical features

Patients with thyroid eye disease usually present with swelling around the eyes, grittiness, redness, retro-orbital pain, excessive watering, photophobia, double vision and blurred vision. Patients may have one or more of the following signs (**Figure 5.2a**):

- eyelid swelling and erythema
- conjunctival redness
- chemosis
- exophthalmos (proptosis)
- restricted eye movement and squint
- corneal ulceration
- decreased colour vision
- decreased visual acuity

The signs of acute inflammation are present in the early phase of the disease, i.e. active thyroid eye disease. Residual signs of thyroid eye disease, such as lid retraction, exophthalmos and squint, may persist when the acute inflammation has settled; this state is called inactive thyroid eye disease.

As well as facial disfigurement, thyroid eye disease can cause visual impairment. Diplopia is caused by restricted movement of extraocular muscles, and visual loss results from corneal ulceration or compression of the optic nerve.

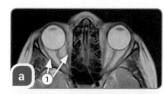
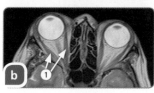

Figure 5.4 Magnetic resonance imaging in thyroid eye disease. (a) Normal. (b) Thyroid eye disease: large extraocular muscles ① and protrusion of the eyeballs (exophthalmos).

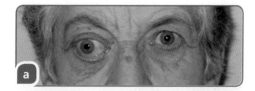

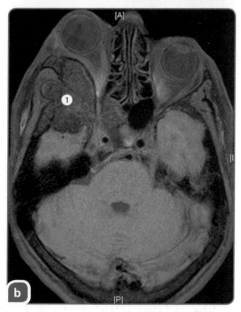

Figure 5.5 (a) Unilateral proptosis left side. (b) MRI showing a large meningioma ① pushing the eyeball forward.

Diagnostic approach

Diagnosis of thyroid eye disease is usually made clinically. In cases of diagnostic uncertainty, CT or magnetic resonance imaging (MRI) is helpful (**Figure 5.4**). For example, thyroid eye disease may need to be confirmed in the presence of unilateral exophthalmos possibly caused by a retro-orbital tumour (**Figure 5.5**).

Management

General management of thyroid eye disease includes smoking cessation, maintenance of euthyroidism, selenium supplement and use of eye lubricants. Diplopia may be addressed by the use of prism lenses.

Patients with severe and active thyroid eye disease receive systemic immunosuppressive therapy, for example using intravenous methylprednisolone. Some of these patients also require orbital radiotherapy or orbital decompression.

Rehabilitative surgery to improve facial disfigurement and visual impairment is done when the disease is inactive.

Hypothyroidism

In hypothyroidism, the thyroid gland secretes an inadequate amount of thyroid hormones. Hypothyroidism caused by diseases of the thyroid gland is called primary hypothyroidism. When it results from pituitary or hypothalamic disorders, it is known as secondary hypothyroidism.

Epidemiology

Primary hypothyroidism is one of the commonest endocrine disorders, affecting about 4% of the general adult population. It is more common in women, in whom the annual incidence is about 4 per 1000; in men, the incidence is about 0.6 per 1000.

Aetiology

Causes of hypothyroidism are shown in **Table 5.6**. Autoimmune thyroiditis is the commonest cause of primary hypothyroidism in high-income countries, but iodine deficiency remains a major cause in many parts of the world. Autoimmune thyroiditis associated with goitre is called Hashimoto's thyroiditis. Hypothyroidism caused by subacute or post-partum thyroiditis is usually transient.

Clinical features

Without thyroid hormone replacement, patients who have undergone total thyroid-ectomy rapidly develop symptoms of hypothyroidism. However, patients with autoimmune hypothyroidism tend to develop symptoms insidiously over many months or years. These symptoms range from non-specific tiredness to a serious life-threatening condition called myxoedema coma (see Chapter 11).

Causes of hypothyroidism	
Category	Causes/pathogenesis
Autoimmune thyroiditis	Autoimmune destruction of thyroid follicular cells
Treatment of thyrotoxicosis	Thyroidectomy and radioiodine ablation
Thyroiditis	Subacute thyroiditis (also called de Quervain's thyroiditis), silent thyroiditis and post-partum thyroiditis
Certain drugs	Thionamides, iodine, amiodarone, lithium and interferon
Congenital	Thyroid aplasia and dyshormonogenesis
Iodine deficiency	Lack of adequate dietary iodine
Disorders of the pituitary gland or hypothalamus (secondary hypothyroidism)	Decreased TSH secretion due to pituitary or hypothalamic disorders

Table 5.6 Causes of hypothyroidism

The most common symptoms and signs of hypothyroidism are shown in **Table 5.7** and **Figure 5.1**).

Diagnostic approach

Patients with severe hypothyroidism have the typical facial appearance and characteristic physical signs of the condition. However, such late presentation is increasingly rare. Now, most patients with hypothyroidism present with non-specific symptoms such as tiredness, lethargy, weight gain and depression.

These symptoms are all common in the general population. Therefore symptoms alone are insufficient for a diagnosis of hypothyroidism; it must be confirmed by biochemical tests.

Investigations

The diagnosis of primary hypothyroidism is confirmed by increased serum TSH concentration and low free T_4 concentration. In subclinical hypothyroidism, also known as mild hypothyroidism, TSH is increased but free T_4 is normal. Measurement of serum free T_3 concentration is unhelpful in the diagnosis, because it is usually normal, even in severe hypothyroidism.

Clinical features of hypothyroidism	
Symptoms	Signs
Tiredness	Periorbital puffiness
Lethargy	Cold hands
Cold intolerance	Bradycardia
Weight gain	Weight gain
Constipation	Dry skin and hair
Depression	Slow-relaxing reflexes
Poor memory	Carpal tunnel syndrome
Muscle weakness	Impaired consciousness (myxoedema coma)
Menstrual irregularities	Ascites, pleural effusion and pericardial effusion (rare)
Hoarseness of voice	

Table 5.7 Clinical features of hypothyroidism

Many patients with untreated hypothyroidism also have:

- hyponatraemia (thought to be caused by decreased free water excretion from the kidneys)
- hypercholesterolaemia (thought to be a consequence of decreased clearance of low-density lipoproteins from the liver)

Thyroid peroxidase antibodies are present in > 90% of cases of autoimmune thyroiditis.

In secondary hypothyroidism, free T_4 concentration is low and TSH is inappropriately normal or low (as pituitary or hypothalamic disorder means that pituitary is unable to secrete more TSH despite low free T_4 concentration). There may also be evidence of deficiency of other pituitary hormones.

Management

Management of hypothyroidism consist of thyroid hormone replacement.

Medication

Levothyroxine (T_4) is the treatment of choice for hypothyroidism. As liothyronine (T_3) has short half-life, it requires multiple doses in a day. It is also difficult to monitor and adjust the dose of liothyronine, therefore it is not a preferred treatment for hypothyroidism. Most cases of hypothyroidism are permanent so patients generally need life-long treatment with levothyroxine.

It is safe to start most patients on a full replacement dose of levothyroxine based on body weight. A daily dose of 1.6 µg/kg body weight is, for example, given as 100 µg daily for a 65 kg person. The exceptions to this are:

- patients with ischaemic heart disease
- patients older than 60 years, who may have undiagnosed ischaemic heart disease

Levothyroxine can precipitate severe angina or even myocardial infarction in these groups of patients by increasing heart rate. Therefore the dose of levothyroxine starts low (25 µg or even 12.5 µg daily) and is titrated very gradually.

> The thyroid gland secretes both T_4 and T_3, but patients who need thyroid hormone replacement receive levothyroxine (T_4) alone. Levothyroxine therapy is sufficient, because T_4 is converted to T_3 by deiodinase enzymes in the body.

Advise patients to take levothyroxine on an empty stomach, because food can affect its absorption. Certain drugs also interfere with levothyroxine absorption. Calcium, iron, aluminium hydroxide and colestyramine must be taken at least 4 h before or after levothyroxine.

Levothyroxine has a long half-life (7 days), so it is taken once daily.

Monitoring thyroid hormone replacement therapy

In patients with primary hypothyroidism, serum TSH concentration is high at diagnosis and returns to reference range with adequate levothyroxine replacement. Therefore the dose of levothyroxine is adjusted to keep serum TSH in the reference range. Annual checks of serum TSH are adequate in patients with stable primary hypothyroidism.

In contrast to primary hypothyroidism, serum TSH concentration is persistently low in secondary hypothyroidism. Therefore serum TSH is unsuitable for determining the dose of levothyroxine. Instead, the levothyroxine dose is titrated to keep the serum concentration of free T_4 at the upper end of the reference range.

> The long half-life of levothyroxine means that the patient does not feel unwell if a dose is missed, and their thyroid function test results may be normal. However, if doses are frequently missed, serum TSH starts to increase even if serum free T_4 remains normal.

Thyroid hormone replacement therapy in pregnancy

Thyroid hormones are essential for the neurological development of the fetus. However, the fetal thyroid gland does not start producing thyroid hormones until about 14 weeks of gestation. Until then, the fetus must rely on maternal thyroid hormones.

Hypothyroidism diagnosed during pregnancy is treated promptly with a full replacement dose of levothyroxine. The dose of levothyroxine needs to be increased in hypothyroid women who become pregnant. During pregnancy, they require monitoring with regular thyroid function tests.

> In most hypothyroid women receiving thyroid hormone replacement, levothyroxine dose needs to be increased by 30–50%. The increase is necessary because of increased urinary iodine excretion, transplacental transfer of thyroid hormones to the fetus, and the metabolism of thyroid hormones by placental deiodinase enzymes.

Thyroid hormone replacement therapy in subclinical hypothyroidism

The use of levothyroxine to treat patients with subclinical hypothyroidism is controversial. This is particularly true in the elderly, who tend to have an age-related increase in serum TSH. Furthermore, some cases of subclinical hypothyroidism reverse spontaneously.

The exception is pregnant women with subclinical hypothyroidism. In these patients, the use of levothyroxine is recommended because maternal subclinical hypothyroidism in pregnancy is associated with impaired neuropsychological development of the offspring and other adverse pregnancy outcomes, such as miscarriage and premature birth.

Prognosis

Hypothyroidism of most causes, including autoimmune thyroiditis, is generally a lifelong condition. However, it is easily treatable with levothyroxine. A small minority of patients have persistent symptoms and reduced quality of life despite biochemically adequate levothyroxine dose.

Thyroiditis

Thyroiditis is inflammation of the thyroid gland. It is a heterogeneous condition with several causes. Clinical manifestations depend on the cause.

Autoimmune thyroiditis

Autoimmune thyroiditis, called Hashimoto's thyroiditis when associated with goitre, is the commonest cause. Over 90% of patients with this condition have thyroid peroxidase antibodies. Many develop hypothyroidism and therefore require long-term thyroid hormone replacement with levothyroxine therapy.

Subacute thyroiditis

Subacute thyroiditis, also called de Quervain's thyroiditis, usually occurs after a viral upper respiratory tract infection. The thyroid is characteristically tender, but not in all cases; in 'silent thyroiditis', the gland is neither painful nor tender.

Thyrotoxicosis may result from release of preformed thyroid hormones in the early phase of the condition, followed by transient hypothyroidism and then euthyroidism (**Figure 5.6**). However, about 10% of patients develop permanent hypothyroidism.

Investigations include:

- erythrocyte sedimentation rate or plasma viscosity (both increased)
- radionuclide uptake scan (uptake in the thyroid is absent or minimal) (**Figure 5.3b**)

> **In thyrotoxicosis caused by thyroiditis, thionamide antithyroid drugs, which decrease thyroid hormone synthesis, are ineffective.** This is because the thyrotoxicosis in thyroiditis arises not from excessive thyroid hormone synthesis but from the release of preformed thyroid hormones from inflamed thyroid follicles. The condition resolves spontaneously.

Management is usually limited to use of a beta-blocker to control the symptoms of thyrotoxicosis. Some patients need non-steroidal anti-inflammatory drugs, and rarely oral steroids, to control pain.

Post-partum thyroiditis

Post-partum thyroiditis occurs within 12 months of delivery of a baby. The pattern of changes in thyroid function is thyrotoxicosis followed by transient hypothyroidism and then euthyroidism (**Figure 5.6**). There is an absence of radionuclide uptake in the thyroid (**Figure 5.3b**), and the treatment of thyrotoxicosis in this condition is similar to that for subacute thyroiditis.

The chance of recurrence of post-partum thyroiditis in subsequent pregnancies is very high (about 75%). More than half of women with post-partum thyroiditis are found to have developed permanent hypothyroidism on long-term follow-up.

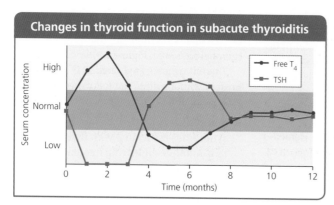

Figure 5.6 Typical sequence of changes in thyroid function in subacute thyroiditis. Serum free thyroxine (T_4) concentration is high in the early phase. This is followed by a transient decrease before a return to normal. There are reciprocal changes in serum thyroid-stimulating hormone (TSH) concentration. A similar pattern of changes in thyroid function occurs in post-partum thyroiditis.

Acute suppurative thyroiditis

Acute suppurative thyroiditis resulting from bacterial infection is rare. Staphylococcus aureus is the most common causative organism.

The condition is associated with fever, rigor, sweating, tachycardia and neck pain. Thyroid function is usually normal. Treatment consists of antibiotics and sometimes drainage of pus.

Invasive fibrous thyroiditis

Invasive fibrous thyroiditis (Riedel's thyroiditis) is extremely rare. Its cause is unknown.

The condition is characterised by dense fibrosis of the thyroid gland and surrounding tissues. Patients present with a hard goitre, which can mimic thyroid cancer. Invasive fibrous thyroiditis is treated with systemic steroids.

Goitre

Generalised or localised swelling of the thyroid gland is called goitre. Most of these are benign, although a small minority are malignant.

Epidemiology and aetiology

Goitre is very common in the general population. In the UK, about 6% of adult population have goitre, with a four-fold higher prevalence in women than in men. In some parts of the world with severe iodine deficiency, the prevalence of goitre is much higher. The causes of goitre are shown in **Table 5.8**. Iodine deficiency is the commonest cause of goitre worldwide. In the UK, autoimmunity (Hashimoto's thyroiditis and Graves' disease) is the most common cause. Thyroid carcinoma is a rare cause of goitre.

Clinical features

Features associated with goitre are listed in Table 2.10. However, most goitres grow insidiously over many years and are asymptomatic. Some patients present with symptoms of hypothyroidism or thyrotoxicosis if there is thyroid dysfunction (e.g. symptoms of hypothyroidism in Hashimoto's thyroiditis or symptoms of thyrotoxicosis in Graves' disease).

Large retrosternal goitre may be detected incidentally on a chest X-ray (**Figure 5.7**). However, a patient with a large goitre may also present with obstructive symptoms, including breathlessness, a choking sensation, stridor and difficulty swallowing (**Figure 5.8a**). When

Causes of goitre	
Cause	Example(s)
Iodine deficiency	Inadequate dietary iodine intake
Multinodular goitre	Toxic multinodular goitre, euthyroid nodular goitre
Autoimmune	Hashimoto's thyroiditis, Graves' disease
Thyroiditis	Subacute (de Quervain's) thyroiditis, post-partum thyroiditis, Riedel's thyroiditis
Neoplasm	Benign thyroid adenoma, thyroid carcinoma (papillary, follicular, anaplastic and medullary)
Ingestion of goitrogens	Cassava, a staple food in many low- and middle-income countries
Infiltrative diseases	Sarcoidosis, amyloidosis and histiocytosis

Table 5.8 Causes of goitre

asked to raise both arms, the patient may develop facial flushing because of compression of vascular structures in the thoracic inlet (Pemberton's sign; **Figure 5.9**).

Thyroid cancers (see page 211) sometimes present with a goitre. The following 'red flags' raise suspicion of malignancy:

- family history of thyroid cancer or syndromes associated with thyroid cancer (e.g. multiple endocrine neoplasia type 2)
- exposure to radiation (e.g. history of neck radiotherapy or of having lived in an area affected by an accident at a nuclear power plant)

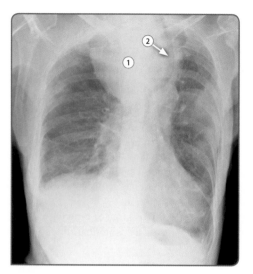

Figure 5.7 Chest X-ray showing incidental retrosternal goitre ①. The tracheal is deviated to the left ② because of the goitre.

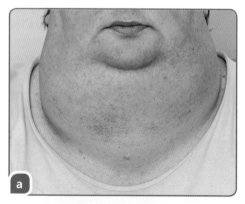

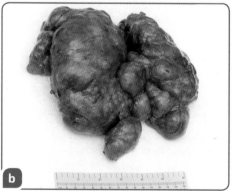

Figure 5.8 (a) Huge multinodular goitre causing obstructive symptoms and cosmetic problem and (b) macroscopic appearance of the goitre after surgical resection.

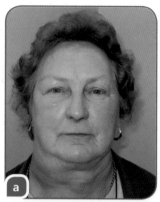

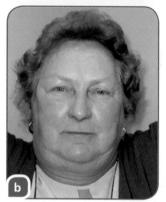

Figure 5.9 Pemberton's sign. (a) Large multinodular goitre. (b) Facial flushing with elevation of both arms.

- extremes of age
- a goitre that is rapidly increasing in size
- a hard, fixed goitre
- lymphadenopathy
- hoarseness of voice

Diagnostic approach

The three key aims of diagnostic work-up for a patient with a goitre are to assess:

- if the goitre is associated with abnormal thyroid hormone levels
- if the goitre is causing clinically significant compression of the trachea and other mediastinal structures
- if the goitre is malignant

Investigations

Assessment of thyroid function, with measurement of serum TSH and free T_4 levels, and ultrasound examination of the thyroid are the two key initial investigations for a patient presenting with a goitre.

Tests for thyroid antibodies can be useful to establish autoimmunity as the cause of a goitre:

- thyroid peroxidase antibodies (in hypothyroid patients or those with normal thyroid function)
- TSH receptor antibodies (in hyperthyroid patients)

In cases of goitre associated with thyrotoxicosis, radionuclide uptake scan can help distinguish between different causes (**Figure 5.3**).

Thyroid ultrasound is required. It shows whether the goitre is diffuse or nodular, and whether the nodule or nodules are cystic or solid, or have features suspicious of malignancy. Fine-needle aspiration cytology carried out under ultrasound guidance is necessary to examine suspicious nodule or nodules. If obstructive symptoms are suspected, flow volume loop and CT scan are done to investigate tracheal compression (**Figure 5.10**).

Management

Asymptomatic benign euthyroid goitre in most cases requires no treatment. Treatment of goitre associated with thyrotoxicosis is described on page 200.

Surgery for euthyroid goitre is indicated in the following circumstances:

- when malignancy is confirmed or suspected based on the results of fine-needle aspiration cytology
- when the patient has symptoms or signs of trachael obstruction
- when the goitre is large or growing rapidly, causing a cosmetic problem (**Figure 5.8**)

Radioiodine is also used occasionally to reduce the size of non-toxic benign goitres.

Prognosis

A goitre itself does not alter life expectancy. If the goitre compresses the airway, it needs to be removed. If there is cancer within the goitre, this sometimes alters life expectancy (page 212).

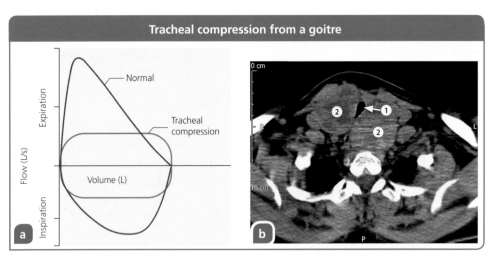

Figure 5.10 Tracheal compression from a goitre. (a) The flow volume loop shows decreased expiratory and inspiratory volume because of upper airway obstruction by the goitre. Blue line, normal flow volume; red line, flow volume in tracheal compression. (b) Computerised tomography scan showing ①marked tracheal compression by the goitre ②.

Thyroid nodule

A thyroid nodule is a localised abnormal growth of thyroid cells resulting in a lump. They are very common. About 5% of people are estimated to have at least one, although ultrasound studies suggest that the prevalence of thyroid nodules is much higher (up to 25%). Thyroid nodules are more common in women and in the elderly.

Clinical features

A thyroid nodule is often discovered incidentally. It is sometimes detected through imaging for another condition, for example MRI for cervical spinal disorders or positron emission tomography for a malignancy elsewhere in the body.

Most patients with a thyroid nodule are asymptomatic. A thyroid nodule is occasionally confused with other neck swelling, such as lymphadenopathy or thyroglossal cyst. A thyroglossal cyst (a cyst in the remnant of embryonic thyroglossal duct) characteristically lies in the midline and moves upwards when the tongue is protruded (see page 18).

About 5% of palpable thyroid nodules are malignant. Occasionally a thyroid nodule autonomously secretes excessive thyroid hormones, resulting in thyrotoxicosis.

Fine-needle aspiration cytology under ultrasound guidance is the investigation of choice to exclude malignancy (**Figure 5.11**). Thyroid function tests must also be done; if the biochemical results show hyperthyroidism, a radionuclide uptake scan is done to confirm a toxic thyroid nodule (**Figure 5.3c**).

Management

Asymptomatic benign thyroid nodules in most cases require no specific treatment. Malignant or suspicious thyroid nodules are treated with surgery. Radioiodine is the treatment of choice for a benign toxic thyroid nodule.

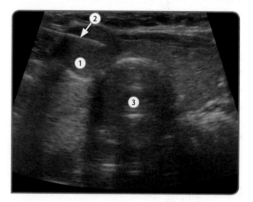

Figure 5.11 Ultrasound-guided fine-needle aspiration of a thyroid nodule ① in the left lobe of the thyroid. Note the needle ② used to aspirate the nodule and the shadow of trachea ③.

Thyroid cancer

Thyroid cancer is the most common endocrine malignancy.

Epidemiology

Thyroid cancer has an annual incidence of about 50 new cases per million in the general population. The incidence is three times higher in women than in men.

Risk factors for thyroid cancer are female sex, advancing age, family history of thyroid cancer and exposure to radiation.

Classification

Thyroid cancer is classified by histology and clinical course as follows:

- papillary thyroid carcinoma
- follicular thyroid carcinoma
- anaplastic thyroid carcinoma
- medullary thyroid carcinoma

Papillary, follicular and anaplastic carcinomas originate from thyroid follicular epithelium. Papillary and follicular carcinomas are also called differentiated cancer. This term distinguishes them from anaplastic carcinoma, which is undifferentiated and follows a more aggressive course.

- Papillary thyroid carcinoma is the commonest type (70% of all thyroid cancers)
- About 20% of thyroid cancers are follicular
- Only 5% are anaplastic

Medullary thyroid carcinoma originates from calcitonin-secreting parafollicular C cells. It accounts for about 5% of all thyroid cancers. This type of cancer can be sporadic or familial; the latter occurs either as a component of familial medullary thyroid carcinoma syndrome or as multiple endocrine neoplasia type 2 syndrome (see Chapter 10).

As well as the four major classes of thyroid cancer, other malignancies may arise in the thyroid. These include lymphoma and metastasis from primary carcinomas, particularly of breast, lung, colon, kidney and melanoma.

Clinical features

Most thyroid cancers present as a single thyroid nodule. Others manifest as a rapidly enlarging goitre with hoarseness and other obstructive symptoms (see page 208). Cervical lymphadenopathy and other evidence of metastasis may be present.

Investigations

Thyroid ultrasound with fine-needle aspiration cytology is usually the first investigation when a patient presents with a thyroid lump suspected to be malignancy. If thyroid cancer is confirmed, further imaging (e.g. chest X-ray, CT, MRI or positron emission tomography) is carried out for staging of the cancer. Serum calcitonin is a useful tumour marker in cases of medullary thyroid carcinoma.

Imaging with contrast-enhanced CT is avoided in patients with differentiated thyroid cancer. The iodine in the contrast medium can result in saturation of thyroid tissues with iodine. This can impair the uptake of radioiodine, used in diagnostic scanning or therapy, by normal thyroid cells or thyroid cancer cells for several months.

Management

Surgery is the mainstay of treatment for all operable thyroid cancers.

Thyroid-stimulating hormone stimulates the growth of both normal and cancerous thyroid cells, and suppression of TSH has been shown to be associated with lower recurrence in patients with differentiated thyroid cancers (papillary and follicular thyroid carcinoma). These patients are treated with levothyroxine at a dose high enough to suppress TSH concentration towards the lower limit of the reference range.

Papillary and follicular thyroid cancers

Differentiated (papillary and follicular) thyroid cancer cells take up radioiodine. Therefore radioiodine is used to ablate any residual malignant cells in these cancers after thyroidectomy. Radioiodine ablation is also used in metastasis and recurrence of differentiated thyroid cancers.

Some patients with advanced differentiated thyroid cancers are treated with external beam radiotherapy and chemotherapy.

Anaplastic thyroid cancers

Most anaplastic thyroid cancers are not curable with surgery. Treatment is in most cases limited to palliative radiotherapy and chemotherapy.

Medullary thyroid cancers

These cancers are treated with total thyroidectomy. Radiotherapy is not very effective against this type of cancer. Tyrosine kinase inhibitors have some efficacy for treating advanced medullary thyroid carcinoma. Serum calcitonin is a useful tumour marker for monitoring disease progression or relapse in patients with medullary thyroid cancer. About a quarter of cases are associated with a mutation in the *RET* proto-oncogene.

Prognosis

Papillary and follicular thyroid cancers generally have a good prognosis; 90% of people with papillary and 80% of people with follicular cancer will be alive after 10 years. Young age and limited spread of the cancer are also good prognostic features. The prognosis for medullary thyroid cancer depends how much it has spread. If the cancer has spread, the prognosis is about 40% survival at 5 years. Anaplastic thyroid cancer usually has a survival time of 2–6 months.

> **All patients with medullary thyroid cancer should be tested for mutations in the *RET* gene.** If a mutation is detected, the patient's family members can be tested and offered prophylactic thyroidectomy if the result is positive.

Answers to starter questions

1. It has long been suggested that emotional stress can cause autoimmune hyperthyroidism (Graves' disease). Many patients report major negative life events in the year before the diagnosis of Graves' disease and studies suggest that stress may play a role in its pathogenesis. It is thought that stress modulates the immune system to trigger Graves' disease. However, the exact mechanism remains uncertain.

2. Many thyroid disorders, including autoimmune hypothyroidism and Graves' disease, are more common in women. Two possible causes are genetic and hormonal factors. Women are thought to inherit predisposing genes via their sex chromosomes. Oestrogen, which has higher concentrations in women, modulates the immune system causing autoimmune thyroid diseases. Some thyroid disorders are also related to hormone changes in pregnancy (e.g. gestational hyperthyroidism) and child birth (e.g. post-partum thyroiditis).

3. Thyroid storm is a rare but life-threatening condition caused by very high thyroid hormone levels. Risk factors for this condition in patients with thyrotoxicosis include poor treatment compliance, surgery, infection and trauma. Thyroid storm has a 10% mortality rate, making treatment of the condition a matter of urgency.

4. Although most thyroid lumps are benign, malignancy should be suspected if the lump is rapidly increasing in size, and is hard or fixed. The presence of lymphadenopathy and hoarseness of voice are other worrying signs. A past history of exposure to radiation and family history of thyroid cancers should also raise suspicion.

Chapter 6
Pituitary disease

Starter questions

Answers to the following questions are on page 237.

1. Why does breastfeeding often prevent pregnancy?
2. Can benign pituitary tumours still be dangerous?
3. How do pituitary hormones influence a person's height?

Introduction

The pituitary gland is a major hormonal control centre. Problems with pituitary hormonal secretion are congenital or acquired; they are usually caused by a pituitary mass or the absence or reduction of pituitary tissue. Masses usually arise from within the gland, as in cases of benign pituitary adenoma, or they occasionally infiltrate the gland, as with metastases. They range from masses smaller than 1mm to large masses causing visual disturbance and invading the surrounding structures.

Patients with pituitary disease commonly present in four distinct ways:

- with a mass effect (volume of tissue causing symptoms) causing headache, cranial nerve palsy or visual field defect
- with hormonal excess (e.g. prolactinoma, Cushing's disease, acromegaly and thyrotropinoma)
- with hormonal deficiency
- with an incidental finding on imaging

The main indications for operating on a pituitary tumour are a threat to vision, removal of a secretory tumour and, occasionally, for diagnostic biopsy. However, all tumours can grow over time, so patients require regular reviews.

Case 5 Headaches and change in facial appearance

Presentation

Jeff, who is 55 years old, attends the orthopaedic clinic with tingling in his fingers. The surgeon notices that Jeff has fleshy hands and an enlarged tongue, and suspects that he has acromegaly.

Initial interpretation

The diagnosis of acromegaly is often a 'spot' diagnosis. A new physician meeting the patient for the first time is more likely to make the diagnosis than the patient's regular clinician, who may miss subtle changes that develop over a long time.

The tingling in Jeff's fingers suggests carpal tunnel syndrome. Carpal tunnel syndrome is common in the general population, but its association with acromegaly is well recognised. Looking for other clues suggesting active acromegaly help make the diagnosis.

Further history

On further questioning, Jeff admits that he has suffered from headaches for months. His shoe size has gone up from 9 to 11 over the past few years, and he no longer wears his wedding ring because it is too tight.

Jeff has had regular visits to the dentist as two false teeth have become loose. His friends find it difficult to believe that the picture on his driving license is of him as his facial features are more coarse; his nose bigger and his brow more prominent. His diet-controlled diabetes and hypertension (treated with ramipril) were diagnosed 5 years ago.

Examination

Jeff has the typical features of acromegaly with increased soft tissue of the hands (leading to carpal tunnel syndrome), enlarged feet, headaches and change in appearance. He is hypertensive, with a blood pressure of 160/90 mmHg. Confrontation test detects no visual field defect.

Interpretation of findings

Acromegaly is often a spot diagnosis. However, it is also necessary to consider this condition in patients who present

Common conditions associated with acromegaly	
Common symptom or sign	Cause(s)
Hypertension	Sodium retention
	Volume expansion
	Sympathetic nervous system activity
Diabetes mellitus	Growth hormone causes insulin resistance
Sleep apnoea	Enlargement of soft tissues of the pharynx and tongue
Carpal tunnel syndrome	Enlargement of soft tissues of the hand, causing compression of the median nerve
Osteoarthritis	Thickening of articular cartilage
	Widening of joint spaces
Headache	Stretching of the dura mater (the outermost meningeal layer surrounding the brain)
	Erosion of the pituitary fossa by a tumour
Left ventricular hypertrophy	Cardiac muscle hypertrophy
Colonic polyps or cancer	Probably growth-stimulating effect of insulin-like growth factor-1,

Table 6.1 Common conditions associated with acromegaly

Case 5 *continued*

with the more common conditions associated with acromegaly (**Table 6.1**). Tests are arranged to confirm the clinical suspicion biochemically.

Investigations

Jeff's growth hormone concentration fails to be suppressed during a glucose tolerance test. His serum insulin-like growth factor-1 is increased. Haemoglobin A1c value is mildly increased, and serum calcium is at the upper end of the normal range. Magnetic resonance imaging (MRI) shows a 2-cm pituitary lesion.

Diagnosis

Acromegaly is confirmed by the biochemical results and by the lesion in the pituitary.

The tumour is removed surgically by transsphenoidal hypophysectomy.

The possible complications of pituitary surgery must be clearly described to the patient before they give their consent.

- Common risks are infection, bleeding, hypopituitarism, cerebrospinal fluid leak and failure to remove all the tumour
- Uncommon risks are complications from the anaesthetic agents, including myocardial infarction (heart attack) and stroke
- The rare but devastating consequences of intracranial bleed (from damage to the internal carotid arteries) and death

Case 6 Weight gain and easy bruising

Presentation

Jackie Drury, aged 30 years, attends her general practitioner (GP) feeling miserable because she has gained weight over the past 2 years, despite her best efforts to diet. Recently, she has noticed incidental bruising, and that her ankles are swollen at the end of the day. This is the second time she has seen her GP in 3 months, which is unusual for her.

Initial interpretation

Weight gain is a common complaint. Simple obesity is the commonest cause; other causes are shown in **Table 6.2**. Whenever a common condition such as hypertension or obesity is diagnosed, secondary causes should be considered. Features suspicious of a secondary cause for weight gain are:

- no other overweight family members
- other associated new symptoms appearing at the same time as weight gain (e.g. pink stretch marks, striae)
- no major life changes (e.g. puberty, new job or home, new relationship or marriage, and childbirth)
- easy bruising (commonly reported by many patients, but a recent change may be relevant)
- depression (a non-specific symptom often associated with weight gain)

Further history

Last year, Mrs Drury fractured her arm after tripping on a curb, and during treatment for this, diabetes was diagnosed. She has no family history of diabetes, and the rest of her family are slim.

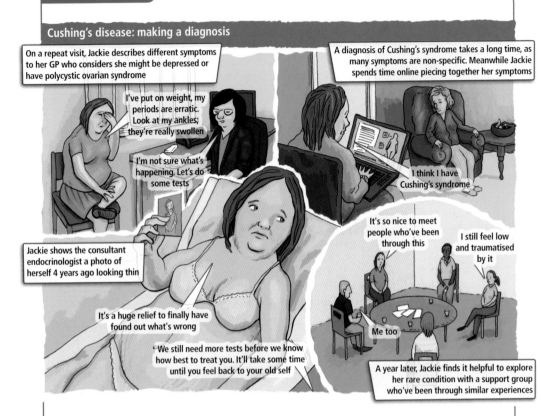

Case 6 *continued*

Cushing's disease: making a diagnosis

On a repeat visit, Jackie describes different symptoms to her GP who considers she might be depressed or have polycystic ovarian syndrome

I've put on weight, my periods are erratic. Look at my ankles; they're really swollen

I'm not sure what's happening. Let's do some tests

A diagnosis of Cushing's syndrome takes a long time, as many symptoms are non-specific. Meanwhile Jackie spends time online piecing together her symptoms

I think I have Cushing's syndrome

Jackie shows the consultant endocrinologist a photo of herself 4 years ago looking thin

It's a huge relief to finally have found out what's wrong

We still need more tests before we know how best to treat you. It'll take some time until you feel back to your old self

It's so nice to meet people who've been through this

I still feel low and traumatised by it

Me too

A year later, Jackie finds it helpful to explore her rare condition with a support group who've been through similar experiences

Mrs Drury works in a shop but has recently struggled to lift boxes on to the top shelf. She has started to look on the internet to find what could be the cause of her symptoms. She is not on any regular medication, and she uses no over-the-counter creams or tablets.

> **Patients frequently use the Internet for self-diagnosis.** It is not uncommon for patients to suspect that they have Cushing's syndrome or hypothyroidism, but only a minority actually do.

Examination

Mrs Drury has central adiposity (abdominal fat accumulation) with proximal myopathy (muscle weakness) in the arms and legs, an interscapular fat pad, a round face

with flushed cheeks, pink striae and mild ankle oedema. She has a large bruise from a blood test last week, and her skin is thin. Her blood pressure is 146/90mmHg, and she has a trace of glucose on urinalysis.

Interpretation of findings

Mrs Drury has many symptoms:

- fracture after minimal trauma
- proximal myopathy (she is unable to lift things above her head)
- persisting ankle oedema
- atypical weight gain
- diabetes and hypertension without a family history of these conditions

However, these symptoms are occurring in unusual circumstances at a young age. The combination of clinical findings suggests Cushing's syndrome.

Case 6 *continued*

Causes of weight gain	
Category	Cause(s)
Simple obesity	Unhealthy diet, sedentary lifestyle, or both
Endocrine	Hypothyroidism
	Cushing's syndrome
	Hypothalamic damage
	Insulinoma (pancreatic neuroendocrine tumour)
	Growth hormone deficiency
Certain drugs	Steroids
	Insulin
	Some oral hypoglycaemic agents (e.g. sulfonylurea)
	Psychotropics
	Antidepressants
	Oral contraceptive pill
	Anticonvulsants
Genetic disorder or syndrome	Leptin deficiency
	Prader–Willi syndrome
	Down's syndrome
	Turner's syndrome
Psychiatric disease	Depression

Table 6.2 Causes of weight gain

Investigations

Mrs Drury's 24-h urinary cortisol is three times the upper limit of normal, and her cortisol fails to suppress on a low-dose dexamethasone suppression test (see page 108). Her haemoglobin A1c and cholesterol are mildly increased, and a dual-energy X-ray absorptiometry (DEXA) bone scan shows osteopenia.

Further tests showed increased adrenocorticotrophic hormone (ACTH) and a 1-cm lesion on pituitary MRI.

Diagnosis

A diagnosis of pituitary-dependent Cushing's disease is made as she has autonomous (not regulated by feedback) cortisol production due to excessive ACTH with a pituitary lesion on MRI. She is referred for transphenoidal surgery after discussion at the endocrine MDT. She will have a close liason with the endocrine specialist nurse as she will need a lot of support to help her recover physically and emotionally even if cured at operation.

Acromegaly

Acromegaly is a condition of growth hormone excess. In children, growth hormone excess causes tall stature and is called gigantism, but in adults it causes characteristic physical changes that lead to a 'spot' (instant) diagnosis. Because it is uncommon and physical changes occur slowly, it can take up to 12 years for the condition to be diagnosed.

Epidemiology

Acromegaly is caused by excessive growth hormone. The condition is rare: the incidence is estimated at three or four cases per million people in USA annually. Mean age at diagnosis is 40–45 years. Both sexes are affected equally.

Aetiology

Acromegaly is usually sporadic. However, about 5% of cases are associated with syndromes such as multiple endocrine neoplasia type 1 (Chapter 10; page 295) or familial acromegaly. Familial acromegaly is an autosomal dominant disease (leading to a 50% chance of inheriting the defective gene from a parent) but it has incomplete penetrance, which means that even if the gene is inherited you may not develop the disease. Patients usually develop it in their teens or early adulthood and often the tumours co-secrete prolactin.

Pathogenesis

Acromegaly is caused by somatotroph adenomas of the pituitary. Somatotroph cells account for 50% of the pituitary hormone secreting cells. Very occasionally, acromegaly is caused by growth hormone secretion from non-pituitary tumours (ectopic growth hormone secretion) or by growth hormone-releasing hormone secreted by tumours outside the hypothalamus (e.g. by a neuroendocrine tumour in the lung).

Growth hormone binds mainly to receptors in the liver to stimulate production of insulin-like growth factor-1 (**Figure 6.1**). Insulin-like growth factor-1 has a role in cell division and cell death. It has effects mainly on

bone increasing osteoprogenitor cells (osteoblasts and osteoclasts) to maintain bone, adipose tissue to help reduce fat mass and muscle inducing protein synthesis (see page 32).

Clinical features

Gigantism is the name of growth hormone excess presenting in childhood; at this stage of life, the long bones have not fused and so the child continues to grow in response to excess growth hormone.

The symptoms adults with acromegaly have are:

- arthralgia
- sweating
- polyuria and polydypsia (due to diabetes and mild hypercalcaemia)
- menstrual irregularity or impotence (due to hypogonadism)
- tingling fingers or muscle wasting (due to carpal tunnel syndrome)
- daytime drowsiness (due to obstructive sleep apnoea)

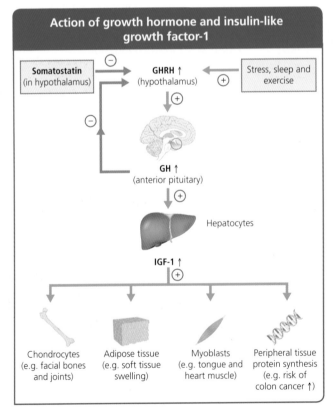

Figure 6.1 Action of growth hormone (GH) and insulin-like growth factor (IGF-1) on tissues. GHRH, growth hormone releasing hormone.

The clinical signs are shown in **Figure 6.2** and **Figure 6.3**.

The initial presentation of acromegaly result from:

- a mass effect from the pituitary tumour causing headache or visual field defect
- symptoms of another pituitary hormone deficiency
- the effects of excessive growth hormone on visceral tissues and bone (**Figure 6.1** and **6.2**)

When acromegaly is treated, the visceral soft tissue features improve but the bony features remain. Excessive growth hormone is associated with colonic polyps and cancer as it may act as a growth factor stimulating cell growth, proliferation and differentiation (division of cells).

Diagnostic approach

Acromegaly is often a spot diagnosis made by a physician on first meeting the patient (**Figures 6.2** and **6.3**). When seeing patients with hypertension, diabetes or carpal tunnel syndrome, it is necessary to consider acromegaly.

Investigations

The diagnosis is confirmed by a growth hormone measurement that fails to be suppressed with glucose tolerance testing (see page 108), as well as increased insulin-like growth factor-1. Insulin-like growth factor-1 is produced in the liver, so altered hepatic function can lead to a false negative result.

A normal result on random growth hormone measurement does not exclude the diagnosis of acromegaly, because growth hormone is secreted in pulses. At least 20% of growth hormone–secreting adenomas cosecrete prolactin, so serum prolactin is also checked.

The rest of the pituitary functions are checked to exclude hypopituitarism. Once the biochemical diagnosis is made, MRI of the pituitary is done.

Management

The aims of treatment for acromegaly are shown in **Table 6.3**. Treatment options are surgery, drug therapy and radiotherapy.

Surgery

Transsphenoidal surgery (**Figure 6.4**) is the treatment of choice to remove the pituitary

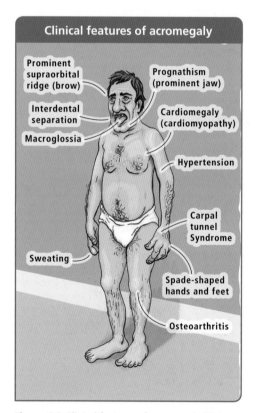

Clinical features of acromegaly

Prominent supraorbital ridge (brow)

Prognathism (prominent jaw)

Interdental separation

Macroglossia

Cardiomegaly (cardiomyopathy)

Hypertension

Carpal tunnel Syndrome

Sweating

Spade-shaped hands and feet

Osteoarthritis

Figure 6.2 Clinical features of acromegaly. There is also enlargement of the soft tissues of the nose (not shown).

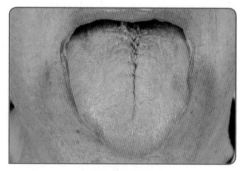

Figure 6.3 Macroglossia in acromegaly.

Aims of treatment for acromegaly

Aim	Consequence
Remove the tumour	Relieves pressure (mass) effects and normalises growth hormone
Relieve clinical symptoms	Reduces headaches and clinical symptoms
Normalise insulin-like growth factor-1 and growth hormone concentration	Reduces risk of death
Prevent recurrence	Reduce need for additional treatment
Treat long-term complications	Persisting arthritis (unresolved by normalisation of growth hormone and insulin-like growth factor 1)

Table 6.3 Aims of treatment for acromegaly

tumour and thus normalise IGF-1 concentration by removing the excessive growth hormone. Possible complications of transsphenoidal surgery are:

- cerebrospinal fluid leak (usually repaired at the time of operation)
- meningitis
- diabetes insipidus (either temporary or permanent)
- hypopituitarism
- loss of vision (because of possible damage to the nearby optic chiasm)

- stroke (a rare but devastating consequence possible because of the close proximity of the internal carotid arteries to the pituitary)

Medication

The three types of drug therapy available for acromegaly are:

- somatostatin analogues
- dopamine agonist
- growth hormone receptor antagonist

Somatostatin analogues are usually given by monthly injection and inhibit growth hormone release from the pituitary. However, these drugs also inhibit pancreatic and gastrointestinal function, so a minority of patients have intolerable diarrhoea.

Oral cabergoline, a dopamine agonist, is a cheaper option and is effective in approximately 10% of patients (usually with mild growth hormone excess).

Other more expensive options, such as the growth receptor antagonist pegvisomant, are reserved for patients whose symptoms are not controlled on other treatments.

Medication is used for the following indications:

- to reduce soft tissue swelling and sometimes help shrink the tumour preoperatively (e.g. with somatostatin analogues)
- for patients who are unfit for surgery
- for patients who cannot be cured by surgery

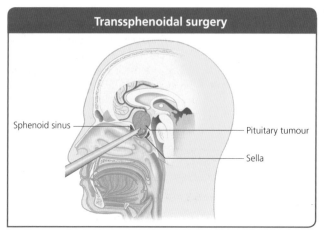

Transsphenoidal surgery

Sphenoid sinus
Pituitary tumour
Sella

Figure 6.4 Transsphenoidal surgery can be done using direct visualisation with a microscope or an endoscope. The approach is through the upper lip or nose and through the sphenoid bone.

Radiotherapy

This is frequently used to control growth hormone excess. However, the effects of radiotherapy take many years to reduce growth hormone and commonly leads to hypopituitarism.

Prognosis

Active acromegaly confers a two-fold increase in mortality, mainly because of higher rates of cardiovascular disease (e.g. ischaemic heart disease and cardiomyopathy), respiratory disease (e.g. obstructive sleep apnoea), complications of diabetes and neoplasia (particularly colon cancer). Mortality is normalised after restoration of normal growth hormone or insulin-like growth factor-1.

The size of the tumour and experience of the surgeon determine the chances of cure with surgery alone. Even when acromegaly is cured, many patients suffer joint problems and the consequences of long-term hypopituitarism.

Patients whose acromegaly has been cured are frequently invited to examinations, because they are well and in long-term follow-up. Examiners are impressed by an ability to show the difference between active acromegaly (excessive soft tissue, e.g. doughy hands and sweaty palms) and treated acromegaly (bony features only). Do not forget to look for a visual field defect.

Prolactinoma

Prolactinomas are the commonest benign (non-cancerous) secretory pituitary tumours. They can be treated medically obviating the need for surgery in the majority of cases. Although the gonadotrophins are usually suppressed at diagnosis when the prolactin is high (causing erectile dysfunction and amenorrhoea), these usually spontaneously resolve as the prolactin is treated.

Epidemiology

Prolactinomas account for about 25–30% of all pituitary adenomas. Microprolactinomas (<1 cm) are more common in women than macroprolactinomas, which are more common in men. Microprolactinomas may go unnoticed in men, because they are frequently late to report erectile dysfunction and are less likely to develop galactorrhoea.

Aetiology

Prolactinomas usually occur in isolation. However, as with all other pituitary tumours, they occasionally form part of multiple endocrine neoplasia type 1 (see Chapter 10).

Prolactinomas are stimulated by oestrogen. Microprolactinomas usually go into remission

at menopause, when ovarian oestrogen production ends. Prolactinomas need to be monitored carefully during pregnancy, because the increased oestrogen in pregnancy may stimulate their growth.

Pathogenesis

Prolactinomas arise from the lactotroph cells of the pituitary. They can be the size of a pinhead and difficult to visualise on MRI, or they can be extensive, expanding into the cavernous sinuses and pressing on the optic chiasm (**Figure 6.5a**).

Serum prolactin concentration gives some indication of the likely size of the lesion. Prolactin is sometimes measured at several thousand times above the normal range, and the tumour spreads widely beyond the pituitary fossa. Dopamine, produced from the hypothalamus, inhibits prolactin release. Any drugs that inhibit dopamine release (e.g. antiemetics or antipsychotics) will stop the inhibition and lead to a rise in prolactin.

Clinical features

Increased prolactin usually leads to suppressed gonadotrophin levels. Therefore, in

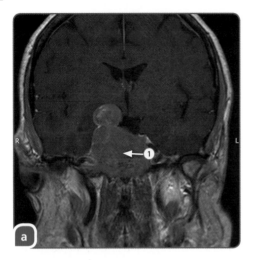
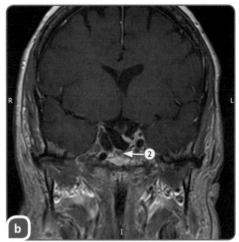

Figure 6.5 Prolactinoma. (a) Before treatment ① Prolactinoma. (b) After treatment ② Reduction in prolactinoma.

women, prolactinoma often presents during infertility investigations. The clinical features of prolactinomas are shown in **Table 6.4**.

The level of prolactin does not always correlate with the likelihood of galactorrhoea (expression of milk from the breasts). A tumour pressing on the optic chiasm usually causes a visual field defect (**Figure 6.6**).

| Left Eye | Right Eye |

Figure 6.6 Visual field perimetry test showing bitemporal hemianopia in a patient with a large pituitary tumour.

Diagnostic approach

The diagnostic approach to increased prolactin or galactorrhoea is as follows.

- Exclude possible local malignant breast causes for discharge from the breast
- Exclude non-pituitary causes of increased prolactin such as stress of venpuncture or drugs through history, examination and blood tests
- Arrange MRI of the pituitary if no other cause is identified
- Look for other associated hormone changes, particularly changes in the concentration of other pituitary hormones

The differential diagnoses of an increased serum prolactin concentration are extensive

Clinical features of prolactinoma	
Women	Men
Oligomenorrhoea or amenorrhoea	Erectile dysfunction
Features of low oestrogen (such as hot sweats)	Loss of libido
Vaginal dryness	
Dyspareunia (painful sexual intercourse)	
Infertility	Infertility
Galactorrhoea (30-80% of women)	Galactorrhoea (< 30% of men)
Headaches and visual disturbances	Headaches and visual disturbances
Low bone density	Low bone density
Hypopituitarism	Hypopituitarism

Table 6.4 Clinical features of prolactinoma in women and men

(**Table 6.5**). Common physiological and pharmacological causes need to be ruled out. Once these are excluded, it is necessary to distinguish between the following:

- endogenous prolactin production from lactotrophs
- suppressed dopamine level (leading to increased prolactin), caused by interruption of the pituitary stalk (disinhibition) by a large pituitary mass

Unilateral blood-stained nipple discharge is considered a malignant breast lesion until proven otherwise.

Investigations

Further investigation is necessary only if the prolactin concentration remains high after stopping potentially causative medication. The stress of venepuncture may cause prolactin to increase; a normal result may be obtained if the sample is drawn through a cannula 1 hour after insertion. All female patients of reproductive age require a pregnancy test. Thyroid and renal function are routinely checked.

If a patient has no symptoms suggesting increased prolactin, the assay is used to test for the inactive 'macroprolactin' molecule. Macroprolactin is a dimer of prolactin. It is rarely physiologically active but may register with certain assays to cause a falsely increased prolactin concentration.

If other causes have been excluded, an MRI is required. The size of the lesion on MRI correlates to the serum prolactin (the higher the prolactin the larger the prolactinoma). Therefore MRI, combined with prolactin measurement can help differentiate between a prolactinoma and an incidental non-functioning tumour causing disinhibition of the pituitary stalk (where the prolactin is usually below 2000 mU/L). For example, a large lesion on MRI:

- with a prolactin concentration > 5000 mU/L is likely to be a prolactinoma
- with a prolactin concentration < 1000 mU/L suggests a pituitary tumour with disinihibition of the pituitary stalk

It is necessary to distinguish the two conditions, because they require different treatment.

Other aspects of pituitary function need to be checked. Suppression of gonadotrophins is common. This effect leads to the failure to ovulate and amenorrhoea in female patients, and erectile dysfunction in men. The larger the tumour, the more likely that other hormones of the pituitary axis are affected.

Management

Prolactinoma is the only pituitary tumour that is usually cured with medication alone.

Medication

First-line treatment is with dopamine agonists such as cabergoline and bromocriptine. The symptoms and the mass lesion usually reduce as prolactin concentration normalises

Causes of increased serum prolactin concentration	
Category	**Causes**
Physiological	Pregnancy
	Breastfeeding
	Stress (e.g. venepuncture, surgery and hypoglycaemia)
Pharmacological	Antiemetic drugs (e.g. metoclopramide and domperidone)
	Antidepressant drugs (e.g. tricyclic antidepressants)
	Antipsychotic drug (e.g. risperidone)
	Antiepileptic drugs
	Oral contraceptive pill
	Opiates
Pathological	Prolactinoma
	Pituitary tumour with disinhibition of the pituitary stalk
	Hypothyroidism
	Chronic renal failure
Assay interference	'Big' or 'macro' prolactin (inactive)

Table 6.5 Causes of increased serum concentration of prolactin

with these medications (**Figure 6.5b**). Treatment is given for a minimum of 2 years for a microprolactinomas, but it is sometimes lifelong for larger tumours. The adverse effects of nausea or depression may limit the use of these drugs.

Gonadotrophins, and therefore fertility, are more likely to be restored in patients with microadenoma than in those with macroadenoma. Prolactin concentration is normalised in 85–90% of patients whose microadenomas is treated with medication. Within 1 month of starting therapy, a regular menstrual cycle is restored in about 25% of patients; this figure increases to 80% by 10 months. Treatment is stopped in most cases when a patient becomes pregnant. Other pituitary hormones sometimes recover, but this is less likely.

Surgery

Surgical resection is considered for patients who are unable to tolerate dopamine agonist therapy, as well as or for those who are resistant to it.

Macroprolactinomas treated with dopamine agonists show reduction in both prolactin concentration and tumour size on MRI. In cases of tumour compressing the pituitary stalk (not prolactinomas), dopamine agonists also normalise prolactin concentration but the tumour will not be shown to have shrunk on MRI.

Prognosis

Prolactinomas are almost always benign; they have no effect on life expectancy. However unrecognised prolactinomas commonly affect fertility, and hypogonadism has long-term deleterious effects on bone mineral density.

In men, testosterone replacement therapy is delayed after prolactinoma treatment. This is because there is frequently a spontaneous recovery of testosterone levels and the ability to attain an erection.

Cushing's syndrome

Cushing's syndrome is a state of pathological cortisol excess. It most commonly results from exogenous glucocorticoid administration (excessive use of steroid medicines). It is also caused by excessive endogenous secretion of cortisol from:

- ACTH-secreting pituitary tumour (Cushing's disease)
- Adrenal tumour secreting cortisol (see Chapter 7)
- Ectopic ACTH secretion (see Chapter 10)

Epidemiology

Most cases of Cushing's syndrome are secondary to exogenous glucocorticoid administration. Endogenous Cushing's syndrome is less common, with an annual incidence of about 2.5 cases per million people in the USA.

Pituitary-dependent Cushing's syndrome is known as Cushing's disease. This condition accounts for 60–80% of all cases of endogenous Cushing's syndrome.

Pituitary Cushing's disease and adrenal Cushing's syndrome are usually diagnosed between the ages of 25 and 40 years. The low incidence and frequently insidious onset of Cushing's syndrome often mean that it is diagnosed late.

Aetiology

Most cases of Cushing's syndrome are sporadic and can occur in anyone. However, the condition is occasionally linked with endocrine syndromes such as multiple endocrine neoplasia type 1 (see page 295). In these cases Cushing's syndrome is usually caused by Cushing's disease or ectopic Cushing's syndrome resulting from a carcinoid tumour.

The causes of endogenous Cushing's syndrome are shown in **Table 6.6**.

Pathogenesis

The pathogenesis of Cushing's syndrome depends on the origin of the cortisol excess:

- Cushing's disease originates in the corticotroph cells of the anterior pituitary. The tumour is usually small (can be the size of a pinhead)
- Adrenal Cushing's syndrome is secondary to an adenoma or carcinoma originating from the adrenal cortex
- Ectopic Cushing's syndrome is secondary to the secretion of ACTH from neuroendocrine cells e.g. lung carcinoid tumour.

Clinical features

Cushing's syndrome has many symptoms and signs (**Figures 6.7** and **6.8**).

In addition to the clinical signs, patients frequently have:

- Fatigue
- Depression, anxiety and irritability
- Amerorrhoea or erectile dysfunction
- Proximal myopathy (weakness and wasting of proximal muscles)
- Diabetes
- Hypertension

Florid Cushing's syndrome is difficult to miss. However, mild or periodic excessive secretion of cortisol, called 'cyclical Cushing's syndrome', is less phenotypically obvious but can still cause morbidity.

The speed of onset of symptoms gives a clue as to the likely aggressiveness of the lesion. For example, adrenal carcinoma or ectopic ACTH syndrome from a small-cell lung cancer usually has a short history, over weeks, with extremely high cortisol secretion. In contrast, patients with Cushing's disease may present after many years of symptoms.

Patients who have aggressive Cushing's syndrome with very high serum cortisol often have disturbance of their mental state. It is essential to assess their capacity to make decisions about their health. Relationships are frequently put under strain when patients have active disease due to altered behaviour.

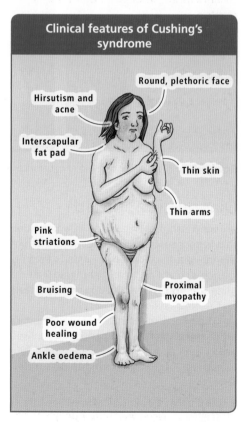

Clinical features of Cushing's syndrome

Round, plethoric face

Hirsutism and acne

Interscapular fat pad

Thin skin

Thin arms

Pink striations

Bruising

Proximal myopathy

Poor wound healing

Ankle oedema

Figure 6.7 Clinical features of Cushing's syndrome.

Main causes of endogenous Cushing's syndrome	
ACTH-dependent	**ACTH-independent**
Cushing's disease	Adrenal adenomas
Ectopic ACTH syndrome	Adrenal carcinomas
■ Small-cell lung cancer (> 25% of ectopic cases) ■ Lung carcinoid ■ Thymomas ■ Pancreatic islet cell ■ Medullary cancer thyroid	Bilateral macronodular adrenal hyperplasia
ACTH, adrenocorticotrophic hormone.	

Table 6.6 Main causes of endogenous Cushing's syndrome

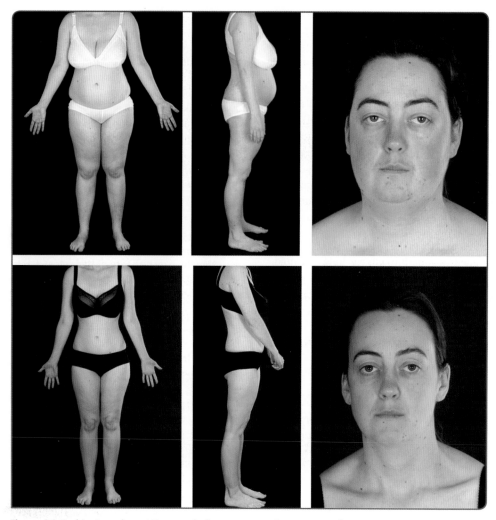

Figure 6.8 Cushing's syndrome. Top row: before treatment. Bottom row: after treatment.

Diagnostic approach

Pseudo-Cushing's syndrome is a condition that is not caused by a disorder of the hypo-thalmo–pituitary–adrenal axis. Patients with this condition have cushingoid features and false positive results on screening tests for Cushing's syndrome.

Common causes of pseudo-Cushing's syndrome are severe depression, alcoholism, anxiety and obesity. The general approach to a diagnosis of Cushing's syndrome is as follows:

- Ensure that the clinical features fit with a diagnosis of Cushing's syndrome

- Confirm cortisol excess by two separate tests
- Measure ACTH, because the results help direct further imaging
- Use imaging studies to identify potential sources
- Carry out petrosal sinus sampling if the diagnosis is still unclear

Investigations

Patients usually present with the clinical features of Cushing's syndrome, but occasionally they present with a pituitary or adrenal mass incidentally identified on imaging. Routine screening of all obese patients for Cushing's syndrome is not advisable, because the rarity of Cushing's syndrome and the high frequency of false positive tests lead to a very low yield of detection of actual cases.

Cortisol tests

Various tests are used to diagnose cortisol excess (see pages 104 and 108). The first-line test is often 24-h urinary cortisol, but samples are difficult to collect reliably in children and the elderly. Low-dose and overnight dexamethasone suppression tests are carried out as a first- or second-line test (after urinary cortisol) to confirm increased serum cortisol.

All tests have false positives and false negatives. Suppressed cortisol after low-dose dexamethasone, or normal urinary cortisol, excludes Cushing's syndrome in about 95% of cases (meaning a 5% false negative rate). Causes of false positives include pseudo-Cushing's syndrome, enzyme-inducing drugs (enzymes metabolise the dexamethasone), non-compliance (with the dexamethasone test) and acute illness.

Midnight cortisol (serum or salivary) is increased in patients with Cushing's syndrome (cortisol is undetectable in normality).

Adrenocorticotrophic hormone test

Once a diagnosis of Cushing's syndrome has been made, ACTH is measured to distinguish between adrenal and pituitary or ectopic disease.

- Suppression of ACTH confirms an adrenal source of excessive cortisol (feeding back to suppress the ACTH from pituitary)
- If ACTH is not suppressed, the patient is most likely to have pituitary Cushing's disease, but they may also have ectopic ACTH production

If ACTH is normal or increased, patients next require pituitary MRI

Petrosal sinus sampling

If the lesion in the pituitary is very small or not visible, petrosal sinus sampling (see page 110) is used to differentiate between a pituitary-dependent Cushing's disease and Cushing's syndrome from an ectopic source of ACTH.

Other tests

High-dose dexamethasone suppression test and corticotrophin-releasing hormone test occasionally provide additional information as to the source of the ACTH.

Management

It is imperative that the planning of treatment for Cushing's syndrome should be done by a multidisciplinary team. Surgery remains first-line treatment, but medication and radiotherapy also have a role in controlling disease, particularly when a cure is not achievable.

Surgery

The definitive treatment for Cushing's disease is transsphenoidal surgery (**Figure 6.4**). When done by experienced surgeons, it can achieve remission in up to 90% of patients with microadenomas. However, larger tumours require additional treatment after surgery around 50% of the time.

If the source of Cushing's syndrome is not identified despite extensive investigation, a bilateral adrenalectomy is considered. This operation cures Cushing's syndrome but does not treat the underlying cause.

Medication

Several drug treatments are available for Cushing's syndrome. These lower cortisol and are used if the patient is unsuitable for an operation or if an operation has failed to control the cortisol excess.

Metyrapone inhibits the enzyme 11β-hydroxylase in the final stages of cortisol synthesis, leading to a build-up of precursors of cortisol. These precursors include adrenal androgens, so women become hirsute (hairy) over time.

The antifungal drug ketoconazole used to be a common treatment for Cushing's syndrome, because it suppresses cortisol at high dose, however it may prove difficult to obtain in the future as it is no longer first line for fungal infections (its main use) and therefore the supply is limited.

In emergency situations, an anaesthetic agent called etomidate is used to achieve rapid control of excess cortisol.

> An abrupt change in hormone concentrations, such as the large decrease in cortisol after pituitary surgery for Cushing's disease, frequently leads to difficult psychological problems. Presurgical anxiety and depression are usually replaced post-operatively by exhaustion, aches and pains, and continuing mood disturbance despite hydrocortisone replacement. Some surgeons tell patients that if they feel dreadful after the operation, it is a good sign that they are cured.

Radiotherapy

This treatment is usually used as an adjunct if patients with Cushing's disease are not cured by transsphenoidal surgery. However, radiotherapy usually takes many years to normalise cortisol concentration.

Prognosis

Untreated Cushing's syndrome is associated with significant mortality from vascular disease (e.g. myocardial infarction), uncontrolled diabetes and sepsis. Normalising the cortisol is thought to restore life expectancy to normal, however morbidity usually continues even after cure. Even mild cortisol excess increases the risk of diabetes and hypertension.

Patients with pituitary-dependent Cushing's disease have a high rate of relapse and therefore require lifelong follow-up.

Hypopituitarism

Hypopituitarism refers to complete or partial failure of secretion of anterior or posterior pituitary homones, or both. Onset may be in childhood or adult life. The condition is generally permanent and requires one or more specific hormone replacements.

Epidemiology

The prevalence of hypopituitarism is 300–450 per million. Pituitary hormonal deficiencies may develop over many years, particularly if the patient has had cranial radiotherapy. Alternatively, they may all occur simultaneously after a sudden event such as surgery, trauma or pituitary haemorrhage (pituitary apoplexy).

Aetiology

Hypopituitarism may arise as a result of:

- congenital pituitary defects
- acquired pituitary or hypothalamic disease
- lesions in the infundibulum (pituitary stalk), which interfere with hypothalamic control of the pituitary

The main causes of hypopituitarism are shown in **Table 6.7**. Sudden loss of pituitary hormones occasionally occurs when blood supply to the pituitary is interrupted, as in serious head injury. Pituitary apoplexy occurs when there is a bleed, an infarction, or both, of the pituitary gland. This is usually associated with a sudden severe headache, similar to that caused by a subarachnoid haemorrhage. Pituitary apoplexy frequently causes cranial nerve palsies, particularly of the 3rd, 4th and 6th cranial nerves, which lie adjacent to the pituitary gland.

Sheehan's syndrome is post-partum necrosis and infarction of the pituitary gland associated with severe blood loss and hypotension during and after childbirth. The condition is seen less frequently with modern obstetric care.

Radiotherapy of head and neck cancers can include the pituitary in the radiation field and lead to hypopituitarism. The treatment usually have different effects depending on the dose administered and the patient's age at the time of therapy.

Pathogenesis

Hypopituitarism classically develops in sequential order: the impaired secretion of growth hormone, then gonadotrophins, then

Main causes of hypopituitarism	
Category	Cause
Neoplastic	Pituitary adenoma
	■ Secretory (e.g. in Cushing's disease, acromegaly and prolactinoma)
	■ Non-secretory (non-functioning)
	Metastases (e.g. breast, renal and bronchial)
	Peripituitary
	■ Craniopharyngioma
	■ Germ cell tumours
	■ Meningiomas
Inflammatory	Lymphocytic hypophysitis
Infectious	Tuberculosis
	Syphilis
Infiltrative	Haemochromatosis
	Sarcoidosis
Vascular	Sheehan's syndrome
	Pituitary apoplexy
Cystic	Rathke's cleft cyst
Post-irradiation	Pituitary radiotherapy
	Head and neck radiotherapy with pituitary in the field (some radiation affects the pituitary as an unwanted consequence of radiation to a wider area)
Miscellaneous	Traumatic brain injury
	Empty sella

Table 6.7 Main causes of hypopituitarism

thyroid-stimulating hormone and ACTH. Antidiuretic hormone deficiency is almost never a primary feature of pituitary adenomas.

Clinical features

The clinical features of hypopituitarism depend on the patient's age when symptoms develop and the number of hormones affected (**Table 6.8**). For example, growth hormone deficiency in childhood results in reduced height for age, whereas deficiency developing after fusion of the epiphyses in adulthood (when no further bone growth can occur) reduces psychological well-being and decreases muscle mass and bone strength.

Diagnostic approach

Baseline and stimulation tests (see pages 102 and 106) define the extent of pituitary failure and include the following:

- Adrenocortical axis: serum cortisol (9 a.m.), short synacthen or insulin stress test and ACTH
- Thyroid axis: free T_4 and thyroid-stimulating hormone
- Gonadal axis: luteinising hormone and follicle stimulating hormone
  - Women: oestradiol
  - Men: testosterone (9 a.m.)

- Prolactin
- Insulin-like growth factor-1 and insulin stress test for growth hormone
- Paired serum and urine osmolality, and water deprivation test

In addition, a pituitary MRI helps define the cause of pituitary failure.

Management

Replacement therapy is usually achieved through the target hormone, e.g. hydrocortisone in ACTH deficiency, levothyroxine in thyroid-stimulating hormone deficiency and oestradiol (in women) or testosterone (in men) in luteinising hormone and follicle-stimulating hormone deficiency.

However, growth hormone is the hormone used for replacement (rather than the target hormone of insulin-like growth factor 1).

Medication

The aim of hormone replacement is to alleviate symptoms by titrating the dose of hormones to replicate normal physiology as closely as possible.

Hydrocortisone

Hydrocortisone (cortisol) is usually taken on waking, at lunchtime and in the early evening to best replicate normal physiological variation. In times of illness, doses need to be increased to compensate for the inability of the body to mount a stress response. If patients have diarrhoea or vomiting, they may not absorb oral hydrocortisone and will require a parenteral injection

Clinical features of hypopituitarism		
Hormone deficiency	Clinical features in adults	Clinical features in children
Adrenocorticotrophic hormone	Fatigue	Same as in adults, but hypoglycaemia is more prominent
	Weakness	
	Dizziness	
	Nausea	
	Vomiting	
	Weight loss	
	Myalgia	
	Hypoglycaemia	
Thyroid-stimulating hormone	Fatigue	Growth retardation
	Cold intolerance	Learning difficulties and delayed skeletal maturation
	Constipation	
	Weight gain	
	Dry skin	
Growth hormone	Impaired psychological well-being	Growth retardation
	Increased fat mass	
	Reduced muscle mass	
	Increased cardiovascular risk	
Luteinising hormone and follicle-stimulating hormone	Impaired fertility and amenorrhoea (women)	Delayed puberty
	Erectile dysfunction (men)	
	Anaemia	
	Reduced muscle mass and bone density	
Prolactin	Failure of lactation (women)	
Antidiuretic hormone	Nocturia	Enuresis (bed-wetting)
	Polyuria	
	Polydipsia	

Table 6.8 Clinical features of hypopituitarism

(usually intramuscular) to ensure that they have adequate systemic cortisol.

Hydrocortisone should always be replaced before levothyroxine. If levothyroxine is replaced before hydrocortisone it can precipitate a life-threatening adrenal crisis (see page 315).

The aims of treatment are to improve energy and well-being and to prevent adrenal crisis. The mineralocorticoid function of the adrenal gland is preserved in patients with hypopituitarism. Therefore, patients do not need fludrocortisone replacement (unlike in cases of primary adrenal failure).

If a patient forgets to take their hydrocortisone tablets when well, it is often inconsequential. However, if the patient is unwell, missing tablets usually leads to adrenal crisis.

Testosterone

Testosterone is usually replaced transdermally or intramuscularly, and oestrogen orally or transdermally with a patch. If fertility is desired, gonadotrophins or gonadotrophin-releasing hormones are used to restore spermatogenesis or ovulation. Aside from erectile function and libido, sex hormone replacement helps maintain bone integrity, muscle mass and normal erythropoiesis.

Growth hormone

Growth hormone replacement is given by subcutaneous injection. In children, the treatment is given to improve their final height. In adulthood, after the bones have fused, growth hormone also improves psychological well-being and increases muscle mass and bone density.

Levothyroxine

Thyroxine replacement is discussed in Chapter 5. In hypopituitarism (secondary hypothyroidism), serum thyroid-stimulating hormone is low, and its measurement is not helpful when titrating the dose of levothyroxine. Instead, serum free T4 is monitored to adjust the dose of levothyroxine in this condition. There is no clinical indication to replace prolactin.

Prognosis

Mortality in patients with hypopituitarism used to be significantly higher than in the general population. However, this is felt to have been the consequence of over-replacement with steroids and an association with growth hormone deficiency and increased mortality.

It is thought that patients on full pituitary hormone replacement may have approaching normal life expectancy, all be it with daily medication and regular medical reviews. They need medically supervised additional hormonal manipulation, particularly if they wish to achieve fertility (ovulation or spermatogenesis) and when they are unwell.

Non-functioning pituitary tumours

Non-functioning benign adenomas make up about half of all pituitary tumours. They are commonly an incidental finding when a scan is performed for another reason and may not require treatment. Although they don't produce excessive hormones (unlike prolactinomas, Cushing's disease and acromegaly) they can compress the normal pituitary, leading to deficiency of hormones (hypopituitarism).

Epidemiology

The incidence of pituitary tumours is increasing, because of their more frequent detection at the time of brain imaging for other reasons. At autopsy, about 10% of people are shown to have pituitary adenomas of up to 6 mm. Pituitary macroadenomas are defined as pituitary tumours > 1 cm.

The prevalence of pituitary adenomas is around 19–28 per 100,000 people in the UK. The reporting of incidence and prevalence depends on the amount of imaging done in different countries (as many are incidental findings), but pituitary adenomas have been found as an incidental finding in up to 27% of people.

Aetiology

A diagnosis of a non-functioning pituitary adenoma is often reached after excluding other secretory pituitary tumours and masses around the pituitary. A mass may be associated with normal pituitary function, or the patient may be hypopituitary.

Craniopharyngiomas are tumours deriving from the embryological tissue of the hypothalamus. They need to be differentiated from pituitary adenomas as they tend to require more radical surgery and radiotherapy than pituitary adenomas. This is particularly important in children and young adults when the brain is especially vulnerable and the minimum amount of treatment necessary to achieve a cure is indicated.

Pathogenesis

A non-functioning pituitary adenoma is usually an isolated finding. However, it is occasionally part of an inherited syndrome such as multiple endocrine neoplasia type 1 (see page 295) or familial pituitary adenomas.

Clinical features

Patients with non-functioning pituitary tumours may present with a visual field defect. The defect is usually bitemporal hemianopia caused by compression of the optic chiasm by an enlarging pituitary mass.

Alternatively, patients may have hormonal insufficiency (see page 230), have headaches or an incidental finding on brain imaging.

Investigations

Investigations are carried out to find out if hormones are deficient and whether the size of the lesion warrants surgical removal. The investigation has three parts:

- tests of pituitary function
- visual field tests
- MRI

Pituitary function is tested at baseline and when stimulated (see pages 102 and 106). Baseline tests are: prolactin, 9am cortisol, luteinising hormone and follicular stimulating hormone and oestradiol/testosterone, growth hormone and insulin-like growth factor 1, thyroid stimulating hormone and thyroxine and serum and urine osmolarity.

Stimulated tests are used for cortisol if the 9am cortisol is not sufficient to rule out deficiency. Stimulation tests are rarely used for the other pituitary hormones as basal (baseline) levels are sufficient to make a diagnosis.

Visual field testing is done to check for a visual defect. Such defects develop because of compression of the optic chiasm.

Magnetic resonance imaging of the pituitary gland is necessary to visualise the extent of the lesion and to guide surgery. Regular scans are done to detect any tumour growth.

Management

In cases of non-functioning pituitary adenoma, surgery is needed only to relieve the consequences of a mass effect, such as a threat to vision from compression of the optic chiasm (apparent either at presentation or during follow-up surveillance). In the absence of optic atrophy, vision is frequently restored postoperatively, so it is essential to assess patients quickly.

As well as normalising vision, resection of a non-functioning tumour occasionally improves hormonal function. Therefore patients' pituitary function should be retested postoperatively.

Frequently there is tumour regrowth and radiotherapy is then offered.

Conservative management is common for non-functioning pituitary adenomas. Patients may decide against an operation even if there are signs of progression, that threatens vision, especially if the risks of surgery are considered significant or the patient is very elderly. Patients need to feel informed when making their choice. Some patients still want a physician to make the decision for them.

Prognosis

Patients may be deficient in individual hormones (partial), or all hormones (panhypopituitary). However, these hormones can be replaced and patients should expect to live a normal life (page 231). It is often difficult to remove all the abnormal cells, so there is a chance of tumour regrowth. For this reason, all patients are reviewed annually or more frequently if there is a large amount of residual tumour.

Diabetes insipidus

Diabetes insipidus is characterised by excessive thirst and the passage of large amounts of dilute urine. The patient's body is unable to concentrate the urine if water intake is restricted.

Types and aetiology

Diabetes insipidus is either cranial or nephrogenic.

Cranial diabetes insipidus is caused by decreased secretion of antidiuretic hormone by the neurosecretory cells in the hypothalamus (which is then stored in the posterior pituitary).

Nephrogenic diabetes insipidus results from resistance to the action of antidiuretic hormone in the kidney, which leads to dilute urine. The main causes of the condition are shown in **Table 6.9**. Antidiuretic hormone deficiency is a common presenting manifestation of conditions that infiltrate the hypothalamus or pituitary, such as germ cell tumours, pituitary metastases and granulomatous disorders.

Epidemiology

The annual incidence of diabetes insipidus is 3 in 100,000. The condition affects both sexes equally and can occur at any age.

Pathogenesis

The hypothalamus produces antidiuretic hormone in the supraoptic and paraventricular nuclei. The hormone is transported to the posterior pituitary gland for storage.

Antidiuretic hormone is released in response to increased plasma osmolarity or decreased extracellular fluid volume. It binds to receptors in the collecting tubule of the kidney, thus increasing water permeability and therefore reabsorption. The responses of the baroreceptors and hypothalamus to reduced extracellular fluid volume are shown in **Figure 6.9**.

Diabetes insipidus rarely (incidence of 2 per 100 000 pregnancies) occurs in pregnancy. The condition is thought to arise from the production of vasopressinase in the placenta, because vasopressinase breaks down antidiuretic hormone.

Established diabetes insipidus worsens in pregnancy. To control their symptoms, many women with a diagnosis of diabetes insipidus will need an increase in their desmopressin dose during pregnancy to ensure that their replacement therapy remains adequate.

Clinical features

Diabetes insipidus is characterised by excessive thirst and an inability to concentrate the urine. Therefore the body generates an excessive amount of dilute urine (> 3 L/day).

Nocturia is a common presenting symptom in adults. In children, typical symptoms are enuresis (bed-wetting), fatigue and growth delay.

When taking a history of nocturia, establish the volume of fluid passed and whether the patient is thirsty. If a patient has a condition that increases urine volume, and therefore dehydrates them, they will report drinking large amounts at every opportunity, even at night, to satisfy their thirst.

Main causes of diabetes insipidus	
Cranial	Nephrogenic
Idiopathic	Chronic renal failure
Tumours of the pituitary or hypothalamus	Lithium toxicity
Cranial surgery	Hypercalcaemia
Head trauma	Hypokalaemia
Infections (e.g. meningitis and encephalitis)	Glycosuria (glucose in the urine)
Granulomatous diseases (e.g. neurosarcoid or tuberculosis)	Tubulointerstitial disease

Table 6.9 Main causes of diabetes insipidus

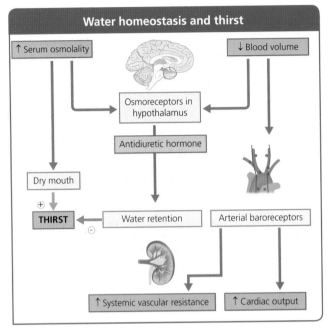

Figure 6.9 Water homeostasis. When dry, signals from the arterial baroreceptors and osmoreceptors in the hypothalamus cause vasoconstriction, increased cardiac output and concentration of the urine (via increased antidiuretic hormone, ADH). Responding to thirst helps to restore the normal equilibrium.

Diagnostic approach

The approach to diagnosis focuses on:

- excluding conditions that cause an osmotic diuresis (e.g. uncontrolled diabetes mellitus)
- establishing if excessive urine volume (>3 L/24 h) is present (not just increased urinary frequency)
- arranging further tests to establish the ability to concentrate urine

The results of these further tests are used to differentiate cranial diabetes insipidus, nephrogenic diabetes insipidus and primary polydipsia (excessive thirst).

Investigations

After establishing that the urine volume is excessive, the key is to see whether a patient is able to concentrate their own urine (if denied water) and if not, whether the addition of desmopressin can help. A 24-h urine volume of >3 L, or a urine output of >200 mL/h for two consecutive hours, is considered excessive. Serum sodium concentration may be at the upper end of the reference range or high, and urea is increased.

Paired urine and serum tests

Concentrated serum osmolarity (>295 mOsm/kg) paired with dilute urine osmolarity (<300 mOsm/kg) strongly suggests diabetes insipidus. Conversely, in primary polydipsia (or psychogenic polydipsia; see Chapter 2), serum and urine osmolarity and sodium are likely to be low.

Water deprivation test

This test is used to confirm a diagnosis of diabetes insipidus and to differentiate between cranial and nephrogenic diabetes insipidus (see page 108). The administration of desmopressin distinguishes between cranial and nephrogenic diabetes insipidus, because patients with the latter condition have very little response to the drug.

Once cranial diabetes insipidus is diagnosed, the cause is investigated with a thorough clinical examination (including breast examination as cancer can metastasise to the pituitary causing diabetes insipidus). Furthermore, MRI is required to identify pituitary or hypothalamic pathology.

Management

Desmopressin is administered subcutaneously, nasally or orally. It has an almost instant effect in cranial diabetes insipidus; it seems to 'switch off' or minimise urine output.

In the presence of normal thirst, the body adapts and regulates its intake. However, severe hypothalamic damage may cause failure of the 'thirst centre'; the resulting loss of thirst in affected patients means that they require a fixed input and output of fluid.

If a patient has nephrogenic diabetes insipidus, the cause must be addressed. For example, any causative drug such as Lithium is discontinued. Nephrogenic diabetes insipidus tends to be resistant to treatment but sometimes responds to indomethacin or bendroflumethiazide.

Prognosis

Cranial diabetes insipidus responds well to desmopressin. However, the underlying pituitary or hypothalamic pathology is what will determine the prognosis.

Answers to starter questions

1. Breastfeeding causes an elevation in serum prolactin which suppresses gonadotrophins and consequently ovulation. However, it is not a reliable method of contraception and many women become pregnant before their menstrual cycles resume.

2. Benign pituitary tumours rarely metastasise, but they can compress normal pituitary tissue causing life-threatening hormone deficiencies. Compression of other surrounding structures can cause visual failure, cerebrospinal fluid leaks (and meningitis) and affect breathing and consciousness. Acutely, large tumours occasionally cause hemorrhage or infarctions (pituitary apoplexy).

3. Final height is mainly determined by genetic factors (particularly the height of the parents), nutrition and chronic disease in childhood. All pituitary hormones play a role in normal growth. Although there are no clear differences in serum concentrations of these hormones between individuals, children with idiopathic short stature usually increase their final height by supplementing growth hormone, even if there is no deficiency detectable. Delaying puberty with hormones also gives extra time for additional height spurts before the bones fuse.

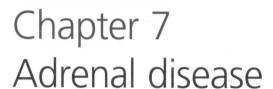

Chapter 7
Adrenal disease

Starter questions

Answers to the following questions are on page 253.

1. How do Cushing's disease and Cushing's syndrome differ?
2. What happens when both adrenal glands are removed?
3. Why is adrenal transplantation not a good treatment for Addison's disease?
4. What is adrenal fatigue?
5. Can adrenal failure due to Addison's disease be prevented?

Introduction

The two adrenal glands are situated at the superior pole of the kidneys. They contain three hormone secreting layers. The adrenal glands produce steroid hormones (i.e. cortisol, aldosterone, androgens) and catecholamines (adrenaline and nor-adrenaline) that are essential for normal development and the maintenance of health.

Congenital absences of enzymes of the steroid synthesis pathway, such as in con-genital adrenal hyperplasia, can cause life-threatening illness at birth. In later life, hypo- and hyperproduction of cortisol can result in Addison's disease and Cushing's syndrome, respectively. Benign and malignant tumours can arise from the adrenal glands, and both types can secrete an excessive amount of adrenal hormones. For example, phaeochromocytomas secrete excess adrenaline (epinephrine).

Case 7 Headaches and profuse sweating

Presentation

Mrs Adams, aged 45 years, is referred to the endocrinology outpatient clinic with a 6-month history of intermittent episodes of headaches associated with profuse sweating. Her general practitioner notes that she has also developed hypertension.

Initial interpretation

There are several different causes of excessive sweating (**Table 7.1**) and headaches for a woman in her forties. The symptoms need to be explored further.

Headaches in association with sweating rarely indicate a less common diagnosis, such as phaeochromocytoma or intracranial tumour. The association with hypertension raises the suspicion of an endocrine cause for these symptoms.

Sweating associated with weight loss and fatigue raises the possibility of thyrotoxicosis, malignancy or chronic infection. The absence of weight loss potentially narrows down the differential diagnosis.

Further history

Mrs Adams explains that she has had episodes of headaches and sweating for many months that occur together. At these times, she also feels anxious and can feel her heart racing. The episodes are unpredictable and can occur day or night.

Since the headaches and sweating started, she has not experienced any weight loss or other symptoms of infection. However, she says that she has some abdominal pain and occasionally diarrhoea. She is still having regular menstrual periods and has two adult children, both of whom are well.

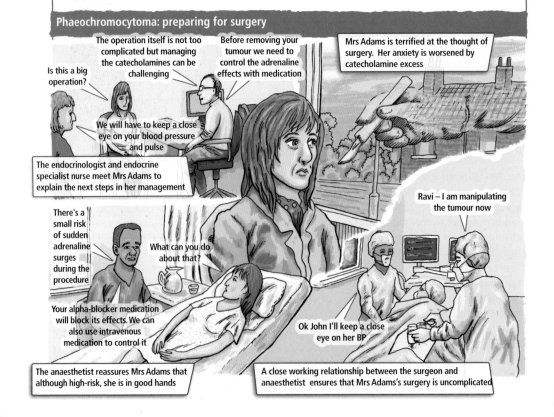

Phaeochromocytoma: preparing for surgery

Is this a big operation?

The operation itself is not too complicated but managing the catecholamines can be challenging

Before removing your tumour we need to control the adrenaline effects with medication

Mrs Adams is terrified at the thought of surgery. Her anxiety is worsened by catecholamine excess

We will have to keep a close eye on your blood pressure and pulse

The endocrinologist and endocrine specialist nurse meet Mrs Adams to explain the next steps in her management

Ravi – I am manipulating the tumour now

There's a small risk of sudden adrenaline surges during the procedure

What can you do about that?

Your alpha-blocker medication will block its effects. We can also use intravenous medication to control it

Ok John I'll keep a close eye on her BP

The anaesthetist reassures Mrs Adams that although high-risk, she is in good hands

A close working relationship between the surgeon and anaesthetist ensures that Mrs Adams's surgery is uncomplicated

Case 7 *continued*

Causes of sweating	
Endocrine	**Non-endocrine**
Thyrotoxicosis	Infection (e.g. tuberculosis and infective endocarditis)
Menopause	Haematological malignancy (e.g. lymphoma)
Phaeochromocytoma	Solid organ malignancy (e.g. renal cell carcinoma)
Hypoglycaemia (e.g. insulinoma, exogenous insulin and use of oral hypoglycaemic drugs)	Certain drugs (e.g. selective serotonin reuptake inhibitors and opiates)
Acromegaly	Autonomic neuropathy (e.g. secondary to excessive alcohol intake or diabetes mellitus)
Carcinoid syndrome	Psychiatric disorder (e.g. anxiety)
Obesity	Idiopathic hyperhidrosis

Table 7.1 Endocrine and non-endocrine causes of sweating

Mrs Adams has no noteworthy past medical history and is on no regular medication. She drinks a bottle of wine per week and does not smoke. Her father had a 'kidney tumour' that was removed in middle age.

She had initially put her symptoms down to stress at work. However, her husband has been worried about her, so she sought help.

Examination

The results of examination are unremarkable except for tachycardia at rest (110 beats/min) and high blood pressure (172/96 mmHg). There is no tremor, and thyroid examination is normal.

Interpretation of findings

Hyperthyroidism is common in women of Mrs Adams's age and can cause sweating and tachycardia. However, the condition

is usually associated with tremor, weight loss and oligomenorrhoea, none of which are present in this case.

The maintenance of regular periods excludes menopause and makes thyrotoxicosis unlikely. Her family history of a kidney tumour is relevant as some forms of phaeochromocytoma are familial. Both of her children, however, are well and not affected. She is not taking any medication or alcohol, both of which could have been causing her symptoms as a side-effect.

The most likely diagnosis is phaeochromocytoma, because of the combination of headaches, profuse sweating, palpitations and new onset hypertension. Simple tests to rule out inflammatory conditions (full blood count and

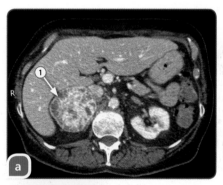

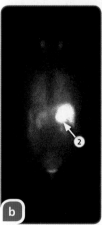

Figure 7.1 Phaeochromocytoma. (a) Computerised tomography shows a 6-cm right adrenal mass ① just anterior to the upper pole of the right kidney. (b) The same right adrenal mass ②, with avid tracer uptake in an iodine-131 meta-iodobenzylguanidine (MIBG) scan (posterior view).

Case 7 *continued*

measurement of C-reactive protein concentration) would be helpful. Other endocrine conditions to exclude are the menopause and carcinoid syndrome.

Investigations

Metadrenaline (metanephrine) and normetadrenaline (normetanephrine) are the breakdown products of adrenaline (epinephrine) and noradrenaline (norepinephrine), respectively. Mrs Adams has elevated plasma and urinary concentrations of metadrenaline and normetadrenaline which is highly specific for phaeochromocytoma and confirm its diagnosis. Full blood count, C-reactive protein and thyroid function tests are normal.

Computerised tomography (CT) of the adrenal glands is performed to discover if there is evidence of an adrenal tumour and shows a 6-cm lesion in the right adrenal (**Figure 7.1a**). The activity of this mass is confirmed by avid uptake of tracer in an iodine-131 meta-iodobenzylguanidine (MIBG) scintiscan (**Figure 7.1b**).

Diagnosis

The diagnosis of phaeochromocytoma resulting from an adrenal medulla tumour is confirmed by the presence of excess catecholamines and the active adrenal tumour on imaging. The next step is to commence her on alpha-blocker medication and prepare her for a right adrenalectomy.

Addison's disease

Addison's disease, also called primary adrenal insufficiency, is a disorder of the adrenal glands. It is caused by total or near-total destruction of the adrenal cortex by various pathological processes. The resulting deficiency of cortisol (a glucocorticoid) and aldosterone (a mineralocorticoid) leads to clinical disease characterised by weight loss, fatigue, hypotension and addisonian crisis.

Epidemiology

The prevalence of Addison's disease is about 100 per million people in Western Europe and the USA. Its worldwide incidence is unknown.

Aetiology

Causes of Addison's disease are shown in **Table 7.2**. Before the advent of antibiotics and immunisation programmes, the commonest cause of Addison's disease was adrenal cortex destruction by tuberculosis (**Figure 7.2**).

Since the 1950s, the commonest cause in high-income countries has been autoimmune adrenalitis.

In autoimmune adrenalitis, the body has an autoimmune response to the adrenal cortex and the enzymes it produces. The precipitant for the autoimmune reaction is unknown but there is a genetic element as autoimmune endocrinopathies tend to run in families. Autoimmune adrenalitis occurs in isolation or in association with other endocrinopathies.

Pathogenesis

Cortisol and aldosterone deficiency can occur gradually. Therefore Addison's disease may go unrecognised and untreated for years.

A stressful event may precipitate acute addisonian crises in a patient with the condition (see Chapter 11). The stress is often infection but can also be any severe physiological or psychological stress, including surgery or trauma.

Causes of Addison's disease	
Type	**Examples**
Autoimmune	Isolated autoimmune Addison's disease
	Autoimmune polyglandular syndrome type 1: ■ hypoparathyroidism ■ mucocutaneous candidiasis ■ type 1 diabetes ■ autoimmune hypothyroidism
	Autoimmune polyglandular syndrome type 2: ■ type 1 diabetes ■ autoimmune thyroid disease ■ primary ovarian failure
Infective or inflammatory	Tuberculosis
	Histoplasmosis
	AIDS-associated infections (e.g. cytomegalovirus)
Adrenal haemorrhage	Clotting disorders or over-anticoagulation
	Waterhouse-Friderichsen syndrome (secondary to meningococcal septicaemia)
Adrenal destruction	Bilateral adrenalectomy
	Bilateral adrenal metastases
	Bilateral adrenal infarction (associated with antiphospholipid syndrome)
Genetic or developmental	Congenital adrenal hyperplasia
	Adrenoleucodystrophy
	Adrenal hypoplasia congenita

Table 7.2 Causes of Addison's disease

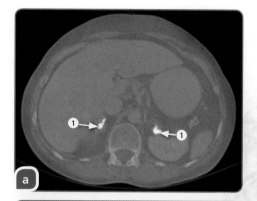

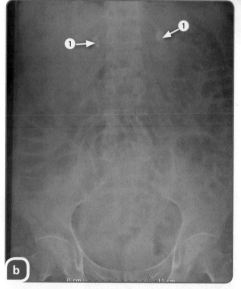

Figure 7.2 (a) Transverse section of computerised tomography and (b) anteroposterior plain X-ray of ① adrenal calcification in a patient with Addison's disease secondary to adrenal tuberculosis.

The stress results in acute cortisol deficiency. Cortisol deficiency, in turn, leads to circulatory collapse, shock, organ hypoperfusion and ultimately death. Cortisol deficiency resulting from adrenal failure releases the hypothalamus and pituitary gland from negative feedback, so more adrenocorticotrophic hormone (ACTH) is produced (**Figure 7.3**).

Clinical features

The clinical features of Addison's disease include manifestations of chronic glucocorticoid and mineralocorticoid deficiency:

■ fatigue
■ weight loss
■ muscle weakness
■ reduced appetite
■ salt craving
■ abdominal pain
■ nausea and vomiting

Postural hypotension is often present because of whole body water depletion. Postural hypotension causes the symptoms of dizziness on standing up from a sitting or supine position.

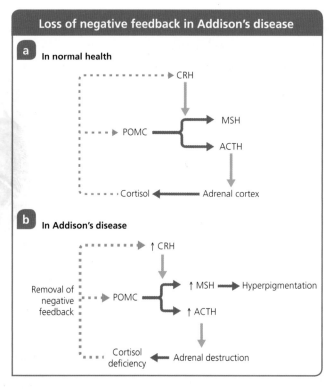

Figure 7.3 Loss of negative feedback in Addison's disease. (a) In normal health, corticotrophin-releasing hormone (CRH) stimulates the conversion of pro-opiomelanocortin (POMC) to melanocyte-stimulating hormone (MSH) and adrenocorticotrophic hormone (ACTH). ACTH stimulates adrenal cortex to secrete cortisol, which has negative feedback on the pituitary and hypothalamus. (b) Adrenal cortex destruction in Addison's disease leads to the loss of negative feedback to the hypothalamus and pituitary gland, resulting in excess CRH and ACTH production. MSH is cosecreted in excess, causing hyperpigmentation.

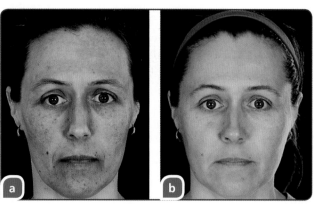

Figure 7.4 Hyperpigmentation in Addison's disease. (a) Before treatment. (b) After treatment with hydrocortisone for cortisol replacement.

A by-product of excess ACTH production is melanocyte-stimulating hormone (the hormone that controls skin pigment deposition). Therefore patients with Addison's disease appear hyperpigmented (**Figure 7.4**). Hyperpigmentation is most obvious in the palmar creases and buccal mucosa, as well as in old scars (Figure 2.9).

Biochemically, the deficiency of aldosterone is indicated by hyponatraemia, hyperkalaemia and mild metabolic acidosis (although this is not always present). Glucocorticoid deficiency may lead to hypoglycaemia.

Addisonian crisis

This is the term used to describe a life-threatening cortisol deficiency (see page 315). An addisonian crisis results from profound cortisol deficiency, often precipitated by concurrent acute infection. Patients present in shock, which is often refractory to intravenous fluid administration.

An addisonian crisis occurs when steroids suppress the hypothalamic–pituitary–adrenal axis enough to cause adrenal failure. Chronic use of oral, inhaled or parenteral glucocorticoids can cause irreversible adrenal suppression. If therapeutic glucocorticoids are used for a prolonged period at a high dose, the dose must be reduced slowly; abrupt cessation can cause an addisonian crisis.

Diagnostic approach

Addison's disease is often suspected in patients with non-specific symptoms such as fatigue and weight loss, especially when other autoimmune endocrinopathies are present.

When an addisonian crisis is suspected, treatment should be immediate. High-dose hydrocortisone is administered. Definitive investigations can always be done in more controlled conditions at a later date.

Investigations

Cortisol release from the adrenal gland is pulsatile and shows diurnal variation, so random measurement of serum cortisol concentration is not particularly useful in the diagnosis of Addison's disease. Cortisol production peaks early in the morning. Therefore a 9 a.m. serum cortisol concentration >550 nmol/L virtually excludes the diagnosis of adrenal insufficiency, but a value of <100 nmol/L strongly supports it.

Plasma aldosterone concentration is low and plasma renin activity high in Addison's disease, unlike in secondary adrenal deficiency when aldosterone production is preserved.

Adrenocorticotrophic hormone stimulation test

As in other hormone deficiencies, a hormone stimulation test is required to diagnose Addison's disease. The short Synacthen (tetracosactide) test is used (see page 106). In adrenal insufficiency, the cortisol level fails to rise above 550 nmol/L after the tetracosactide stimulation.

Endogenous adrenocorticotrophic hormone (ACTH) is measured concurrently with baseline cortisol.

- A high concentration of ACTH in a patient with adrenal insufficiency is consistent with Addison's disease, because of the loss of negative feedback of cortisol to the pituitary gland and consequent increase in ACTH production
- Low or normal ACTH raises the possibility of secondary adrenal insufficiency resulting from pituitary or hypothalamic disorders

Autoantibody tests

To investigate the cause of Addison's disease, antiadrenal antibodies are measured.

- A positive result confirms autoimmune adrenalitis; antibodies to enzymes in the steroid synthesis pathway and to the adrenal cortex itself are detectable in most patients with the condition
- Alternative diagnoses are considered if the results are negative

Measurement of very–long-chain fatty acid concentration

Adrenoleucodystrophy is ruled out in male patients with a negative result for antiadrenal antibodies. This is done by testing for very–long-chain fatty acid concentrations which are elevated in this condition. This rare, X-linked recessive condition causes adrenal failure and also affects the myelin sheaths of the nerves, with neurological consequences.

Addison's disease is a potentially serious but treatable condition. Although clinical suspicion should be high in patients with non-specific symptoms and hyponatraemia, the vast majority of patients will have normal adrenal function, but Addison's disease is a diagnosis not to be missed.

Management

Addison's disease requires long-term management with corticosteroids and mineralocorticoids.

- Cortisol replacement is typically achieved with hydrocortisone 10 mg on waking, 5 mg at midday and 5 mg in the early evening; this dosage pattern attempts to mimic the normal diurnal release of cortisol
- Mineralocorticoid is replaced by synthetic aldosterone, namely fludrocortisone

The dose of hydrocortisone used for cortisol replacement in Addison's disease is adjusted to the well-being and clinical response of each patient. Measurement of ACTH is not useful when determining the dose (compared to monitoring of thyroid hormone replacement in primary hypothyroidism when TSH measurement is routine).

The lowest dose possible is used, because long-term-over-replacement of corticosteroids leads to adverse metabolic consequences. These include diabetes mellitus, weight gain and hypertension.

Patient education is vital for the self-management of Addison's disease (**Table 7.3**). Patients should be reminded of the the importance of adhering to treatment as well as increasing the dose of glucocorticoid during illness and stress.

For management of addisonian crisis, see Chapter 11.

Prognosis

With adequate hormone replacement, most people with Addison's disease feel well. However, they are reported to have a reduced quality of life, as measured by quality-of-life questionnaires. This may be because cortisol replacement with oral hydrocortisone does not closely mimic natural cortisol production.

Advice for patients with Addison's disease
■ Ensure that you take prescribed corticosteroids every day
■ Carry a MedicAlert bracelet and steroid card to alert others to the diagnosis in emergency situations
■ Double the dose of corticosteroid when unwell (e.g. when you have an infection) until your condition improves
■ Keep a stock of parenteral (intramuscular) steroids to use if your body is unable to absorb oral corticosteroids (e.g. if you are vomiting or have diarrhoea)
■ Always inform healthcare professionals of your diagnosis of Addison's disease
■ Avoid running out of steroids; always have a spare prescription

Table 7.3 Advice given to patients with Addison's disease

Conn's syndrome

Conn's syndrome, also called primary hyperaldosteronism, is aldosterone excess caused by a unilateral benign adrenal adenoma or bilateral adrenal hyperplasia, resulting in hypertension. The excessive production of aldosterone is independent of the usual feedback mechanisms involving renin and angiotensin. Conn's syndrome often goes unrecognised in the huge number of patients with primary hypertension, which has multiple causes (**Table 7.4**).

Epidemiology

Conn's syndrome is thought to affect about one person per million in a year. This figure is likely to be an underestimate, because the condition often goes unrecognised.

Causes of systemic hypertension	
Non-endocrine	Endocrine
Essential hypertension	Conn's syndrome
Renal causes (e.g. polycystic kidney disease and chronic kidney disease)	Phaeochromocytoma
Vascular causes (e.g. vasculitis, renal artery stenosis and coarctation of the aorta)	Cushing's syndrome
Neurological causes (e.g. cerebral tumours)	Some forms of congenital adrenal hyperplasia
Inherited syndromes (e.g. Liddle's syndrome)	Hormone replacement therapy
Certain drugs (e.g. non-steroidal anti-inflammatory drugs and alcohol)	Acromegaly

Table 7.4 Causes of systemic hypertension

Aetiology

The syndrome which was originally described as being caused by a unilateral benign adrenal adenoma, is now also known to be caused by bilateral adrenal hyperplasia or, rarely, adrenocortical carcinomas. The exact prevalence of each of these pathologies is unclear. Excessive aldosterone production causes renal sodium retention, which is balanced by the loss of potassium and hydrogen ions in the distal convoluted tubule of the kidney. Excessive sodium retention leads to extracellular volume expansion and hypertension.

Clinical features

Hypertension is the predominant feature of Conn's syndrome. It may be severe or uncontrolled by multiple drug treatments. Hypokalaemia occurs in only half of cases and is associated with metabolic alkalosis. Other possible complications are those associated with:

- hypertension (e.g. headaches and retinopathy)
- hypokalaemia (e.g. paraesthesia, weakness and cardiac arrhythmias)

Diagnostic approach

Hypertension is common, and an endocrine cause is unlikely for each individual. However, the following features raise the suspicion of Conn's syndrome.

- Severe hypertension: blood pressure > 180/100 mmHg or hypertension that is difficult to control despite the use of multiple anti-hypertensive agents
- Hypertension occurring at a young age (about 20–40 years)
- Hypertension with spontaneous or diuretic-induced hypokalaemia
- Hypertension in patients with coexisting adrenal adenomas or hyperplasia

Routine screening for Conn's syndrome in patients with hypertension has very low detection rates and is not recommended. However, patients with early onset hypertension; severe or treatment resistance hypertension; hypertension and hypokalaemia; or hypertension and adrenal adenoma or hyperplasia should undergo testing for the condition.

Investigations

Conn's syndrome is confirmed by the results of biochemical tests and imaging studies which determine the source of the excess aldosterone.

Blood tests

If Conn's syndrome is suspected, the initial investigation is calculation of the aldosterone:renin ratio, which is increased in patients with the condition. Antihypertensive drugs affect the results, especially beta-blockers and aldosterone antagonists (i.e. spironolactone) which are discontinued several weeks before the test. Furthermore, potassium supplements are used to normalise serum potassium before measurement of aldosterone and renin, because hypokalaemia inhibits aldosterone production. In addition, patients are told not to restrict their salt intake prior to the test and additional salt tablets (or a saline infusion) are occasionally given.

Imaging

If the blood test results show an increased aldosterone:renin ratio, a CT scan of the adrenal glands is done to confirm the presence of an adrenal tumour. If a unilateral adrenal adenoma is found adrenal venous sampling confirms that the mass seen on CT is responsible for the excess production of aldosterone. In this radiological procedure, aldosterone samples are taken from each of the adrenal veins and the peripheral venous blood to determine whether one or both adrenals are secretory.

Management

The treatment of Conn's syndrome is determined by the cause of hyperaldosteronism. Unilateral tumours are treatable with unilateral adrenalectomy. Bilateral disease is managed with medication (as bilateral adrenalectomy would render the patient permanently cortisol and aldosterone deficient).

Medication

This is the first-line treatment for Conn's syndrome:

- when the cause is bilateral adrenal hyperplasia
- in patients with an adrenal adenoma but who are unfit for or unwilling to undergo adrenalectomy

Aldosterone antagonists are effective; spironolactone therapy is the first-line treatment. The dose of spironolactone is often limited by its adverse effects, notably gynaecomastia, which occurs in half of men and is dose-dependent. Other antihypertensive drugs, such as calcium channel blockers, may be required in addition to lifestyle measures such as exercise and weight loss.

Surgery

In cases of unilateral adrenal adenoma, laparoscopic adrenalectomy is curative and therefore the treatment of choice. Aldosterone antagonists are discontinued at the time of surgery.

Prognosis

In bilateral adrenal hyperplasia, the prognosis depends on the adequacy of control of hypertension. Poorly controlled hypertension leads to cardiovascular complications, but the adverse effects of the anti-hypertensives used to treat Conn's disease may also cause morbidity.

Phaeochromocytoma

A phaeochromocytoma is a tumour of the adrenal medulla that secretes excessive catecholamines: adrenaline (epinephrine), noradrenaline (noradrenaline) and, rarely, dopamine. Catecholamine-secreting tumours of the sympathetic and parasympathetic chain have similar clinical presentations and are termed extraadrenal paragangliomas.

Epidemiology

These are rare tumours, with an annual incidence of 2–8 cases per million people in the UK. Phaeochromocytomas occur most commonly in middle age.

Aetiology

Ninety percent of phaechromocytomas are benign. Bilateral phaeochromocytomas are present in 10% of cases.

Recent advances in gene mapping have indicated a hereditary cause for phaechromocytomas in a quarter of cases. Genetic syndromes causing phaeochromocytoma are detailed in **Table 7.5**.

Clinical features

The paroxysmal release of catecholamines causes intermittent signs and symptoms, including:

- anxiety
- headache
- palpitations
- sweating
- hypertension (which may be paroxysmal or absent) and hypertensive crisis
- tachycardia
- pallor

Genetic syndromes associated with phaeochromocytoma	
Syndrome	Other clinical features
Von Hippel-Lindau disease	Cerebral haemangioblastoma
	Renal angiomas and renal cell carcinoma
	Pancreatic tumours
Neurofibromatosis type 1 (von Recklinghausen's disease)	Cutaneous neurofibromas
	Neural fibromas
	Café-au-lait spots
Multiple endocrine neoplasia type 2a	Medullary thyroid carcinoma
	Primary hyperparathyroidism
Multiple endocrine neoplasia type 2b	Marfanoid appearance
	Mucosal neuromas
	Medullary thyroid carcinoma
Paraganglioma syndrome (mutations of the SDHB and SDHD genes)	Paragangliomas (carotid body tumours)

Table 7.5 Genetic syndromes associated with phaeochromocytoma. SDHB, succinate dehydrogenase B; SDHD, succinate dehydrogenase D

> **Not all patients with phaeochromocytoma are symptomatic.** A quarter of cases are discovered during investigation for incidental adrenal adenomas identified through imaging studies done for another reason.

Diagnostic approach

Diagnosis of phaeochromocytoma requires biochemical evidence of plasma or urine catecholamine excess, followed by imaging to localise the tumour.

Investigations

Urine collections for catecholamines or their metabolites (metadrenaline and normetadrenaline) are often used as a first-line screening test for those with clinical features of phaeochromocytoma or those who had had an incidentally-discovered adrenal adenoma through CT imaging of the abdomen.

Biochemical investigations

Urine or plasma samples are used for biochemical tests for the breakdown products of adrenaline (epinephrine) and noradrenaline (norepinephrine), namely metadrenaline (metanephrine) and normetadrenaline (normetanephrine), respectively.

- 24-h urine metadrenaline and normetadrenaline collection is necessary as the production of catecholmaines varies during the day as a result of physiological stress and actively. Total urinary metadrenaline and normetadrenaline levels are elevated in phaeochromocytoma.
- Plasma tests for metadrenaline and normetadrenaline have a higher sensitivity rate than urine metadrenaline and normetadrenaline tests and therefore are a good screening test for cases in which there is a high index of suspicion (e.g. in suspected familial phaeochromocytomas).

Imaging

Most adrenal tumours are identified by CT or magnetic resonance imaging of the abdomen. If no adrenal tumour is detected, imaging of the entire sympathetic chain is necessary to identify paragangliomas (**Figure 7.5**). To confirm the functionality of an identified lesion, functional imaging with iodine-131 MIBG scintiscan is required (Figure 2.31).

Management

Patients with confirmed phaeochromocytoma must be stabilised on medication to prevent hypertensive crisis. Definitive surgical treatment is considered once patients are established on medical treatment.

Medication

Blockade of α-adrenoceptors, with phenoxybenzamine or doxazosin, must be started first to control peripheral vasoconstriction and hypertension. Beta-blockade, with propranolol or bisoprolol, prevents tachycardia and can be started only when adequate alpha-blockade is achieved.

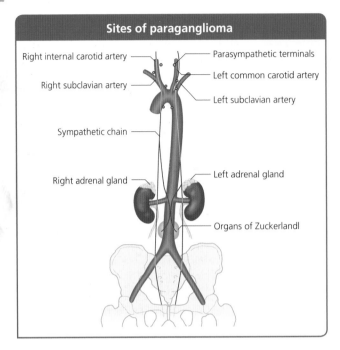

Sites of paraganglioma

Right internal carotid artery

Parasympathetic terminals

Left common carotid artery

Right subclavian artery

Left subclavian artery

Sympathetic chain

Right adrenal gland

Left adrenal gland

Organs of Zuckerlandl

Figure 7.5 Paraganglioma may arise at parasympathetic or sympathetic sites. Therefore imaging must include a view from the skull base to the lower pole of the pelvis.

- Alpha-blockers are used to control blood pressure
- Beta-blockers are used to control pulse rate

> **If beta-blockers were to be started before adequate alpha-blockade, this could lead to massive vasoconstriction and a hypertensive crisis.** The resulting pulmonary oedema or intracranial haemorrhage could be life-threatening.

Surgery

Surgical removal of phaeochromocytomas is risky in patients with inadequate alpha- and beta-blockade because of the potential for massive catecholamine release resulting in a hypertensive crisis. Surgery is either performed by laparoscopic or open approaches, depending upon the size of the tumour.

Prognosis

Untreated and undiagnosed phaeochromocytomas can cause life-threatening complications, such as:

- hypertensive crisis
- stroke
- cardiac complications (e.g. arrhythmia, cardiac failure and myocardial infarction)

Surgical resection is usually curative. However, long-term clinical and biochemical surveillance is necessary because of the 10% risk of malignancy, which is often difficult to determine histologically.

Congenital adrenal hyperplasia

Congenital adrenal hyperplasia (CAH) is a group of autosomal recessive conditions in which varying degrees of enzyme deficiency in the steroid synthesis pathway result in deficiency of cortisol or aldosterone, or both, as well as androgen excess. The most common form of congenital adrenal hyperplasia is a consequence of 21-hydroxylase deficiency and accounts for 90% of cases.

Epidemiology

Congenital adrenal hyperplasia affects about 1 in 18,000 newborn babies in the UK population. The worldwide prevalence varies greatly depending on the ethnic groups such as Ashkenazi Jews in whom non-classical CAH occurs in 1 in 27.

Clinical features

Complete enzyme deficiency (classical congenital adrenal hyperplasia) results in cortisol and aldosterone deficiency occurring soon after birth. This is termed a salt-wasting crisis and manifests as:

- dehydration
- hypotension
- tachycardia
- hyponatraemia

Partial enzyme deficiency results in simple virilising disease. This presents as androgen excess in females, leading to virilisation (development of clitoromegaly due to the effects of excessive androgens) and ambiguous genitalia but without salt wasting.

Non-classical congenital adrenal hyperplasia (mild partial enzyme deficiency) can present with hirsutism or subfertility in adolescence or adulthood.

> **Non-classical congenital adrenal hyperplasia is sometimes diagnosed during the investigation of primary amenorrhoea or subfertility.** The condition is characterised by increased plasma 17-hydroxyprogesterone.

Diagnostic approach

The diagnosis of congenital adrenal hyperplasia is based on increased concentrations of adrenal hormone precursors, such as 17-hydoxyprogesterone. This finding may be combined with biochemical signs of cortisol and aldosterone deficiency (hyperkalaemia and hyponatraemia) in classical congenital adrenal hyperplasia.

Management

In salt-wasting classical congenital adrenal hyperplasia, corticosteroid, mineralocorticoid and fluid replacement are the mainstays of emergency treatment and are life-saving. Corticosteroid replacement suppresses natural adrenal corticosteroid synthesis (by suppressing ACTH stimulation), thereby reducing the supraphysiological androgen production (page 38).

> **Testicular adrenal rest tumours (TART) arise in embryonic remnants of adrenal tissue. They occur in the testes** of adults with CAH and are usually bilateral. These tumours are benign and shrink with an increased dose of glucocorticoids. However, if unrecognised, they can be mistaken for testicular malignancy, resulting in unnecessary orchidectomy.

Medication

Glucocorticoid replacement is administered in the form of hydrocortisone, prednisolone or dexamethasone. Aldosterone replacement is given in the form of fludrocortisone to reduce postural hypotension and maintain replete sodium stores.

Surgery

Reconstructive urological surgery is performed in individuals in whom CAH has resulted in the formation of ambiguous genitalia or virilisation.

Prognosis

This depends on the balance between achieving adequate androgen suppression and minimising the effects of excess glucocorticoid replacement. Short stature, caused by premature fusion of the epiphyses, and infertility are common in all but non-classical forms of congenital adrenal hyperplasia. Men with inadequate suppression may develop testicular adrenal rest tumours, which can decrease fertility.

Patients with congenital adrenal hyperplasia are offered genetic and prenatal counselling to discuss the detection of affected fetuses in utero. Treatment with corticosteroids of women carrying an affected female foetus can reduce the degree of infant virilisation at birth.

Cushing's syndrome

Cushing's syndrome is a disease characterised by excess cortisol production. Adrenal disorders causing excessive cortisol production include an adrenal adenoma or adrenocortical carcinoma. When cortisol over-secretion is caused by an ACTH-secreting pituitary adenoma it is termed Cushing's disease.

Clinical features

The clinical features of Cushing's syndrome are identical to those of Cushing's disease (see page 227).

Diagnostic approach

Once hypercortisolaemia is confirmed by measurement of urinary free cortisol, or a dexamethasone suppression test, serum ACTH concentration must be checked. Suppressed ACTH implies that there is an adrenal Cushing's syndrome, independent of ACTH control (page 41). Adrenal CT or magnetic resonance imaging is used to identify an adrenal adenoma or carcinoma.

Management

Medical treatment is used prior to surgery to minimise the adverse metabolic effects of excess cortisol. Adrenalectomy is the ultimate goal of treatment.

Medication

Medical treatment for Cushing's syndrome mirrors that for Cushing's disease. Preoperative metyrapone is used to normalise cortisol and therefore help wound healing and reduce infection. Postoperative mitotane therapy improves survival in patients with Cushing's syndrome due to adrenocortical carcinoma.

Surgery

Adrenalectomy is the definitive treatment. The procedure is done laparoscopically or through an open approach for larger tumours.

Prognosis

Patients may require postoperative corticosteroid replacement if prolonged hypothalamic–pituitary–adrenal axis suppression has occurred. If unilateral adrenal tumours are resected, prognosis is good. However, with malignant or metastatic adrenocortical carcinoma the prognosis is poor.

Adrenal adenomas

The widespread use of CT imaging of the abdomen leads to identification of adrenal masses of uncertain significance. Most are benign and non-hormone producing ('nonfunctioning'), but endocrinologists attempt to identify functioning and malignant tumours. It is the malignant or functioning tumours that are harmful and require treatment.

The prevalence of adrenal adenomas increases from 1% to 7% from young to old age.

Clinical features

Patients are screened for symptoms and signs of functional tumours, i.e. Cushing's syndrome, phaeochromocytoma and Conn's syndrome. Relevant screening tests are required if any condition is suspected.

The likelihood of a malignant lesion depends on its CT appearance and larger size. A lesion >6 cm has a 25% chance of being malignant.

Management

Non-functioning tumours of benign appearance require no treatment and patients can be reassured. If a tumour is functioning or of high malignant potential then specific medical and surgical treatment is required.

Surgery

Adrenal masses >4 cm or those of malignant appearance on CT are excised by adrenalectomy. Secretory tumours are managed as described on page 252.

Prognosis

Small non-functioning tumours with low probability of malignancy may be followed up with interval imaging and appropriate endocrine testing. There is little evidence to suggest that these non-functioning tumours change over time.

Answers to starter questions

1. Cushing's disease is characterised by raised cortisol levels caused specifically by an ACTH-secreting pituitary tumour. Cushing's syndrome is a term that covers all the causes of excess cortisol, including cortisol-secreting adrenal tumours, other cortisol-secreting tumours, ACTH-secreting pituitary tumours, ectopic ACTH secretion (not from the pituitary gland) and exogenous glucocorticoid administration.

2. Removing both adrenal glands results in cortisol and mineralocorticoid deficiencies which require immediate replacement. Other adrenal hormones, such as catecholamines and adrenal androgens, are less vital to survival and their replacement is not required.

3. Adrenal transplantation is not used to treat Addison's disease, mainly because it is relatively easy to replace the deficient hormones compared to other diseases such as type 1 diabetes. Transplanted adrenal glands would also be at risk of autoimmune destruction if this was the initial cause for the disease.

4. Adrenal fatigue is a theory put forward by some alternative health practitioners. It asserts that chronic physical and mental stress cause reduced adrenal gland function, resulting in chronic fatigue. There is no scientific proof that this condition exists. It is very distinct from adrenal insufficiency, where a deficiency in cortisol production can be shown by low cortisol levels. Patients who identify with adrenal fatigue can do themselves considerable harm by taking unproven adrenal supplements in an attempt to treat themselves. For example, by self-medicating with cortisol replacement, patients can cause Cushing's syndrome.

5. It is difficult to prevent Addison's disease because adrenal cortex destruction is often advanced at the time of clinical presentation and there is currently no method of reversing it. Clinical trials of immunosuppressive treatments aimed at arresting the progression of adrenal failure and maintaining adrenal function are ongoing.

Chapter 8
Calcium homeostasis and metabolic bone disease

Starter questions

Answers to the following questions are on page 271.

1. Why are women more likely to develop osteoporosis?
2. Why do some patients with hyperparathyroidism have no symptoms?
3. Can low vitamin D levels cause cancer?
4. Can our lifestyles affect the risk of developing osteoporosis?

Introduction

Extracellular calcium homeostasis is vital for the control of a range of processes, including:

- regulation of voltage-gated ion channels in neurons and muscle
- mineralisation and strengthening of bone
- facilitation of blood clotting

Disorders of calcium homeostasis have various pathological effects. In severe cases, serum calcium excess or depletion causes diverse symptoms. Minor abnormalities in serum calcium concentrations are usually asymptomatic. Abnormalities in calcium metabolism occur if there is dysregulation in:

- parathyroid hormone production
- vitamin D production
- renal dysfunction
- metabolic bone disease
- gut dysfunction and dietary deficiency of calcium, phosphate or magnesium

Case 8 Sharp pain in the back and tiredness

Presentation

Mrs Gupta, aged 46 years, presents to the emergency department with sudden onset of lower back pain after bending over to pick up a shopping bag. She has not had back pain before, but did have some loin pain last year when she had a kidney stone. An X-ray of the lumbar spine shows a crush fracture of the 4th lumbar vertebra (L4).

Initial interpretation

Low-trauma fractures occur in demineralised bone, in most cases because of osteoporosis. The condition is most commonly found in post-menopausal women, in whom it is the result of oestrogen deficiency. Osteoporosis is also common in people with alcoholism (due to abnormal vitamin D and calcium metabolism) and anorexia nervosa (due to oestrogen deficiency).

Pathological fractures also occur in diseases of the bone, such as:

- primary hyperparathyroidism
- Paget's disease
- severe vitamin D deficiency (particularly common in dark-skinned people living far from the equator)
- multiple myeloma with secondary bone deposits in malignancy

Further history

Mrs Gupta reports that she has recently been feeling tired, and that she has become constipated and had some abdominal pain. On direct questioning, she admits that she is always thirsty and feels the need to drink water while in bed at night. Consequently, she rises several times overnight to pass urine. Also, her mood has been low.

Hyperparathyroidism: parathyroidectomy

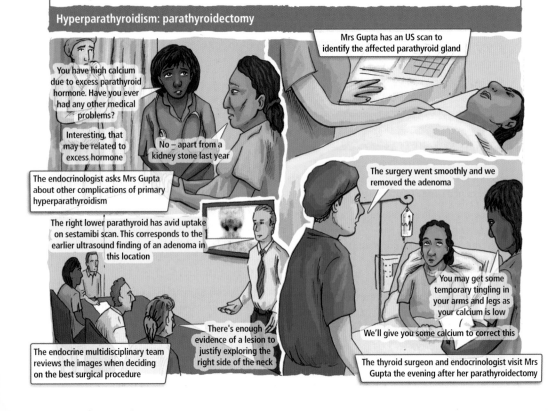

She has a normal menstrual cycle and has four children. Her diet is healthy, and she takes no regular medication. She does not smoke or drink alcohol. There is no family history of osteoporosis.

Examination

No significant abnormalities are found on physical examination. Mrs Gupta has a healthy body mass index of 24 kg/m².

Interpretation of findings

Mrs Gupta has a low-impact vertebral fracture and symptoms that suggest hypercalcaemia: fatigue, constipation, abdominal pain, polydipsia, polyuria and low mood.

The key investigations are measurements of corrected serum calcium, parathyroid hormone and 25-hydroxy vitamin D concentration.

- Serum calcium is measured to verify if her symptoms are due hypercalcaemia.
- Parathyroid hormone measurement will determine the source of the excessive calcium (elevated in hyperparathyroidism)
- 25-hydoxyvitamin D is frequently deficient in those of Asian origin living in the northern hemisphere and is commonly low in hyperparathyroidism
- A full blood count demonstrating anaemia raises the suspicion of an underlying malignancy
- Serum creatinine concentration, if increased, would indicate renal failure, which can cause a deficiency in activated vitamin D
- A dual-energy X-ray absorptiometry (DEXA) scan is also done to measure bone mineral density as she has had a fracture after minimal trauma

Investigations

Blood tests show normal full blood count and renal function, as well as adequate 25-hydroxy vitamin D concentration. However, the following are abnormal.

- High corrected serum calcium: 2.95 mmol/L (reference range, 2.05–2.55 mmol/L)
- Low serum phosphate: 0.65 mmol/L (reference range, 0.8–1.5 mmol/L)
- Parathyroid hormone: 8.5 pmol/L (reference range 1.6–6.9 pmol/L)

Mrs Gupta's 24-h urinary calcium concentration is increased.

The DEXA scan confirms osteoporosis, with a T-score of −3.8 (T-score <−2.5 is diagnostic of osteoporosis).

Diagnosis

Increased serum calcium associated with inappropriately normal (in the context of elevated serum calcium, the production of PTH should be suppressed due to negative feedback on the parathyroid glands) or increased parathyroid hormone is consistent with the diagnosis of primary hyperparathyroidism. If hypercalcaemia were independent of the parathyroid glands, for example with malignancy, the parathyroid hormone would be suppressed by the negative feedback effects of calcium (see Figure 1.12).

The diagnosis of primary hyperparathyroidism and consequential osteoporosis is explained to Mrs Gupta. The next step is to try to localise the adenoma that is secreting the excess parathyroid hormone. This is done with a combination of ultrasound and parathyroid scintigraphy (see page 263). If an overactive parathyroid gland is identified, then minimal invasive surgery is performed to remove the gland. If an adenoma is not identified on imaging, venous sampling is sometimes carried out to identify the source of excessive parathyroid hormone or both sides of the neck are explored surgically to visualise the abnormal gland directly and remove it.

Case 9 Leg pain while walking

Presentation

Mr Stockwell, a 45-year-old white man, presents to his general practitioner with a chronic history of discomfort and cramps in the back of his legs while walking or standing for prolonged periods. He was previously well. He has no risk factors for peripheral vascular disease (e.g. diabetes, smoking, hyperlipidaemia) and no back pain or injury. He mentions that he has had twitching and contractions of the muscles in his face and arms.

Initial interpretation

Peripheral vascular disease and spinal stenosis are both causes of pain in the the legs when standing or walking due to muscle ischaemia and nerve compression respectively. The problem could also be a consequence of neuromuscular disease. Hypocalcaemia is also considered in patients with these symptoms as it can cause muscle cramps and muscle twitching.

Further history

A year ago, Mr Stockwell underwent total thyroidectomy for a large multinodular goitre. He now receives thyroxine replacement.

Examination

Neurovascular examination is normal except for occasional muscular twitching. Chvostek's and Trousseau's signs are both positive (see page 87).

Interpretation of findings

The history and examination suggest hypocalcaemia. He has typical symptoms of hypocalcaemia; muscle cramps and muscle twitching and spasms. There is

is also a plausible mechanism for him to develop hypocalcaemia from damage to the parathyroid glands during previous thyroid surgery.

A complication of thyroid surgery is hypoparathyroidism. This diagnosis should be considered, because of Mr Stockwell's thyroidectomy. Electrocardiography is performed as hypocalcaemia is a cause of cardiac arrhythmias.

Investigations

The results of investigations are listed in **Table 8.1**. Electrocardiography shows prolongation of the corrected QT interval.

Diagnosis

The biochemical results show that Mr Stockwell has hypocalcaemia and decreased parathyroid hormone. If the parathyroid gland was functioning normally, low serum calcium would cause an increase in PTH levels thus normalising

Blood test results for a patient with leg pain while walking		
Measurement	Result	Reference range
Corrected calcium concentration (mmol/L)	1.86	2.05–2.55
Inorganic phosphate concentration (mmol/L)	1.52	0.8–1.5
Magnesium concentration (mmol/L)	0.84	0.7–1.0
Parathyroid hormone concentration (pmol/L)	0.5	1.6–6.9
Estimated glomerular filtration rate (mL/min/1.73 m²)	90 (normal)	> 90
25-hydroxy vitamin D concentration (pmol/L)	58 (sufficient)	50–75

Table 8.1 Blood test results for a patient with leg pain while walking

Case 9 *continued*

the serum calcium. Therefore primary hypoparathyroidism, secondary to damage to parathyroid glands from previous thyroid surgery, is the cause of his symptoms.

The commonest cause of primary hypoparathyroidism is surgery or radiotherapy to the neck. Autoimmune primary hypoparathyroidism is a rare cause that can occur as part of autoimmune polyglandular syndrome type 1 (see page 298). This syndrome can include autoimmune Addison's disease.

Mr Stockwell is given intravenous calcium gluconate and his symptoms resolve rapidly. He is commenced on long-term oral alfacalcidol (an analogue of vitamin D), to maintain a serum calcium just below normal range.

Hypercalcaemia

Hypercalcaemia is a condition characterised by increased serum calcium concentration. **Table 8.2** shows the causes of hypercalcaemia.

Clinical features

This common biochemical abnormality causes:

- polydipsia and polyuria
- fatigue and lethargy
- anorexia, nausea, abdominal pain and constipation
- weakness, depression, confusion and rarely coma
- renal calculi (stones)

Investigations

The key test for identifying the cause of hypercalcaemia is measurement of serum parathyroid hormone concentration. Hypercalcaemia with a low parathyroid hormone suggests a parathyroid hormone–independent cause and raises the possibility of malignancy with lytic bony metastases (**Table 8.2**).

Some malignancies secrete parathyroid hormone-related peptide (PTHrP) which is not detected by the parathyroid hormone assay and suppresses the natural parathyroid hormone. Common malignancies that produce PTHrP include:

- breast
- lung
- head and neck squamous cancer
- renal
- bladder
- cervix
- uterus
- ovary

Resecting the PTHrP-secreting tumour normalises serum calcium.

Causes of hypercalcaemia	
Mechanism	Parathyroid hormone
Hyperparathyroidism	
Primary	↑ or normal
Tertiary	↑
Malignancy (bony metastases and tumours secreting parathyroid hormone–related peptide)	↓
Multiple myeloma	↓
Bone diseases (rarely hypercalcaemia occurs when a patient with Paget's disease is immobilised)	↓ or normal
Familial hypocalciuric hypercalcaemia	Mildly elevated or high-normal
Vitamin D toxicity	↓
Certain drugs (lithium and thiazides)	↓ (but may be normal in lithium-induced hypercalcaemia)
Sarcoidosis	↓

Table 8.2 Causes of hypercalcaemia

> **Some tumours produce parathyroid hormone–related peptide, a mimic of parathyroid hormone.** Parathyroid hormone–related peptide stimulates the parathyroid hormone receptor, causing an increase in serum calcium and a decrease in serum parathyroid hormone.

Management

Hypercalcaemia, if mild (corrected calcium 2.55–2.9 mmol/L), often needs no immediate treatment apart from encouraging the patient to maintain a good oral fluid intake. Severe hypercalcaemia causes dehydration and acute kidney injury therefore rehydration with intravenous fluid is required. Bisphosphonates are used to reduce serum calcium once the patient is rehydrated (see page 136). Once the calcium has stabilised, attention is given to treating the underlying cause.

Hyperparathyroidism

Hyperparathyroidism occurs when the regulation of parathyroid hormone secretion is disrupted. When this happens, excessive quantities of parathyroid hormone are secreted from the parathyroid glands, which usually results in hypercalcaemia. Hyperparathyroidism is classified into three groups (**Table 8.3**).

Epidemiology

Primary hyperparathyroidism is the commonest cause of hypercalcaemia. Its incidence increases with age; the condition is usually diagnosed in patients in their forties. Women are 2.5 times more likely than men to develop primary hyperparathyroidism (although the reason for this is unknown). In the UK, the prevalence is 6 per 1000 people aged > 20 years.

Secondary hyperparathyroidism is common in patients with moderate to severe chronic kidney disease, and tertiary hyperparathyroidism (with autonomous hypersecretion of parathyroid hormone) develops in less than 10% of them.

Aetiology

Different pathologies underlie each type of hyperparathyroidism (**Table 8.3**).

Most cases of primary hyperparathyroidism are caused by a single functional

Pathologies underlying hyperparathyroidism	
Type of hyperparathyroidism	Pathology
Primary	Autonomous production of excessive parathyroid hormone by an adenoma of a single parathyroid gland (sporadic cases or as part of genetic syndromes such as MEN type 1 and 2a)
	Multiple parathyroid gland hyperplasia (sporadic cases or as part of genetic syndromes such as MEN type 1 and 2a)
Secondary	Renal failure increasing serum phosphate concentration
	Renal failure or vitamin D deficiency resulting in a deficiency in activated vitamin D, which causes a compensatory increase in parathyroid hormone production to maintain serum calcium concentration (calcium concentration is usually low or normal)
Tertiary	Autonomous hypersecretion of parathyroid hormone in some cases of persistent secondary hyperparathyroidism, which results in hypercalcaemia and often hyperplasia of all four parathyroid glands

Table 8.3 Pathologies underlying hyperparathyroidism

parathyroid adenoma. Another cause is parathyroid gland hyperplasia and parathyroid carcinoma.

Primary hyperparathyroidism can occur sporadically or as part of multiple endocrine neoplasia types 1 and 2a (see page 296).

Clinical features

Primary hyperparathyroidism is usually asymptomatic. The clinical symptoms of the resulting hypercalcaemia that it does cause (**Table 8.4**) can be remembered by the following rhyme.

- Bones: pain
- Stones: renal stones
- Abdominal groans: abdominal pain, constipation and anorexia
- Psychic groans: depression and anxiety

Other common symptoms of hypercalcaemia include: polydipsia, polyuria, fatigue, muscle weakness and cardiac arrhythmia (**Table 8.4**).

The degree and duration of hypercalcaemia correlate with the severity of symptoms. Chronic excessive urinary excretion of calcium leads to its deposition in the kidneys. Calcium deposition produces renal stones, nephrocalcinosis (calcium deposition in renal parenchyma) and renal failure (even in the absence of renal stones). Parathyroid hormone excess demineralises bone, causing osteoporosis and thus increasing the risk of fractures.

Brown tumours , also known as osteitis fibrosa cystica, are benign changes that occur rarely in the bones of patients with hyperparathyroidism. They are produced by osteitis fibrosa cystica, a non-malignant process in bone that occurs in chronic primary hyperparathyroidism or secondary hyperparathyroidism. The tumours form through increased osteoclastic activity, which results in bone resorption and fibrosis around bone trabeculae.

Brown tumours may be multiple and usually occur in the ribs, pelvis and long bones. The bone changes are visible on radiographs and bone scans in association with hypercalcaemia, so it is important to distinguish these tumours from bony metastases (**Figure 8.1**).

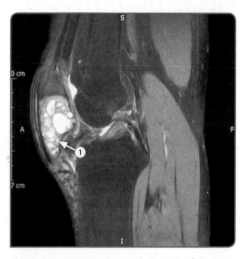

Figure 8.1 Magnetic resonance imaging of the knee (sagittal view) demonstrating ① increasing signal uptake in the patella indicating a Brown's tumour.

Symptoms of primary hyperparathyroidism		
Cause	Organ system	Symptoms
Hypercalcaemia	Urinary (renal diuresis)	Polydipsia, polyuria and nocturia
	Gastrointestinal	Constipation, abdominal pain and anorexia
	Central nervous system	Lethargy, weakness, confusion and coma
	Cardiovascular	Palpitations and syncope
Calcium deposition	Urinary (renal calculi)	Abdominal and flank pain
Skeletal demineralisation	Skeletal (fragility fractures)	Bone pain

Table 8.4 Symptoms of primary hyperparathyroidism

> **Primary hyperparathyroidism is usually discovered incidentally on checking serum calcium concentration.** Mild disease with no symptoms or complications progresses slowly and may be difficult to distinguish from normal ageing. It may never require active treatment.

Diagnostic approach

The diagnostic algorithm for hypercalcaemia is shown in **Figure 8.2**. The characteristics of primary hyperparathyroidism include:

- hypercalcaemia
- hypophosphataemia
- increased or inappropriately normal parathyroid hormone concentration. In a normal individual, an elevated serum calcium would produce a cessation of PTH release due to negative feedback on the parathyroid glands. A PTH concentration within the normal range is therefore an 'inappropriately elevated' concentration
- normal or increased urinary calcium excretion

> **Mildly increased parathyroid hormone and hypercalcaemia occur in familial hypocalciuric hypercalcaemia as well as in primary hyperparathyroidism.** Familial hypocalciuric hypercalcaemia is an uncommon inherited autosomal dominant condition caused by a mutation of calcium-sensing receptors in the parathyroid glands. The mutation increases the threshold calcium concentration at which these receptors are activated.

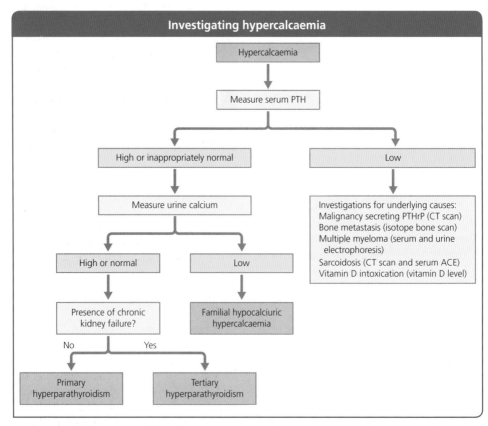

Figure 8.2 Investigations used in patients with hypercalcaemia. ACE, angiotensin-converting enzyme; PTH, parathyroid hormone; PTHrP, parathythroid hormone-related protein.

Investigations

Once primary hyperparathyroidism has been confirmed by the results of serum parathyroid hormone, serum calcium and urinary calcium excretion tests, the cause and complications of the condition can be investigated. Investigations include:

- ultrasound scan of the parathyroid glands to identify an adenoma (**Figure 8.3a**)
- parathyroid scintigraphy, which shows increased tracer uptake in an adenoma (**Figure 8.3b**)
- DEXA scan, which shows osteoporosis secondary to bone demineralisation
- renal tract ultrasound scan to show any asymptomatic renal calculi

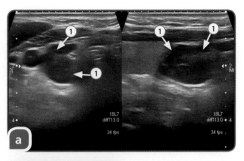

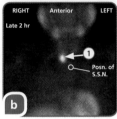

Figure 8.3
Parathyroid adenoma.
(a) Ultrasound identifies an adenoma ① in the right inferior parathyroid gland. (b) Parathyroid scintigraphy confirms increased uptake of tracer in the hyperactive gland ①.

Management

Primary hyperparathyroidism is treated by surgical removal of the affected gland (if it is caused by a single adenoma). If multiple parathyroid glands are involved, total parathyroidectomy is necessary. The indications for parathyroidectomy are:

- symptomatic hypercalcaemia
- asymptomatic hypercalcaemia (calcium concentration 0.25 mmol/L above the upper limit of the normal range)
- osteoporosis
- chronic kidney disease
- renal stones

Secondary hyperparathyroidism caused by renal failure is treated with activated vitamin D. This addresses the activated vitamin D deficiency resulting from the inability of the kidneys to hydroxylate 25-hydroxycholecalciferol to 1,25-dihydroxycholecalciferol in patients with chronic renal failure.

Tertiary hyperparathyroidism is managed with total parathyroidectomy.

Medication

The initial treatment of acute severe hypercalcaemia is rehydration with intravenous fluids. Once the patient is rehydrated (may require 4–6 L), bisphosphonates are used to treat severe acute hypercalcaemia. Bisphosphonates work by inhibiting bone resorption by osteoclasts. However, bisphosphonates are not effective for long-term control of hypercalcaemia as once the osteoclasts are maximally inhibited there is no additional benefit to repeated bisphosphonate administration.

Cinacalcet may be used to reduce the high serum calcium caused by hyperparathyroidism in patients who are unsuitable for parathyroidectomy (e.g. if they are too frail or unfit for surgery). This drug is a calcimimetic; it activates calcium-sensing receptors, thus inhibiting parathyroid hormone production.

> **Cinacalcet is not the first-line treatment for primary hyperparathyroidism.** The drug is effective but also expensive, and parathyroidectomy is curative in most patients with primary hyperparathyroidism.

Surgery

For single adenomas, parathyroidectomy is done with either open surgery or a minimally invasive, laparoscopic procedure. In cases of primary hyperparathyroidism with four-gland hyperplasia, the removal of all four glands is indicated in patients with:

- a strong family history of primary hyperparathyroidism
- multiple endocrine neoplasia type 1 tertiary hyperparathyroidism

Prognosis

Removal of a single adenoma in primary hyperparathyroidism is curative. With calcium and vitamin D replacement, bone mineral density slowly improves.

Hypocalcaemia

Hypocalcaemia (low serum calcium) is common in patients who have been admitted to hospital.

Clinical features

Clinical manifestations are listed in **Table 8.5**. The condition has multiple causes, including:

- hypomagnesaemia
- hypoalbuminaemia
- renal failure
- severe sepsis
- vitamin D deficiency
- refeeding syndrome (the metabolic disturbance that occurs when feeding is commenced after a period of severe malnutrition)
- hyperphosphataemia
- adverse drug effects (e.g. of bisphosphonates and cisplatin)
- hypoparathyroidism

Clinical features of hypocalcaemia	
Symptoms	Signs
Muscle cramps	Tetany
Fatigue	Chvostek's sign*
Anxiety or mood disturbances	Trousseau's sign*
Paraesthesia	
Reduced seizure threshold	

*For a description of these signs, see page 85.

Table 8.5 Clinical features of hypocalcaemia

Investigations

Investigations include determination of corrected calcium (protein-bound) and ionised calcium (free calcium), phosphate and parathyroid hormone. In hypocalcaemia, parathyroid hormone is increased, except in cases of hypoparathyroidism, in which parathyroid hormone is low or inappropriately low-normal.

Management

Mild hypocalcaemia (1.9–2.05 mmol/L) can be managed by administration of oral calcium supplements. Vitamin D supplementation is indicated if there is vitamin D deficiency and helps to enable calcium absorption form the gut.

Intravenous calcium replacement is indicated in severe hypocalcaemia (1.9–2.05 mmol/L) or symptomatic hypocalcaemia, if there are ECG abnormalities (e.g. prolonged corrected-QT interval) or if the patient is unable to tolerate oral replacement due to vomiting or malabsorption.

If magnesium is deficient this should also be replaced as magnesium is required for the production and bioactivity of parathyroid hormone.

> **Severe symptomatic hypocalcaemia requires immediate treatment with intravenous preparations of calcium.** Electrocardiographic monitoring is also necessary because of the risk of cardiac arrhythmias.

Hypoparathyroidism

Hypoparathyroidism is caused by a deficiency of parathyroid hormone, which results in hypocalcaemia. The condition has various causes:

- surgical removal of a parathyroid adenoma, leading to transient hypoparathyroidism as the normal glands recover from suppression
- surgical removal of all parathyroid glands at the time of thyroidectomy or neck dissection
- irradiation of the neck causing parathyroid gland failure
- autoimmune hypoparathyroidism
- congenital hypoparathyroidism (rare)

During extensive thyroid surgery (e.g. neck dissection for thyroid cancer), parathyroid tissue is identified and reimplanted into the neck to permit normal parathyroid function. However, patients occasionally develop permanent hypoparathyroidism because an inadequate amount of parathyroid tissue is retained unintentionally.

Clinical features

The signs and symptoms of hypoparathyroidism are due to hypocalcaemia (**Table 8.5**).

Management

The aims of management of hypoparathyroidism are to:

- maintain serum calcium concentration at the lower end of the normal range
- ensure that patients are symptom-free

For patients on calcium replacement, if the serum calcium level is maintained too high there is a risk of developing hypercalciuria and subsequent renal stones or nephrocalcinosis.

Medication

Recombinant parathyroid hormone is available to address the parathyroid hormone deficiency in hypoparathyroidism, but this is an experimental treatment and not in common use in clinical practice. Therefore, most patients are treated with oral calcium supplementation in combination with activated vitamin D (as PTH is required to activate vitamin D and therefore inactivated vitamin D would not be an effective treatment) (see Figure 1.13).

Prognosis

Hypoparathyroidism after removal of a parathyroid adenoma is usually transient, resolving when the remaining parathyroid glands are released from the inhibition of the dominant, hyperfunctioning adenoma. However, most cases of primary hypoparathyroidism resulting from other causes are permanent.

Pseudohypoparathyroidism

Pseudohypoparathyroidism is characterised by an inherited dysfunction of parathyroid hormone receptor signal transmission, resulting in hypocalcaemia, hyperphosphataemia and elevated parathyroid hormone levels. The condition has other phenotypical features, for example:

- short stature
- overweight
- intellectual impairment
- short 4th and 5th metacarpal bones
- calcium deposition under the skin
- poor dentition

Pseudopseudo hypoparathyroidism

In pseudopseudohypoparathyroidism, the phenotypical features of pseudohypoparathyroidism are present but without the dysfunction in parathyroid hormone signalling. Therefore patients have normal calcium biochemistry and PTH levels.

Osteoporosis

Osteoporosis is characterised by reduced mineralisation of bone; the bone becomes more fragile, with a propensity to fracture. The condition is usually asymptomatic, so a fragility fracture is commonly the first presenting feature.

Osteoporosis is termed primary osteoporosis if no secondary cause (e.g. rheumatoid arthritis or Cushing's syndrome) is identified. The condition has multiple causes (**Table 8.6**); in women, the commonest of these is oestrogen deficiency after the menopause.

Epidemiology

Osteoporosis is the most common metabolic bone disease worldwide. The condition affects about 6% of the UK population, a figure likely to increase as the population ages. In the UK, about 300,000 fragility fractures are treated each year.

Aetiology

Bone turnover is a continuous process of resorption of old bone and production of new bone. Osteoclasts break down bone, and osteoblasts synthesise new bone.

Bone mass develops during childhood and adolescence, and into early adulthood. Peak bone mass is reached in the mid-twenties. In later life, osteoporosis develops when osteoclastic activity exceeds osteoblastic activity.

Clinical features

Osteoporotic fractures (fragility fractures) occur in characteristic bones:

- the distal radius (known as a Colles' fracture)
- the hip (the neck of the femur)
- lumbar vertebrae
- the pelvis

Low-impact trauma can cause fractures. The elderly are more at risk of falls and therefore the risk of sustaining fragility fractures.

Diagnostic approach

A low-impact fracture at a common site indicates that the bone is reduced in strength and therefore osteoporotic.

Causes of osteoporosis		
Category	Cause	Patient characteristics or examples
Primary	Post-menopausal oestrogen deficiency	Women aged > 50 years
	Old age	Men and women aged > 70 years
Secondary	Hypogonadism	Turner's syndrome, Klinefelter's syndrome , testosterone deficiency in men, and anorexia nervosa
	Endocrine disease	Cushing's syndrome, acromegaly, thyrotoxicosis, Addison's disease and hyperparathyroidism
	Deficiency states	Malabsorption, malnutrition and vitamin D deficiency
	Inflammatory disease	Rheumatoid arthritis, systemic lupus erythematosus and ankylosing spondylitis
	Neoplastic disease	Myeloma, lymphoma and leukaemia
	Reduced physical activity	Reduced weight-bearing exercise
	Genetic factors	Patients with a family history of osteoporosis
	Certain drugs	Corticosteroid, antiretroviral, antipsychotic and chemotherapeutic drugs; nicotine (smoking) and excessive alcohol

Table 8.6 Causes of osteoporosis

Investigations

Dual-energy X-ray absorptiometry (**Figure 8.4**) is the investigation of choice for confirming that bone is osteoporotic (see page 112). Other tests to exclude secondary causes of osteoporosis are necessary and depend on any suggestive history.

- Full blood count: anaemia is seen in secondary causes of osteoporosis (e.g. myeloma) and elevated white blood cells are seen in some forms of leukaemia (e.g. chronic myeloid leukaemia)
- Renal profile: to exclude renal failure
- Bone profile (calcium, phosphate and alkaline phosphatase): to rule out primary hyperparathyroidism and Paget's disease
- Thyroid function tests: because hyperthyroidism can cause osteoporosis
- Vitamin D concentration: to exclude deficiency

In addition, testosterone concentration is checked in young men who develop osteoporosis; this is done to rule out hypogonadism. For the same reason, a menstrual history is taken from women to detect oligomenorrhoea or amenorrhoea, both of which are symptoms of hypogonadism.

Management

Management is of the fracture itself, as well as risk factor modification and the use of medication that improves bone strength. The decision to start treatment for osteoporosis is based on the FRAX score. This is a diagnostic tool that allows evaluation of the 10-year probability of a bone fracture and integrates results from DEXA scans and clinical risk factors.

Medication

Calcium and vitamin D supplementation are simple treatments to address dietary deficiency and reduced sunlight exposure (causing vitamin D deficiency), which are common, especially in the elderly. Maintenance of adequate vitamin D concentration is essential in all patients with osteoporosis.

Bisphosphonates are administered orally or intravenously. This class of drug inhibits bone breakdown by reducing the action of osteoclasts, and are effective at increasing bone mineral density. Common adverse effects are nausea and oesophageal reflux. There have also been reports of bisphosphonates causing osteonecrosis of the jaw.

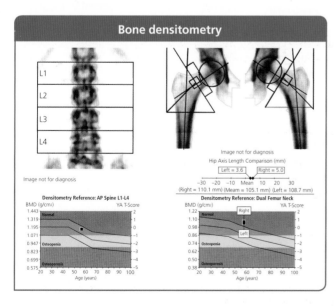

Figure 8.4 Dual-energy X-ray absorptiometry scanning (densitometry) categorises bone as normal, ostopenic or osteoporotic as shown in the lower panels. This patient's spinal and femoral neck bone density is normal (and high for this age group).

Other treatment options are as follow.

- Strontium ranelate: stimulates bone formation and inhibits its resorption
- Selective oestrogen receptor modulators (including raloxifene): stimulate the oestrogen receptor and can be used to treat osteoporosis in post-menopausal women
- Human recombinant parathyroid hormone: an anabolic stimulator of bone, which is administered in daily subcutaneous pulses; however, this is an expensive and rarely used treatment for osteoporosis
- Denosumab: a monoclonal antibody that binds specifically to cell surface receptors on osteoclasts to inhibit osteoclast-mediated bone resorption

Hormone replacement therapy is no longer used to treat osteoporosis in post-menopausal women, because of the increased risk of thromboembolism, cardiovascular disease and breast cancer. However, hormone replacement therapy reduces the risk of osteoporosis in women taking it to relieve the symptoms of menopause.

> **Concordance with bisphosphonates is frequently poor.** This is because these drugs can have disruptive adverse effects, such as oesophageal irritation, that make them hard to tolerate.

Prognosis

The improvements in bone mineral density that come with medical therapy can be monitored by serial DEXA scans, and therapy is tailored to the individual patient.

Paget's disease

Paget's disease is a metabolic bone disorder of unknown aetiology. It is common, with a prevalence rate in the UK of 0.8%, but is much rarer in some ethnic groups such as Asians. Paget's disease is frequently unrecognised as it is usually asymptomatic.

The condition causes a localised increase in bone turnover, which results in the production of structurally imperfect bone (woven bone). Woven bone is usually deformed, weaker, less compact and highly vascular.

Clinical features

Most patients with Paget's disease are asymptomatic, and the peak age of diagnosis is 65 years. Typical clinical features include bone pain and deformity (**Table 8.7**).

Investigations

Results of biochemical investigations include:

- increased serum bone-specific alkaline phosphatase
- normal calcium and phosphate concentration (unless the patient is

Clinical features of Paget's disease	
Symptoms	Signs
Bone pain (commonest symptom)	Sabre tibia and skull enlargement (bossing)
Bone deformity (bowing of a limb)	Increased skin temperature over affected bone
Bone heat	Muscle weakness and sensorineural deafness
Nerve compression	Joint deformity
Osteoarthritis (in periarticular Paget's disease)	High-output cardiac failure

Table 8.7 Clinical features of Paget's disease

immobile when serum calcium and phosphate rise)

Plain X-ray is done to evaluate abnormal bone and detect fractures. Bone scans show increased uptake of isotope. This is a sensitive but non-specific finding that distinguishes between Paget's disease and other bone disorders, such as myeloma.

Paget's disease is commonly detected by the incidental finding of an isolated raised alkaline phosphatase concentration. If the patient is otherwise asymptomatic, no further investigation is needed.

Management

Many patients do not require active treatment unless there are complications (fractures) or periarticular disease.

Medication

Bisphosphonates are the mainstay of treatment, because of their ability to reduce osteoclastic activity in bone. These drugs also help reduce pain. Patients with a diagnosis of Paget's disease are encouraged to take calcium and vitamin D supplements.

Surgery

Orthopaedic surgery, such as total hip replacement, may be indicated when Paget's disease causes severe refractory joint pain from osteoarthritis. Spinal surgery is offered to patients with nerve compression symptoms caused by vertebral hyperplasia and spinal stenosis.

Prognosis

Osteosarcoma, primary cancer of the bone, is a rare complication of Paget's disease. It is thought to occur because of increased bone turnover and malignant transformation of cells within the bone.

Vitamin D deficiency

Vitamin D is essential for the formation of strong mineralised bones and for proper functioning of several other systems, including the cardiovascular and neurological systems.

Vitamin D deficiency is associated with:

- bone deformity or rickets in children
- osteomalacia in adults

Studies have also suggested a possible link between vitamin D deficiency and higher rates of malignancy, neurological and psychiatric disorders, and type 1 diabetes mellitus.

Epidemiology

Vitamin D deficiency is a common problem worldwide. There is a predominance of vitamin D deficiency in low- and middle-income countries. However, it is also prevalent in European and other high-income countries, particularly those in which exposure to sunlight is limited. In the UK, half the population have inadequate vitamin D, and 20% have severe deficiency (increasing to 90% of people of Asian origin).

Aetiology

Vitamin D is obtained from the diet, but most is synthesised by the skin when it is exposed to sunlight (see page 19). Deficiency can arise from:

- inadequate synthesis of vitamin D
- dietary deficiency
- failure to meet increased requirements

Inadequate synthesis of vitamin D

People with inadequate exposure to sunlight are prone to develop vitamin D deficiency. Populations living farther from the equator are most at risk. Dark skin pigmentation and covering of the skin (with clothes or high skin-protection-factor sunblock) reduce the ability to synthesise vitamin D. The elderly and housebound are also at risk of reduced sunlight exposure and consequent vitamin D deficiency.

The latitude of the UK means that there is sufficient sunlight for the skin to synthesise vitamin D for only 6 months of the year. Some experts argue for routine vitamin D supplementation of certain foods, such as cereals.

Chronic kidney failure results in an inability to activate vitamin D by enzymatic metabolism, resulting in deficiency.

Dietary deficiency

Foods that contain vitamin D include:

- oily fish (mackerel, herring, sardines, salmon and tuna)
- eggs
- fortified foods (margarine, milk and breakfast cereals)

Vitamin D malabsorption is caused by bowel disease, such as inflammatory bowel disease and coeliac disease.

Failure to meet increased requirements

People in high-demand states are most at risk of vitamin D deficiency. This group includes:

- growing children
- pregnant women and breastfeeding mothers

Clinical features

The clinical features of vitamin D deficiency are more severe in the developing and growing bones of infants and children.

Vitamin D deficiency in children

Rickets is the consequence of vitamin D deficiency in children. This disabling condition causes abnormal development of bones and bowing of the weight-bearing bones of the skeleton, i.e. the femur and tibia. These are the effects of reduced bone mineralisation.

Skeletal deformity can cause bone pain and an increased tendency to fracture. Dental development may fail. Patients with severe vitamin D deficiency occasionally have symptomatic hypocalcaemia, with muscle spasms and tetany.

Vitamin D deficiency in adults

The symptoms of vitamin D deficiency in adults tend to be non-specific and include:

- muscle weakness and pain
- bone pain
- increased risk of fracture
- pseudofractures (visible on X-ray and termed Looser's zones). These are seen as thin lucencies at right angles to the cortex of the affected bone

Many conditions (e.g. cancer, neurological conditions) have been linked with vitamin D deficiency in adults. However, correction of the deficiency has not conclusively proved effective for most of these conditions.

Diagnostic approach

Vitamin D is best measured in the serum in its 25-hydroxy vitamin D form. In patients with chronic kidney disease, the adequacy of vitamin D is assessed through the concentration of parathyroid hormone. Increased parathyroid hormone in the context of chronic kidney disease indicates deficiency of activated vitamin D.

Management

Vitamin D deficiency is managed with oral or parenteral vitamin D replacement.

Medication

Vitamin D is available in several preparations. In patients whose kidneys are functioning normally, treatment with calciferol is indicated. This can be given orally at high dose for several weeks before switching to a maintenance dose (800 IU/day). Alternatively, it can be given by injection, particularly for patients with malabsorption or poor adherence to treatment.

In patients with chronic kidney disease, activated vitamin D in the form of 1α-calcidiol is required due to the fact that that they are unable to activate other forms of vitamin D.

Prognosis

Treatment of vitamin D deficiency results in mineralisation and strengthening of bone. In children with rickets, the bone deformities may persist into adulthood. Other symptoms of vitamin D deficiency improve once serum concentration is sufficient.

Answers to starter questions

1. Postmenopausal women have no circulating sex hormones (particularly oestrogen), which are required to maintain bone mineralisation. Although testosterone levels in men decrease gradually with age, there are usually still adequate levels for maintaining bone mineral density.

2. Hyperparathyroidism is usually mild with a serum calcium level that is only slightly elevated. This means that the patient may have no symptoms or such mild symptoms that they go unrecognised.

3. Although vitamin D deficiency is associated with a number of malignancies, including colorectal cancer, there is no evidence that it is the main cause. To prove it is important in the development of cancer, clinical trials will need to show that treating populations with vitamin D reduces the rate of cancer formation over a long period of time.

4. Many lifestyle factors increase the risk of osteoporosis, including smoking, excessive alcohol consumption, eating disorders and low dietary calcium intake. Conversely, weight-bearing exercise protects against osteoporosis in the long term.

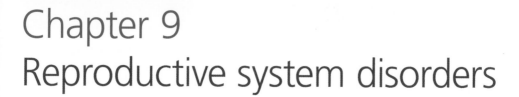

Chapter 9
Reproductive system disorders

Starter questions

Answers to the following questions are on page 291.

1. Why are women with polycystic ovarian syndrome encouraged to lose weight?
2. Can testosterone affect behaviour and mood?
3. Can testosterone be given to women to increase their libido?

Introduction

As well as being essential to reproductive function, sex hormones, primarily testosterone in men and oestrogen in women, have roles in general health. Therefore disorders of sex hormones affect not only fertility but also patients' general and psychological well-being and their long-term metabolic, cardiovascular and bone health.

Diseases of the testes and the ovaries are common causes of reproductive disorders. However, these disorders sometimes also result from diseases of the pituitary gland and hypothalamus, as well as other conditions that disrupt the hypothalamus–pituitary–gonadal axis (see page 215).

Case 10 Complete absence of menstrual periods in a 16-year-old

Presentation

Accompanied by her mother, 16-year-old Emma visits her general practitioner because she has not started her menstrual periods. Emma is worried; all her friends have already started menstruating.

Initial interpretation

The first occurrence of menstruation is known as menarche. The average age of menarche is 13 years in the UK. Genetic factors contribute to determine the age of menarche.

Primary amenorrhoea is the absence of menarche by the age of:

- 16 years in the presence of normal secondary sexual characteristics (such as development of breast, axillary hair or pubic hair)
- 14 years in the absence of secondary sexual characteristics

Secondary amenorrhoea is the absence of menstrual cycles for at least:

- 3 months in women with previously normal menstrual cycles
- 9 months in women with a history of oligomenorrhoea (infrequent periods)

Emma has never menstruated, so she has primary amenorrhoea. There are several causes of primary and secondary amenorrhoea (**Table 9.1**). All causes of secondary amenorrhoea can present with primary amenorrhoea.

Further history

Emma is otherwise well and not on any long-term medications. She denies any cyclical abdominal pain, milk discharge from the breasts, increased facial hair, headaches or visual symptoms. Her weight is steady. She says that she is one of the shorter girls in her class, but that she is still growing and hopes to catch up.

She is doing well at school and does not feel particularly stressed either there or at home. She does not smoke or drink alcohol, and her diet is generally healthy. She does not take part in competitive sports at school but swims twice a week to keep fit.

The family has no history of endocrine or gynaecological disorders. Her mother had menarche at the age of 12 years. Emma has no sisters, but her two elder brothers are well and went through puberty in time.

Examination

Emma's height is 151 cm, putting her in the 10th centile (i.e. 10% of the age-matched female population will be shorter than her). Her body mass index is 26 kg/m² and her blood pressure is 90/60 mmHg. She has no hirsutism (see page 75), acne or goitre. Her sense of smell is intact.

She does not have facial dysmorphia. However, she has a low hairline, and her forearms angle away at the elbows (wide carrying angle or cubitus valgum). Her breasts are small (Tanner stage 3; see page 96) and her nipples widely spaced. There is no galactorrhoea (the spontaneous flow of milk from the nipples).

External examination of the genitalia finds sparse pubic hair (Tanner stage 2; see page 96). There is no clitoromegaly (enlargement of the clitoris) or other abnormalities.

No mass is palpable on abdominal examination. Cardiovascular examination is also unremarkable. Visual fields are full on confrontation test (see page 97).

Interpretation of findings

The absence of galactorrhoea makes hyperprolactinaemia (increased serum

Case 10 *continued*

Causes of primary and secondary amenorrhoea	
Category	**Cause**
Physiological	Pregnancy
	Breastfeeding
Hyperprolactinaemia	Prolactin-secreting pituitary adenoma
	Pituitary adenoma compressing pituitary stalk
	Use of certain drugs (e.g. antipsychotics and antidepressants)
Hypergonadotrophic hypogonadism	Turner's syndrome*†
	Premature ovarian failure (caused by autoimmunity, chemotherapy, pelvic irradiation or mumps)
	Menopause
Hypogonadotrophic hypogonadism	Constitutional growth and pubertal delay*
	Kallmann's syndrome*
	Pituitary and hypothalamic disorders (with or without tumours)
	Sheehan's syndrome
	Functional hypothalamic amenorrhoea (caused by weight loss, intense exercise or severe stress)
Androgen excess	Polycystic ovary syndrome
	Androgen-secreting tumours
	Non-classic congenital adrenal hyperplasia
Outflow tract obstruction	Imperforate hymen*
	Transverse vaginal septum*
Congenital and genetic disorders	Müllerian agenesis*
	Androgen insensitivity syndrome*
Debilitating systemic illnesses	Malignancy, end-stage kidney disease, cystic fibrosis
Other endocrine disorders	Cushing's syndrome
	Thyroid dysfunction

*Typically presents with primary amenorrhoea.

†Can rarely present with secondary amenorrhoea.

Table 9.1 Causes of primary and secondary amenorrhoea in women of reproductive age

prolactin level) unlikely. The lack of hirsutism does not support androgen excess.

External examination of the genitalia helps exclude structural defects such as imperforate hymen and transverse vaginal septum. However, further imaging (such as, ultrasonography or magnetic resonance imaging) would be needed to rule out defects in the urogenital system such as müllerian agenesis, a development defect resulting in the absence of a uterus and malformation of the upper vagina.

Emma's short stature, limited sexual development and primary amenorrhoea could be caused by constitutional growth and pubertal delay. However, they also

Case 10 *continued*

raise the possibility of ovarian failure (hypogonadism).

Ovarian failure may result from defects in the ovaries (primary hypogonadism) or the pituitary gland or hypothalamus (secondary hypogonadism). These two types of ovarian failure are distinguished by measuring gonadotrophin.

■ Gonadotrophin concentration is high in primary hypogonadism, hence its other name, hypergonadotrophic hypogonadism
■ Gonadotrophin concentration is low or inappropriately normal (i.e. normal concentration despite ovarian failure) in secondary hypogonadism, also called hypogonadotrophic hypogonadism

Patients are asked about their sense of smell, because a lack of this sense (anosmia) is a key sign of Kallmann's syndrome. This is a genetic disorder associated with hypogonadotrophic hypogonadism.

The features of low hairline, wide carrying angle and widely spaced nipples are associated with Turner's syndrome (**Figure 9.1**) and warrant further investigation.

Investigations

Blood tests for serum prolactin, thyroid stimulating hormone and testosterone are carried out to exclude hyperprolactinaemia, thyroid dysfunction and androgen excess, respectively. The results of these tests are normal. However serum oestrogen is low at <19 pmol/L, and follicle-stimulating hormone is high at 48 IU/L (in menopause, it is >25 IU/L); these findings (low oestrogen and high follicle-stimulating hormone) are consistent with primary hypogonadism.

Pelvic ultrasound shows a uterus; its presence excludes müllerian agenesis. However, ovaries cannot be detected. Karyotype analysis (visualisation of the chromosomes, see page 115) shows 45X0

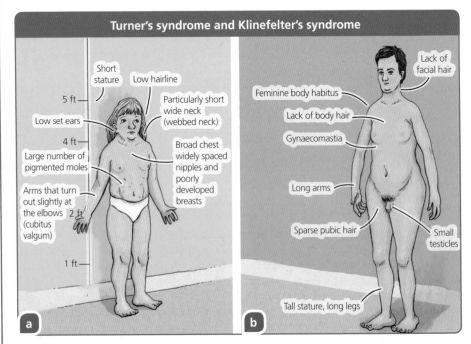

Turner's syndrome and Klinefelter's syndrome

Short stature
Low hairline
5 ft
Low set ears
4 ft
Large number of pigmented moles
Arms that turn out slightly at the elbows (cubitus valgum) 2 ft
1 ft

Particularly short wide neck (webbed neck)
Broad chest widely spaced nipples and poorly developed breasts

Lack of facial hair
Feminine body habitus
Lack of body hair
Gynaecomastia
Long arms
Sparse pubic hair
Small testicles
Tall stature, long legs

a   b

Figure 9.1 Clinical features of (a) Turner's syndrome and (b) Klinefelter's syndrome.

Case 10 *continued*

(absence of an X chromosome from the normal female karyotype), confirming the diagnosis of Turner's syndrome.

Diagnosis

The diagnosis of Turner's syndrome is based on:

- primary amenorrhoea as a consequence of primary ovarian failure (hypergonadotrophic hypogonadism)
- the phenotype of the syndrome and the diagnostic karyotype (45X0)

Emma is started on long-term oestrogen replacement therapy to induce puberty and sexual development.

Case 11 Excessive hair growth

Presentation

Julie, aged 24 years, is referred to the endocrinology clinic with excessive facial hair growth and irregular menstrual periods.

Initial interpretation

Women with hirsutism have excessive growth of terminal hair on their faces and bodies in a male pattern. Hair is present in the beard area, the upper lip, around the nipples and below the umbilicus. The condition is common, affecting about 5% of women in the UK. It is the result of increased androgen concentration or the increased sensitivity of hair follicles to androgen.

The most common cause of hirsutism is polycystic ovary syndrome (PCOS). Julie's irregular menstrual periods support the diagnosis of PCOS, but other causes of hirsutism need to be excluded (**Table 9.2**).

> **Hirsutism must be distinguished from hypertrichosis, a generalised excessive hair growth in both sexes.** Hypertrichosis is not associated with androgen excess, and it is not limited to androgen-sensitive hairs. The condition can be congenital or an adverse effect of several drugs, including minoxidil, cyclosporine and phenytoin.

Causes of hirsutism	
Cause	Associated features
Polycystic ovary syndrome	Obesity, menstrual irregularity, multiple cysts in ovaries
Menopause	Amenorrhoea, menopausal symptoms
Congenital adrenal hyperplasia	Menstrual irregularities, other signs of virilisation (e.g. clitoromegaly), glucocorticoid and mineralocorticoid deficiency
Androgen-secreting adrenal or ovarian tumour	Rapidly progressive, short history of hirsutism and other signs of virilisation (e.g. clitoromegaly)
Cushing's syndrome	Central obesity, proximal myopathy, menstrual irregularity, hypertension, diabetes mellitus
Certain drugs (e.g. androgens or metyrapone)	Positive drug history
Idiopathic	Unknown cause

Table 9.2 Causes of hirsutism

Further history

Julie has been troubled with increased hair growth since her late teens, needing to shave her upper lip on alternate days. She also complains of increased hair around her nipples and abdomen below the umbilicus.

Case 11 *continued*

Her menarche was at the age of 13 years. Since then, her menstrual cycles have always been irregular; more recently, she has been having periods once every 3–4 months. She is not on the oral contraceptive pill and has never been pregnant.

Julie feels well physically, but she is constantly embarrassed and emotionally distressed because of her excessive body hair.

There is no significant medical history. Julie does not take any regular medications. She is a non-smoker and drinks alcohol only occasionally. Neither her mother nor her sisters suffer from similar symptoms.

Examination

Julie is overweight, with a body mass index of 30 kg/m². Her blood pressure is 136/76 mmHg. She has shaved her face but has hair around the nipples, lower abdomen and thighs. The results of the rest of the physical examination are unremarkable.

Interpretation of findings

The combination of long-standing hirsutism, oligomenorrhoea and obesity are consistent with the diagnosis of PCOS.

It is vital to exclude androgen-secreting ovarian and adrenal tumours, which can cause hirsutism. These tumours typically present with a rapidly progressive short history and require treatment without delay.

Cushing's syndrome can also present with hirsutism, as well as weight gain and menstrual disorder. Other typical features of the syndrome are easy bruising, thin skin, purple stretch marks in the abdomen, and proximal muscle wasting and weakness. The absence of these findings does not support the diagnosis of Cushing's syndrome.

Hyperprolactinaemia is also a common cause of irregular menstrual cycles. However, this condition is often associated with galactorrhoea, which Julie does not have.

Investigations

Serum oestrogen, luteinising hormone and follicle-stimulating hormone concentration are normal, but testosterone is mildly increased at 2.8 nmol/L (normal result, < 2.3 nmol/L). Serum prolactin is normal, which excludes hyperprolactinaemia as the cause of Julie's irregular periods. Testing of two 24-h urine samples shows normal free urinary cortisol, excluding the diagnosis of Cushing's syndrome. Serum 17-hydroxyprogesterone is also normal, making the diagnosis of congenital adrenal hyperplasia unlikely.

Pelvic ultrasound shows multiple cysts in both ovaries (**Figure 9.2**).

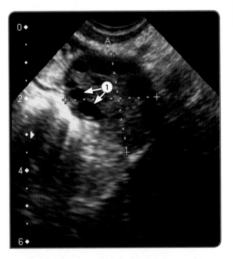

Figure 9.2 Transvaginal ultrasonography showing multiple cysts ① of varying size in the left ovary.

Case 11 *continued*

Diagnosis

The diagnosis of PCOS is based on clinical presentation (hirsutism and oligomenorrhoea), mildly increased serum testosterone and the ultrasound finding of multiple cysts in the ovaries. Julie's GP prescribes an oral combined oestrogen-progesterone pill to regulate her menstrual periods and improve her hirsutism. She is also advised to lose weight through healthy eating and exercise.

Polycystic ovary syndrome

Polycystic ovary syndrome (PCOS) is a common condition associated with hirsutism, irregular menstrual cycles and reduced fertility.

Epidemiology

About 6% of women in the UK have PCOS. It is more prevalent in Mexican-American, Hispanic, Middle Eastern and South Asian populations due to a number of reasons such as genetic make up and prevalence of obesity.

Aetiology

The exact cause of the condition is uncertain. However, genetic factors play a role in the pathogenesis of PCOS, as evidenced by its clustering in families and increased concordance in monozygotic twins compared with dizygotic twins.

Pathogenesis

A cardinal feature of PCOS is the increased secretion of androgens, testosterone in particular, by ovarian theca cells (**Figure 9.3**). The increased androgen secretion is in response to increased pulses of gonadotrophin-releasing hormone secretion from the hypothalamus, resulting in increased pulsatile secretion of luteinising hormone from the anterior pituitary.

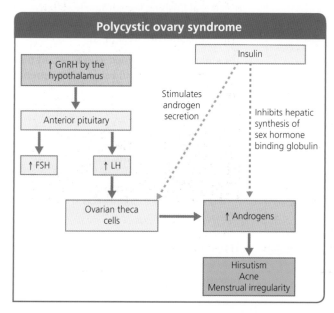

Figure 9.3 Pathogenesis of polycystic ovary sydrome. FSH, follicle stimulating hormone; LH luteinising hormone.

Insulin also contributes to the excessive androgen secretion in PCOS through two mechanisms.

- Insulin acts synergistically with luteinising hormone to stimulate androgen synthesis by ovarian theca cells
- It inhibits synthesis of sex hormone–binding globulin by the liver, resulting in increased free (unbound and therefore biologically active) androgens

Clinical features

Patients with PCOS present with clinical features associated with androgen excess and defects in ovulation (**Figure 9.4**). These include:

- hirsutism
- acne
- androgenic alopecia (male pattern baldness)
- oligomenorrhoea or amenorrhoea
- subfertility or infertility

Obesity, increased visceral adiposity, insulin resistance, type 2 diabetes mellitus and dyslipidaemia are common in patients with PCOS.

Some patients have acanthosis nigricans (see Figure 2.10). These darkened, thickened patches of skin, often in the armpit or around the groin or neck, are a sign of insulin resistance.

Diagnostic approach

The diagnosis of PCOS is made if two of the following three features are present.

- Evidence of androgen excess: clinical features and increased serum testosterone
- Defect in ovulation: history of disturbances in the menstrual cycle
- Polycystic ovaries: multiple ovarian cysts are detected, usually by ultrasonography

Careful clinical history and physical examination often provide clues to the diagnosis. Gradual onset and slow progression of symptoms suggest a benign course, typical of PCOS.

The severity of hirsutism can be assessed using the Ferriman–Gallwey scoring system (**Figure 9.5**). Other signs of virilisation, such as clitoromegaly, deep voice and increased muscularity suggest an androgen-secreting tumour. Examine the patient for:

- galactorrhoea (a sign of hyperprolactinaemia)
- acanthosis nigricans (a sign of insulin resistance)
- signs of Cushing's syndrome (e.g. thin skin, bruises, purple abdominal striae and proximal muscle weakness)

The abdomen is examined to look for any palpable mass, which would suggest an adrenal or ovarian tumour.

> **Always look for signs of a potentially fatal androgen-secreting adrenal or ovarian tumour.** These include rapid-onset severe hirsutism, signs of virilisation (e.g. clitoromegaly) and very high androgen concentration.

Investigations

The following blood tests are required in investigations of PCOS.

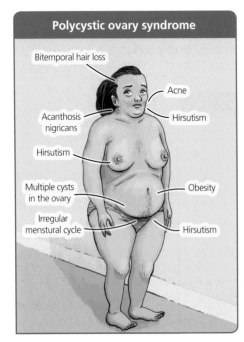

Polycystic ovary syndrome

Bitemporal hair loss

Acne

Acanthosis nigricans

Hirsutism

Hirsutism

Multiple cysts in the ovary

Obesity

Irregular menstural cycle

Hirsutism

Figure 9.4 Clinical features of polycystic ovary syndrome.

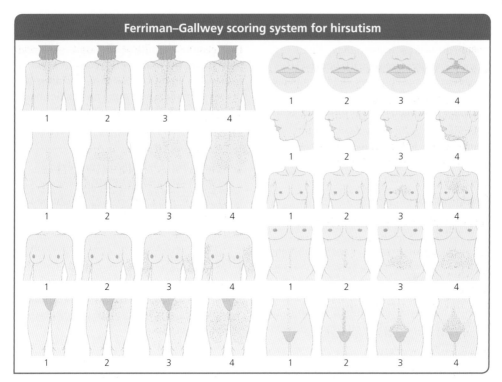

Figure 9.5 The Ferriman–Gallwey scoring system for hirsutism. The extent of excessive hair growth in nine areas of the body is scored from 1 to 4. Normal, total score < 8; mild hirsutism, score 8–15; moderate or severe hirsutism, score > 15.

- Serum testosterone: testosterone concentration is often mildly increased in PCOS
- Prolactin: to exclude hyperprolactinaemia
- Luteinising hormone, follicle-stimulating hormone and oestrogen: to exclude ovarian failure
- Thyroid-stimulating hormone: to exclude thyroid dysfunction
- Serum 17-hydroxyprogesterone: to exclude atypical congenital adrenal hyperplasia
- Haemoglobin A1c and lipid profile: because PCOS is associated with type 2 diabetes mellitus and dyslipidaemia

A 24-h urinary free cortisol test is also needed to exclude Cushing's syndrome if there are other clinical features that suggest this. Urinary cortisol concentration is increased in Cushing's syndrome.

Transvaginal or transabdominal pelvic ultrasound often shows multiple ovarian cysts in patients with PCOS (**Figure 9.2**).

> **Some women with clinical features of PCOS do not have multiple ovarian cysts on ultrasonography.** Conversely, the presence of multiple ovarian cysts on ultrasonography alone is not sufficient for a diagnosis of PCOS.

Management

Management of PCOS is directed towards managing the symptoms rather than curing the disease. It depends on the nature and severity of the presenting symptoms.

Cosmetic treatments for hirsutism in patients with PCOS include bleaching of the hair and hair removal by shaving or waxing. More long-lasting hair removal can be achieved by electrolysis or laser treatment.

Medication

The oral combined (oestrogen–progestogen) contraceptive pill may benefit patients with PCOS.

- Oestrogen suppresses luteinising hormone and therefore reduces androgen secretion from the ovaries. It also reduces free androgens by increasing the hepatic synthesis of sex hormone–binding globulin.
- Some progestogens (for example, cyproterone acetate) have antiandrogenic effects.

The following antiandrogens are sometimes used to improve symptoms resulting from androgen excess in PCOS:

- spironolactone
- finasteride (its use is limited by liver toxicity)
- flutamide (its use is limited by liver toxicity)

The use of glucocorticoids is not recommended in PCOS, because of adverse effects associated with their long-term use (see page 125).

Eflornithine cream can be applied topically to treat hirsutism. Eflornithine inhibits the L-orthinine decarboxylase enzyme involved in hair growth.

Women with PCOS and infertility may need treatment with clomifene, a selective oestrogen receptor modulator, to induce ovulation. Metformin, an oral hypoglycaemic agent, is sometimes in PCOS because the drug improves symptoms and some metabolic abnormalities (such as insulin resistance) associated with PCOS.

> **Weight loss, a healthy diet and exercise often improve symptoms of PCOS.**
> They also reduce the associated higher risk of type 2 diabetes mellitus and cardiovascular disease.

Prognosis

Women with PCOS are at increased risk of type 2 diabetes and cardiovascular disease. These risks can be reduced by weight loss and a healthy lifestyle.

Primary ovarian insufficiency

Primary ovarian insufficiency, also known as primary ovarian failure or premature ovarian failure, is a primary defect of ovarian function resulting in oestrogen deficiency and infertility before the age of 40 years. The condition is characterised by primary or secondary amenorrhoea, oestrogen deficiency and high gonadotrophin concentration.

Epidemiology

Primary ovarian insufficiency is a common condition. It affects about 0.1% of women by the age of 30 years, and about 1% by the age of 40 years.

Aetiology

Primary ovarian insufficiency has diverse causes (**Table 9.3**). The most common of these are chromosomal or other genetic defects, autoimmunity and adverse effects of treatments for other conditions.

Pathogenesis

Primary ovarian insufficiency is a consequence of the depletion or dysfunction of ovarian follicles. Ovarian follicles may be destroyed by an autoimmune response, the effects of certain drugs or infections.

In Turner's syndrome, the lack of one X chromosome results in apoptosis (programmed cell death) of oocytes during fetal life, leading to their depletion. In some genetic causes of primary ovarian insufficiency, such as mutations of the gene for the follicle-stimulating hormone receptor, an adequate number of ovarian follicles are present, but they do not function properly.

Clinical features

The symptoms of primary ovarian insufficiency are variable. They may develop suddenly or gradually over several years.

Causes of primary ovarian insufficiency	
Category	Cause
Chromosomal defects	Turner's syndrome
Single-gene defects	Fragile X syndrome
	Pseudohypoparathyroidism type 1a
	Mutations in follicle-stimulating hormone and luteinising hormone receptor genes
Autoimmune	Autoimmune oophoritis
	As a component of autoimmune polyendocrinopathy type 1 syndrome
	As a component of autoimmune polyendocrinopathy type 2 syndrome
Iatrogenic	Surgery
	Chemotherapy (e.g. with cyclophosphamide)
	Irradiation
Infections	Cyclomegalovirus
	Mumps
Idiopathic	Unknown cause

Table 9.3 Causes of primary ovarian insufficiency

Girls with prepubertal onset of primary ovarian insufficiency usually present with primary amenorrhoea. In addition, there is often evidence of growth retardation and poor pubertal development.

Women with post-pubertal primary ovarian insufficiency present with secondary amenorrhoea. This condition is associated with infertility. Patients may also have menopausal symptoms, such as flushing, night sweats, palpitations, heat intolerance and irritability. Fatigue, vaginal dryness and loss of libido are also common.

Primary ovarian insufficiency (as well as secondary ovarian insufficiency in a young woman) is associated with an increased risk of osteoporosis due to oestrogen deficiency.

Diagnostic approach

Primary ovarian insufficiency is characterised by decreased serum oestrogen, which is associated with high gonadotrophin concentration. Serum follicle-stimulating hormone concentration >30 IU/L in most cases indicates ovarian failure.

Other causes of primary or secondary amenorrhoea (**Table 9.1**) need to be excluded. For example, if there is a history of excessive weight loss or intense exercise, hypothalamic amenorrhoea should be considered (see page 285).

Investigations

Investigations required for a case of primary amenorrhoea are as follows.

- Blood tests for prolactin, thyroid-stimulating hormone, testosterone, oestrogen and follicle-stimulating hormone to investigate if an endocrine dysfunction such as hyperprolactinaemia, thyroid dysfunction, androgen excess or hypogonadism is a cause: patients with primary ovarian insufficiency have low oestrogen and high follicle-stimulating hormone
- Pelvic ultrasound to look for abnormalities of the uterus and ovaries
- Karotype analysis to identify any chromosomal defect
- Ovarian antibody titres to identify autoimmunity as a cause

For women presenting with secondary amenorrhoea, the following investigations are indicated.

- Testing for urinary or serum human chorionic gonadotrophin: to exclude pregnancy

- Measurement of serum oestrogen, luteinising hormone and follicle-stimulating hormone: low oestrogen and high gonadotrophins characterise primary ovarian insufficiency while low oestrogen with low or normal gonadotrophins suggests secondary ovarian insufficiency
- Serum prolactin measurement: to exclude hyperprolactinaemia
- A 24-h urinary free cortisol test: to exclude Cushing's syndrome if clinical features of this condition are present
- Measurement of serum thyroid-stimulating hormone: to exclude thyroid dysfunction
- Serum testosterone measurement and pelvic ultrasound: to exclude PCOS if the patient has clinical features of this condition (see page 280)

Management

Most women with primary ovarian insufficiency are treated with oestrogen replacement. Oestrogen, together with progestogen in a woman with an intact uterus, improves symptoms such as flushing, sweating and vaginal dryness. It also prevents the long-term adverse effects of oestrogen deficiency, osteoporosis in particular. Oestrogen is taken either orally or through the transdermal route.

Management options for infertility associated with primary ovarian insufficiency are limited. Patients may consider egg donation or adoption. With cryopreservation techniques, post-pubertal women who are at high risk of developing ovarian failure (e.g. those undergoing chemotherapy) can preserve their oocytes for future attempts to conceive through in vitro fertilisation.

Prognosis

Both oestrogen deficiency and infertility associated with primary ovarian insufficiency are normally irreversible.

> **Continuous use of oestrogen increases the risk of endometrial cancer.** Women with a functioning uterus who require oestrogen replacement must also be given cyclical progestogen (for ≥ 10 days of a 28-day cycle). The progestogen regularly breaks down the endometrial lining of the uterus and thus prevents endometrial hyperplasia, which is a significant risk factor for endometrial cancer.

Turner's syndrome

Turner's syndrome is the commonest chromosomal anomaly in women causing primary ovarian failure.

Epidemiology and aetiology

The condition affects about 1 in 3000 newborn girls in the general population. It is typically characterised by the absence of an X chromosome from the normal female karyotype (46XX), resulting in the 45X0 karyotype. About 15% of patients with Turner's syndrome have a mosaic karyotype, for example 45X0/46XX, 45X0/46XY or 45X0/47XXX.

Clinical features

The clinical spectrum of Turner's syndrome is variable, but the condition has typical features (**Figure 9.1**).

Newborn babies with Turner's syndrome may have swollen hands and feet, deformed ears and redundant nuchal skin. These features are the result of poor development of the lymphatic channels in fetal life.

As these girls grow, their short stature may become apparent. They may have a webbed neck, low-set ears, a low hairline, a broad chest (sometimes called a 'shield chest'), widely spaced nipples, cubitus valgum (a wide carrying angle of the arms) and multiple skin naevi. Scoliosis (curvature of the spine) may develop.

Pubertal development is poor. Patients have small breasts and amenorrhoea. Most women with Turner's syndrome are infertile.

Patients are more likely to have:

- congenital heart diseases (e.g. coarctation of the aorta, hypoplastic left heart and bicuspid aortic valve)
- congenital kidney diseases (e.g. horseshoe kidneys and a duplicate collecting system)

They are also at increased risk of primary hypothyroidism. Intelligence is usually normal, but specific learning difficulties may be experienced.

Diagnostic approach

Diagnosis of Turner's syndrome is based on the demonstration of typical chromosomal abnormality on karyotype analysis. In addition, adults with this syndrome often show primary ovarian failure on biochemical testing.

Investigations

Biochemical tests often show a low concentration of oestrogen and high concentrations of luteinising hormone and follicle-stimulating hormone in the serum. These results are evidence of primary ovarian failure (hypergonadotrophic hypogonadism).

Ultrasound, magnetic resonance imaging (MRI) or laparoscopy shows the ovaries to be hypoplastic. Histological investigation shows replacement of the ovarian follicles by fibrous streaks ('streak gonads').

Karyotype analysis confirms the diagnosis of Turner's syndrome.

Management

Management consists of oestrogen replacement to treat hypogonadism as well as screening and treatment of associated conditions. Oestrogen replacement is also used for the initiation of puberty. The use of growth hormone may be considered to address patients' short stature.

Patients require periodic screening for:

- thyroid dysfunction (through thyroid function tests)
- cardiac disorders (through echocardiography or cardiac MRI)

Some patients may achieve pregnancy through in vitro fertilisation using donor eggs. However, their pregnancies are at higher risk of miscarriage and maternal complications (such as pre-eclampsia and aortic dissection) than those in the general population.

Many patients with Turner's syndrome need psychological and special educational support but will go on to live independent lives.

Functional hypothalamic amenorrhoea

Functional hypothalamic amenorrhoea is the lack of menstrual periods for > 6 months in the absence of anatomical or organic abnormalities of the hypothalamus, pituitary gland or ovaries.

Epidemiology

The condition is common. About one third of women of reproductive age referred for

investigation of secondary amenorrhoea have functional hypothalamic amenorrhoea.

Aetiology

There are three main causes of functional hypothalamic amenorrhoea: excessive weight loss, excessive exercise and psychological stress (**Table 9.4**).

Main causes of functional hypothalamic amenorrhoea	
Cause	Association(s)
Excessive weight loss	Certain eating disorders such as: ■ anorexia nervosa ■ bulimia nervosa
Excessive exercise	Sports and physical activity requiring low body weight (such as gymnastics, long distance running and ballet dancing)
Severe psychological stress	History of significant stressful life events Obsessive–compulsive personality

Table 9.4 The main causes of functional hypothalamic amenorrhoea

Female athlete triad syndrome is the combination of eating disorder or low energy availability, amenorrhoea and osteoporosis in female athletes. The syndrome is more commonly associated with sports in which low body weight is favourable, for example ballet, gymnastics and long-distance running.

Pathogenesis

Functional hypothalamic amenorrhoea is associated with disruption of the hypothalamic–pituitary–ovarian axis. This is caused by suppression of hypothalamic gonadotrophin-releasing hormone, resulting in decreased pulsatile secretion of luteinising hormone from the anterior pituitary. There is also increased activity of the hypothalamic–pituitary–adrenal axis, with increased secretion of cortisol, adrenocorticotrophic hormone and corticotrophin-releasing hormone.

The exact mechanism leading to suppression of gonadotrophin-releasing hormone in functional hypothalamic amenorrhoea is uncertain. However, the concentration of leptin (a polypeptide primarily secreted by adipocytes) is low in this condition, and normal leptin concentration is necessary for ovulation. Therefore it has been suggested that leptin may mediate metabolic signals arising as a consequence of overall energy deficit and abnormal body weight to inhibit the hypothalamus–pituitary–ovarian axis.

Clinical features

Secondary amenorrhoea, together with associated infertility, is the commonest presenting symptom of functional hypothalamic amenorrhoea. Women with this condition may also have other symptoms and signs of oestrogen deficiency, such as loss of libido, vaginal dryness and mood disturbance. They are at high risk of osteoporosis.

Diagnostic approach

A detailed clinical history and careful physical examination are required to exclude other causes of secondary amenorrhoea (**Table 9.1**). Establish the patient's age at menarche, and if menstrual cycles have been regular in the past. Changes in weight, intensity of exercise and dietary habits may precipitate amenorrhoea. The history may elicit a stressful life event, for example bereavement, divorce or loss of a job. Look for the following signs to exclude other causes of secondary amenorrhoea.

- Galactorrhoea (suggests hyperprolactinaemia)
- Signs of thyroid dysfunction
- Signs of androgen excess, such as hirsutism and acne (suggests PCOS and androgen-producing tumours)
- Absence of sense of smell (suggests Kallmann's syndrome)
- Signs of pituitary or hypothalamic tumours, such as bitemporal visual field defects

Investigations

Biochemical tests include measurement of serum oestrogen, luteinising hormone, follicle-stimulating hormone, prolactin, thyroid-stimulating hormone and thyroxine concentrations. Women with functional hypothalamic amenorrhoea have low oestrogen concentration together with low or inappropriately normal gonadotrophin concentrations. Concentration of serum prolactin tends to be normal.

> **The progesterone challenge test** is sometimes carried out to investigate the cause of amenorrhoea. The patient takes a dosage of medroxyprogesterone orally for 7–10 days. In women who are not oestrogen deficient, withdrawal bleeding occurs within 7 days of stopping the drug. In contrast, women with functional hypothalamic amenorrhoea, because of chronic oestrogen deficiency, will show no withdrawal bleeding.

In some patients, MRI may be necessary to exclude pituitary or hypothalamic tumours.

Management

Treatment of hypothalamic amenorrhoea depends on the cause (**Table 9.5**). Adequate calcium and vitamin D intake is also recommended. Recent studies have shown that replacement therapy with human recombinant leptin may restore menstruation in this condition; however, this treatment is not yet widely used in routine clinical practice.

Prognosis

In hypothalamic amenorrhoea, the prognosis depends on the cause of the condition. Treatment is particularly difficult in cases associated with an eating disorder because psychological and medical interventions to treat eating disorders are often ineffective and patients are often reluctant to have a treatment that will induce a menstrual bleed. If treatment of the primary cause of hypothalamic amenorrhoea is unsuccessful, the associated oestrogen deficiency can be addressed with the use of oral contraceptive pills or hormone replacement therapy. The achievement of fertility for these women is challenging but can sometimes be achieved through in vitro fertilisation.

Management of functional hypothalamic amenorrhoea	
Issues	Management
Excessive weight loss	Screening for eating disorders
	Treatment according to results of screening:
	■ behaviour modification ■ psychotherapy ■ psychiatric treatment
Excessive exercise	Counselling to reduce the amount and/or intensity of exercise
	Provision of advice on:
	■ a healthy diet ■ how to gain weight
Severe psychological stress	Psychological therapy
Persistent amenorrhoea	Oestrogen replacement to help prevent bone loss: ■ oral contraceptive pills ■ hormone replacement therapy

Table 9.5 Management of functional hypothalamic amenorrhoea

Disorders of sex development

Disorders of sex development are a heterogeneous group of conditions associated with abnormal development of the reproductive organs and external genitalia. These disorders were previously known as intersex conditions.

They affect 0.1–2% of the UK population and are caused by a wide range of genetic defects. Disorders of sex development usually present at birth or puberty.

Clinical features

A mix of male and female sexual characteristics is present in the same patient.

Two examples of these disorders are congenital adrenal hyperplasia and androgen insensitivity syndrome.

- In congenital adrenal hyperplasia, a person who is genetically female (with XX sex chromosomes and a uterus and ovaries) presents with a clitoris that resembles a penis; the clitoromegaly is caused by androgen excess.
- In androgen insensitivity syndrome, a person who is genetically male (with XY sex chromosomes) presents with ambiguous or female external genitalia; because of a mutation in the androgen receptor, the body does not respond to androgens and therefore a female phenotype develops.

Management

The key aspects of management of disorders of sex development diagnosed in infancy or adolescence are:

- deciding whether the child is to be raised as a boy or a girl
- reconstructive surgeries and hormone treatment to enhance the chosen sex
- psychological and emotional support for the patient and their parents

Hypogonadism in men

Male hypogonadism is a clinical condition resulting from inadequate secretion of the male sex hormone testosterone. The condition is often associated with male infertility because of defective production of spermatozoa.

Epidemiology

Hypogonadism in men is common, affecting about 5% of middle-aged men in the general population. As these men age, there is a gradual decline in testosterone secretion. Nearly one third of men aged > 75 years have a testosterone concentration below the normal range. However, there is controversy over whether or not this age-related decline in testosterone is pathological and requires treatment.

Aetiology

Male hypogonadism is caused by disorders of one of either of the following.

- The testes: primary hypogonadism or hypergonadotrophic hypogonadism

- Disorders of the pituitary gland or hypothalamus: secondary hypogonadism or hypogonadotrophic hypogonadism

Primary and secondary hypogonadism in men can be either congenital or acquired. Common causes are shown in **Table 9.6**. The most common cause of congenital primary hypogonadism is Klinefelter's syndrome (see page 290).

Infertility associated with secondary hypogonadism can be treated pharmacologically. The drugs used are:

- gonadotrophins

- human chorionic gonadotrophin (which has the biological activity of luteinising hormone)

- gonadotrophin-releasing hormone (in cases of secondary hypogonadism caused by hypothalamic disorders)

These treatments are ineffective in primary hypogonadism because the principal defect is in the ovaries or testes and this is not reversed by these treatments.

Causes of male hypogonadism	
Primary hypogonadism	Secondary hypogonadism
Haemochromatosis	Haemochromatosis
Klinefelter's syndrome	Kallmann's syndrome
Radiation to testes	Radiotherapy involving the pituitary gland and hypothalamus
Certain drugs (e.g. spironolactone and cyclophosphamide)	Certain drugs (e.g. opiates)
Mumps orchitis	Pituitary and hypothalamic tumours
Trauma	Pituitary and hypothalamic surgery
Undescended testes	Congenital hypopituitarism
Autoimmunity	Hyperprolactinaemia
Systemic diseases (e.g. liver failure and renal failure)	Morbid obesity

Table 9.6 Causes of primary and secondary male hypogonadism

Clinical features

The clinical features of male hypogonadism depend on the age of onset. A baby with male sex chromosomes (XY) who develops hypogonadism during fetal development may be born with ambiguous genitalia. Male hypogonadism that develops during childhood often results in delayed or absent puberty.

Clinical features of hypogonadism that develop before puberty and during adulthood are shown in **Table 9.7**.

Kallmann's syndrome is a genetic condition associated with hypogonadotrophic hypogonadism and anosmia (loss of the sense of smell). The syndrome is five times more common in males. Abnormal development of the hypothalamus impairs secretion of gonadotrophin-releasing hormone, leading to decreased secretion of gonadotrophins and testosterone.

Clinical features of male hypogonadism	
Before puberty	During adulthood
Decreased body and facial hair	Decreased body and facial hair
Gynaecomastia	Gynaecomastia
Small testes and penis	Erectile dysfunction
Poor development of muscles	Decreased muscle mass
Reduced libido	Loss of libido
Unclosed epiphyses	Osteoporosis
Eunuchoid body habitus	Fatigue and lassitude
High-pitched voice	Hot flushes
	Depression and mood changes

Table 9.7 Clinical features of male hypogonadism

Diagnostic approach

Male hypogonadism presents with features of androgen deficiency (**Table 5.7**), together with a low early morning serum testosterone concentration.

Investigations

Serum concentrations of gonadotrophins (luteinising hormone and follicle-stimulating hormone) are checked to distinguish between primary and secondary hypogonadism (**Table 9.8**). Primary hypogonadism is characterised by high serum gonadotrophins. Secondary hypogonadism is associated with low or low-normal gonadotrophins.

Further investigations are done to determine the cause of the hypogonadism.

■ Karyotype analysis: Klinefelter's syndrome
■ Serum ferritin: haemochromatosis
■ MRI: pituitary or hypothalamic tumours

Patients with secondary hypogonadism need tests for other pituitary functions (for example serum prolactin, TSH, free T_4, short synacthen test or insulin stress test and IGF1). Patients presenting with infertility require seminal fluid analysis. A bone density scan (dual-energy X-ray absorptiometry)

Hormone level in primary and secondary hypogonadism		
Hormones	Primary hypogonadism	Secondary hypogonadism
Oestrogen (females)	Decreased	Decreased
Testosterone (males)	Decreased	Decreased
LH	Increased	Decreased or inappropriately normal
FSH	Increased	Decreased or inappropriately normal

Table 9.8 Difference in hormone levels in primary and secondary hypogonadism

is necessary if osteoporosis is suspected (e.g. in cases of low-impact fracture).

> **Long-term use of opioid drugs can cause hypogonadotrophic hypogonadism.** It results mainly from the suppression of gonadotrophin releasing hormone from the hypothalamus by opioid drugs.

Management

The aim of management is to improve symptoms by restoring a normal testosterone concentration, usually by testosterone replacement. Testosterone can be delivered through intramuscular, transdermal, oral or sublingual routes, or through implants.

Intramuscular testosterone injections include testosterone enanthate and testosterone propionate; these are short-acting preparations injected every 2–4 weeks. Another option is testosterone undecanoate, a long acting preparation given every 10–14 weeks. It tends to maintain a more steady concentration

of testosterone compared to 2–4 weekly injections, so it is becoming increasingly popular.

Transdermal testosterone is delivered through a gel or patch applied daily. This provides a stable serum testosterone concentration but can irritate the skin.

Oral testosterone (testosterone undecanoate) is of limited use. It has variable absorption, and multiple doses are needed daily.

Sublingual testosterone is rapidly absorbed. However, daily doses are necessary and there is a small risk of local irritation.

Testosterone implants require minor surgery for their insertion and last about 6 months. However, there is a small risk of infection and expulsion of the implant.

Testosterone replacement is contraindicated in some conditions, including:

- prostate cancer
- male breast cancer
- polycythaemia

Adverse effects of testosterone replacement include:

- polycythaemia
- increased risk of prostate cancer
- aggression and emotional lability
- changes in libido

Serum testosterone concentrations of patients treated with the drug are monitored regularly to ensure that the dose of testosterone is correct. In addition, serum prostate-specific antigen is measured for early diagnosis of prostate carcinoma, and haematocrit is done to identify polycythaemia.

Prognosis

Most treatments of male hypogonadism improve quality of life and prevent long-term adverse effects such as osteoporosis. However, the success of treatment of male infertility associated with male hypogonadism is more variable.

Klinefelter's syndrome

Klinefelter's syndrome is the commonest chromosomal anomaly in men causing primary hypogonadism.

Epidemiology and aetiology

The condition affects about 1 in 1000 newborn boys. It is typically characterised by the presence of an extra X chromosome, resulting in a 47XXY karyotype instead of the normal male karyotype (46XY). Some patients have a mosaic karyotype, such as 46XY/47XXY. Others have further additional X chromosomes (e.g. in 48XXXY, 48XXYY or 49XXXXY karyotypes).

Clinical features

Men with Klinefelter's syndrome share certain features (**Figure 9.1**). They are tall, with long legs. They also have a female body habitus, with small testes and gynaecomastia (enlargement of the male breasts).

Infertility is a symptom of the condition. Over 95% of men with Klinefelter's syndrome have azoospermia (absence of sperm in the ejaculate).

They are more likely to have congenital malformations, such as cryptorchidism and cleft palate. They may develop osteoporosis, and are also at increased risk of metabolic syndrome and type 2 diabetes mellitus.

A varying degree of learning difficulties, including an average reduction in IQ by approximately 5-10 points, speech problems and psychological problems, may be present.

Diagnostic approach

Diagnosis of Klinefelter's syndrome involves demonstration of primary hypogonadism with biochemical tests and typical chromosomal abnormality with karyotype analysis.

Investigations

Biochemical investigations show a low concentration of testosterone and high concentrations of luteinising hormone and follicle-stimulating hormone in the serum. These results indicate primary hypogonadism (hypergonadotrophic hypogonadism).

Karyotype analysis confirms the diagnosis of Klinefelter's syndrome.

Management

Testosterone replacement is used to treat hypogonadism in patients with Klinefelter's syndrome.

Fertility may be achieved in some patients with the use of testicular sperm extraction and intracytoplasmic sperm injection.

Many patients with Klinefelter's syndrome require psychological counselling and support for learning.

Answers to starter questions

1. Obesity is common in women with polycystic ovarian syndrome (PCOS) and is associated with increased androgen levels, insulin resistance, glucose intolerance and dyslipidaemia. Weight loss improves symptoms, such as hirsutism and irregular menstrual periods, and metabolic abnormalities associated with PCOS.

2. Testosterone has an important influence on behaviour, mental attitude, sexuality and social interaction in men. These are particularly evident in men with hypogonadism and those on excess testosterone doses. Hypogonadal men often have poor libidos, lethargy and depressive moods, which improve with testosterone replacement. In contrast, high testosterone levels are associated with aggression, although it remains unclear whether it is also associated with antisocial behaviour.

3. Circulating androgens, including testosterone, decrease with age in women, which is associated with reduced sexual drive. Small, randomised controlled trials, have suggested that giving testosterone can improve libido in these women. However, the long-term adverse effects are unknown and the treatment is not routinely recommended.

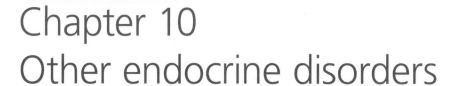

Chapter 10
Other endocrine disorders

Starter questions

Answers to the following questions are on page 304.

1. Why is it important to examine the nails of a patient with autoimmune Addison's disease?
2. Why do 90% of patients with carcinoid tumours have no symptoms of carcinoid syndrome?
3. What is pancreatic cholera?

Introduction

Most endocrine disorders occur sporadically. However, some are inherited and therefore affect many members of a family. Furthermore, several endocrine disorders may coexist in the same patient. For example, a patient may present with one of the multiple endocrine neoplasia (MEN) syndromes with tumours in several endocrine glands.

The MEN syndromes are inherited in an autosomal dominant pattern, so other family members are likely to be affected. Diagnosis of such a disorder in one person prompts screening of members of their family to allow early detection and treatment of the condition.

Some tumours that arise from tissues that do not normally secrete hormones produce ectopic hormones. The ectopic hormones secreted from these tumours cause a range of clinical features, such as those found in Cushing's syndrome caused by a small-cell lung cancer secreting adrenocorticotrophic hormone (ACTH).

Neuroendocrine tumours are tumours arising from cells of neuroendocrine origin and can occur widely in the body. They are a heterogeneous group of tumours that can be benign or malignant and are either secretory or non-secretory (of hormones).

Case 12 Worsening vision and headache

Presentation

Mrs James, aged 29 years, presents to her general practitioner with headaches that have worsened over the past 3 months. The headaches have sometimes woken her from sleep. In the past week, she realised that she also bumps into furniture that she does not notice is there.

Initial interpretation

Headache is a common symptom. The commonest causes are tension headache and migraine. However, it is unusual for headache to wake patients from sleep, so this warrants further investigation. The history of bumping into things points to a problem with vision. This symptom, together with severe headaches, raises a possibility of an intracranial pathology.

Further history

Mrs James is seen in the outpatient clinic for further evaluation. Her headaches are dull and all over the head. They are not associated with visual disturbances, such as flashing lights. Mrs James feels nauseous with her headaches but has not vomited.

She mentions that she has noticed milky discharge from both her breasts for at least 6 months. Lately, her menstrual cycle has become irregular, and she has not had a menstrual period for the past 4 months.

Mrs James is taking omeprazole (a proton pump inhibitor) for acid reflux symptoms. She works as a shop assistant. She does not smoke, and she drinks alcohol only occasionally. She has two daughters and no plans for any more children.

Her father had recurrent stomach ulcers and died in his forties from a pancreatic tumour. Her younger brother recently learned that he has excessive calcium caused by primary hyperparathyroidism.

Examination

Mrs James has bilateral galactorrhoea, with no breast masses. Her visual acuity is normal, but she has bitemporal hemianopia (loss of temporal vision on both sides) on visual field testing. Her abdominal examination is unremarkable.

Interpretation of findings

Headache, secondary amenorrhoea, galactorrhoea and bitemporal hemianopia all point towards the diagnosis of a pituitary macroadenoma with compression of the optic chiasm. The presence of a pancreatic tumour and primary hyperparathyroidism in first-degree relatives raises the suspicion of an inherited syndrome. It is unusual for a young person to have indigestion symptoms strong enough to require treatment with a proton pump inhibitor.

A possible unifying diagnosis is MEN type 1 syndrome, which is an autosomal dominant condition associated with parathyroid, pituitary and pancreatic tumours.

Investigations

A pregnancy test is negative, but serum prolactin is 25,000 mu/L (normal range 102–496). Magnetic resonance imaging (MRI) shows a large pituitary adenoma compressing the optic chiasm (**Figure 10.1**). Serum calcium is 2.8 mmol/L (normal range 2.05–2.55), and serum parathyroid hormone is 9.1 pmol/l (normal range 1.6–6.9); these findings, showing hypercalcaemia together with inappropriately raised serum parathyroid hormone, are consistent with primary hyperparathyroidism.

A sestamibi scan of the parathyroid suggests bilateral parathyroid adenomas. Gastroendoscopy shows two duodenal ulcers. Fasting serum gastrin concentration,

Case 12 *continued*

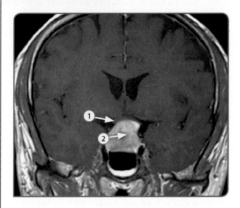

Figure 10.1 Large pituitary adenoma ② compressing the optic chiasm ①.

which is checked after stopping omeprazole for 1 week, is increased to 1500 pg/ml (normal range 0–100). Computerised tomography (CT) shows a 2-cm tumour in the neck of the pancreas.

Diagnosis

These findings suggest a gastrinoma: a gastrin-secreting pancreatic tumour that usually presents with multiple peptic ulcers. Genetic testing identifies a mutation in the *MEN1* gene.

The concurrence of pituitary adenoma, pancreatic tumour and primary hyperparathyroidism in Mrs James, along with the presence of MEN type 1–associated conditions in her family members, are in keeping with the clinical diagnosis of familial MEN type 1. The positive genetic screening test confirms the diagnosis. She starts treatment with cabergoline (a dopamine agonist) for prolactin secreting pituitary adenoma and is referred for parathyroid and pancreatic surgery. Her first degree relatives are offered genetic screening for mutation in the *MEN1* gene.

Multiple endocrine neoplasia syndromes

Multiple endocrine neoplasia syndromes are a group of rare autosomal dominant inherited conditions characterised by the occurrence of tumours of multiple endocrine glands. There are two main types (**Table 10.1**):

- Multiple endocrine neoplasia type 1
- Multiple endocrine neoplasia type 2

Multiple endocrine neoplasia syndrome type 1

Multiple endocrine neoplasia type 1 is a syndrome characterised by a triad of tumours in the parathyroid, pituitary and pancreas (the three P's). Patients occasionally also have

Classification of multiple endocrine neoplasia		
MEN type 1	MEN type 2	
	Type 2a	Type 2b
Parathyroid tumours	Medullary thyroid cancer	Medullary thyroid cancer
Pituitary tumours	Phaeochromocytoma	Phaeochromocytoma
Pancreaticoduodenal tumours	Parathyroid tumours	Characteristic phenotypic features, including marfanoid habitus and mucocutaneous neuromas

Table 10.1 Classification of multiple endocrine neoplasia (MEN) and key associated features

adrenocortical tumours, carcinoid tumours, lipomas, angiofibromas and meningiomas.

Epidemiology

Multiple endocrine neoplasia type 1 is rare. The condition has an annual incidence of one or two cases per 100,000 people in the general population.

Aetiology

MEN type 1 is associated with inactivating mutations in the tumour suppressor gene (*MEN1* gene) on chromosome 11.

Clinical features

The clinical features of MEN type 1 depend on the type of tumours and the hormones that they produce. Over 95% of patients with MEN type 1 develop primary hyperparathyroidism caused by parathyroid adenomas or hyperplasia; this is usually the first condition to become apparent.

Pituitary tumours associated with MEN type 1 include:

- prolactinomas (the commonest)
- Cushing's disease
- acromegaly
- non-functioning adenomas

Pancreaticoduodenal tumours may be gastrinomas, insulinomas, glucagonomas, vipomas or non-secretory tumours.

Diagnostic approach

The clinical diagnosis of MEN type 1 is made if a patient has two out of three main MEN type 1–associated tumours (parathyroid, pituitary and pancreatic). The molecular diagnosis of MEN type 1 can be made by screening for mutations of the *MEN1* gene.

Management

The management of MEN type 1 requires early identification and treatment of individual associated tumours. Patients with this condition tend to develop hyperparathyroidism involving all four glands, so they often need total parathyroidectomy.

Patients are monitored regularly for early detection and treatment of new MEN type 1–associated tumours. If a mutation of the *MEN1* gene is identified in the patient, presymptomatic genetic screening is offered to their first-degree relatives. Relatives with positive genetic mutations also need regular surveillance for development of MEN type 1–related tumours.

> **Counselling of patients with MEN type 1 is essential so that they know what to expect and why continued follow-up is important.** The condition can be associated with a huge economic and psychological burden. Patients are financially disadvantaged by the need to take time off work for treatments and regular tests, as well as the effect on insurance premiums. They are likely to worry about the future, and those who wish to start a family need genetic counselling.

Prognosis

The life expectancy of patients with MEN type 1 is often reduced. Death is usually from metastatic pancreatic tumours.

Multiple endocrine neoplasia syndrome type 2

Multiple endocrine neoplasia type 2 is further classified into MEN type 2a and MEN type 2b (**Table 10.1**). Both conditions are associated with mutations of the *RET* proto-oncogene on the long arm of chromosome 10.

Types

Multiple endocrine neoplasia type 2a is characterised by the presence of medullary thyroid carcinoma and phaeochromocytoma. Primary hyperparathyroidism caused by parathyroid adenomas may also be present. MEN type 2a is rare, with an annual incidence of 2–20 per 100,000 in the general population.

Multiple endocrine neoplasia type 2b is also characterised by the presence of medullary thyroid carcinoma and phaeochromocytoma.

However, it is also associated with a characteristic phenotype. MEN type 2b is much rarer than MEN type 2a, with an annual incidence of about 4 per 100 million in the general population versus 1 in 4 million.

Clinical features

The clinical features of MEN type 2a and MEN type 2b depend on the associated tumours. Medullary thyroid carcinoma is often the initial manifestation in both syndromes, although this occurs much earlier and is more aggressive in MEN type 2b than in type 2a. In addition, patients with MEN type 2b have a characteristic phenotype (**Figure 10.2**), with a marfanoid body habitus, mucosal neuromas (**Figure 10.3**), high-arched palate and thickened corneal nerves.

Diagnostic approach

Investigations for medullary thyroid carcinomas are discussed in Chapter 5 (see page 212),

those for phaeochromocytoma in Chapter 7 (see page 248) and those for primary hyperparathyroidism in Chapter 8 (see page 260). Molecular diagnosis of MEN type 2a and type 2b can be made by screening for mutations of the *RET* gene.

Management

Treatment of MEN type 2 is by surgical excision of associated tumours. In case of inoperable medullary thyroid carcinoma associated with MEN type 2, symptoms can be improved with the use of tyrosine kinase inhibitors, which target vascular endothelial growth factor receptors.

> In patients with MEN type 2, screen for and treat phaeochromocytoma before surgery to remove a medullary thyroid carcinoma. By treating the phaeochromocytoma first, a life-threatening adrenergic crisis is avoided.

If a patient is found to have a mutation of the *RET* gene, genetic screening is offered to

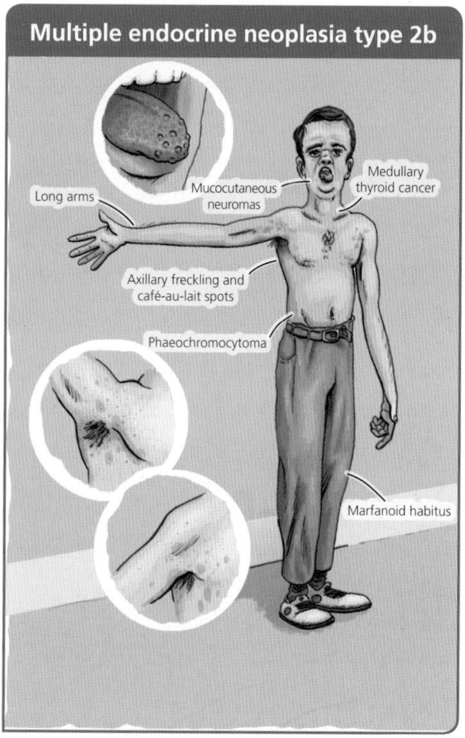

Multiple endocrine neoplasia type 2b

Long arms — Mucocutaneous neuromas — Medullary thyroid cancer

Axillary freckling and café-au-lait spots

Phaeochromocytoma

Marfanoid habitus

Figure 10.2 Clinical features of multiple endocrine neoplasia type 2b.

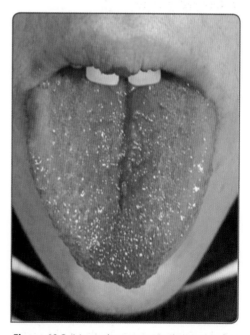

Figure 10.3 Mucosal neuromas in the tongue.

their asymptomatic first degree relatives. Relatives who are mutation positive are strongly advised to undergo prophylactic thyroidectomy, because they have an almost 100% risk of developing a medullary thyroid carcinoma. They also require surveillance for the development of phaeochromocytoma and primary hyperparathyroidism (in cases of MEN type 2a

only because MEN type 2b is not associated with primary hyperparathyroidism).

Prognosis

Prognosis has improved in recent years. Because MEN type 2b is associated with more aggressive medullary thyroid carcinoma, its prognosis is usually worse than MEN type 2a.

Autoimmune polyglandular syndromes

Autoimmune polyglandular syndromes are a diverse group of disorders resulting from coexisting autoimmune disorders of various endocrine glands and other organs. There are two main types: autoimmune polyglandular syndrome type 1 and type 2.

Clinical features

The clinical features of autoimmune polyglandular syndrome type 1 and type 2 are compared in **Table 10.2**.

Comparison of autoimmune polyglandular syndrome types 1 and 2	
Type 1	Type 2
Alternative name(s)	
Autoimmune polyendocrinopathy candidiasis	Schmidt's syndrome
Ectodermal dystrophy syndrome	
Associated autoimmune disorders	
Autoimmune Addison's disease	Autoimmune Addison's disease
Autoimmune hypoparathyroidism	Autoimmune thyroid disease
Chronic mucocutaneous candidiasis	Type 1 diabetes mellitus
Type 1 diabetes mellitus	Primary gonadal failure
Primary gonadal failure	Pernicious anaemia
Pernicious anaemia	Alopecia
Chronic active hepatitis	Vitiligo
Autoimmune hypothyroidism	
Alopecia	
Vitiligo	
Cause	
Monogenic disease caused by mutations in the autoimmune regulator-1 gene in chromosome 21	Complex polygenic disease, with multiple genetic factors (including the HLA genes) affecting susceptibility to the disease
Presentation	
Childhood	Adulthood
Affects both sexes equally	More common in women

Table 10.2 Comparison of autoimmune polyglandular syndromes type 1 and type 2

Management

Individual endocrine disorders associated with both types of autoimmune polyglandular syndrome are managed in the similar way as when these disorders manifest separately.

> **Patients with autoimmune polyglandular syndrome type 1 and type 2** require regular surveillance for development of new autoimmune disorders associated with these syndromes.

Ectopic hormone syndromes

Ectopic hormones are secreted by tumours arising from organs or tissues that do not normally secrete them. Common ectopic hormones and associated clinical syndromes are shown in **Table 10.3**.

The diagnosis of ectopic hormone syndromes is usually made by detecting excessive hormone concentration in the presence of a tumour. These conditions are managed by treating the underlying tumour and relieving the symptoms caused by excessive ectopic hormones.

Clinical features

The clinical features of ectopic hormone syndromes vary depending on the hormone secreted and the nature of the tumour secreting the hormone. For example, a

Tumours producing ectopic hormones and their associated syndromes		
Ectopic hormone	Tumours producing ectopic hormones	Associated clinical syndrome
Adrenocorticotrophic hormone	Small-cell carcinoma of lung	Cushing's syndrome
	Carcinoid tumours (bronchus, thymus, pancreas or gut)	
	Phaeochromocytoma	
	Medullary thyroid carcinoma	
Antidiuretic hormone	Small-cell carcinoma of lung	Syndrome of inappropriate antidiuretic hormone
	Carcinoid tumours (bronchus)	
Human chorionic gonadotrophin	Carcinoma of lung	Gynaecomastia
Parathyroid hormone or parathyroid hormone–related peptide	Squamous cell carcinoma of lung	Hypercalcaemia
	Breast carcinoma	
Growth hormone–releasing hormone	Small-cell carcinoma of lung	Acromegaly
	Carcinoid tumours (bronchus)	
	Pancreatic neuroendocrine tumours	
Insulin-like growth factor 2	Fibrosarcoma	Hypoglycaemia
	Hepatocellular carcinoma	
Corticotrophin-releasing hormone	Small-cell carcinoma of lung	Cushing's syndrome
	Carcinoid tumours	
	Medullary thyroid carcinoma	
Erythropoietin	Renal cell carcinoma	Polycythaemia
	Hepatocellular carcinoma	

Table 10.3 Ectopic hormones, tumours producing ectopic hormones and associated clinical syndromes

small-cell carcinoma of the lung secreting ectopic ACTH presents with Cushing's syndrome. However, the condition of patients with this high-grade cancer often deteriorates rapidly, so they may not survive long enough to develop all clinical features of Cushing's syndrome. These patients have very high concentrations of ACTH and are therefore characteristically hyperpigmented. Hypokalaemia and metabolic alkalosis are also common.

In contrast, a slow-growing carcinoid tumour secreting ectopic ACTH is associated with a more indolent form of Cushing's syndrome. It can sometimes be challenging to differentiate this condition from pituitary-dependent Cushing's disease (see page 226). The carcinoid tumour producing ectopic ACTH can often be smaller than 1 cm, making it difficult to detect by imaging.

Management

The treatment of choice for Cushing's syndrome caused by ectopic ACTH secretion is resection of the tumour; however, this is not possible in many cases. If the tumour is inoperable or undetectable, control of the symptoms of Cushing's syndrome can be achieved by bilateral adrenalectomy or medical treatment (see page 229).

Carcinoid tumours and carcinoid syndrome

Carcinoid tumours are a group of neuroendocrine tumours; neoplasias from a range of neuroendocrine cells that can occur in various parts of the body and cause clinical syndromes (**Table 10.4**).

Carcinoid tumours arise from enterochromaffin cells (a type of neuroendocrine cell) in foregut, midgut and hindgut tumours (**Table 10.5**). Two thirds arise in the gastrointestinal tract, mostly the small intestine. The annual incidence is 20 cases per 1,000,000 in the general population. Most carcinoid tumours grow slowly and are asymptomatic, but about 10% are malignant and lead to debilitating symptoms.

About 10% of patients with a carcinoid tumour present with the classical carcinoid syndrome resulting from an increased secretion of vasoactive peptides into the systemic circulation. Serotonin is the key peptide responsible for this effect; others include kallikrein, histamine and prostaglandins.

Carcinoid syndrome typically occurs with midgut carcinoid tumours with liver metastasis, otherwise the liver metabolises the peptides before they cause the syndrome.

Clinical features

Clinical features of carcinoid syndrome include:

Neuroendocrine tumours and the hormones they secrete	
Neuroendocrine tumour	Hormone(s)
Carcinoid disease	Serotonin
	Kallikrein
	Histamine
	Prostaglandins
Insulinoma	Insulin
Glucagonoma	Glucagon
Gastrinoma (Zollinger–Ellison syndrome)	Gastrin
Vipomas	Vasoactive intestinal peptide
Somatostatinomas	Somatostatin
Phaeochromocytoma	Catecholamines
Paraganglioma	Catecholamines
Medullary thyroid carcinoma	Calcitonin
Small-cell carcinoma of the lung	Adrenocorticotrophic hormone
	Vasopressin
Non-secretory pancreatic neuroendocrine tumours	–

Table 10.4 Neuroendocrine tumours and hormones secreted by the tumours

Classification of carcinoid tumours	
Class	Site
Foregut	Thymus
	Bronchus
	Stomach
	Duodenum
Midgut	Pancreas
	Small intestine
	Appendix
Hindgut	Colon
	Rectum

Table 10.5 Classification of carcinoid tumours based on the location of the primitive gut from where they originate

- episodic flushing
- secretory diarrhoea
- bronchospasm
- pleural fibrosis
- right-sided cardiac valvular lesions (particularly tricuspid incompetence and pulmonary stenosis)
- pellagra

Some patients with carcinoid syndrome develop pellagra, a serious deficiency of niacin. Pellagra presents with skin lesions, diarrhoea, cardiomyopathy and dementia. The deficiency develops because the tumour consumes dietary tryptophan to make serotonin, and tryptophan is needed for the synthesis of niacin.

Diagnostic approach

Carcinoid syndrome is diagnosed if the patient has increased urinary 5-hydroxy-indole acetic acid (5-HIAA), which is the end product of serotonin metabolism in the body. Tryptophan-rich foods may mildly increase urinary 5-HIAA and should therefore be avoided during the test; they include bananas, avocados, aubergines, plums, walnuts and pineapples. The concentration of chromogranin A, a peptide produced by carcinoid and other neuroendocrine tumours, is also often increased.

Carcinoid tumours are often small and difficult to identify with conventional imaging. In addition to ultrasound, CT and MRI, scintigraphy using a radiolabelled somatostatin analogue (octreoscan) are used to identify primary carcinoid tumours and metastasis. Metaiodobenzylguanidine (MIBG) and positron emission tomography scans are also occasionally used for localising these tumours.

Management

The management of carcinoid syndrome consists of controlling symptoms and treating the underlying disease.

Somatostatin analogues prevent release of vasoactive peptides, leading to relief of symptoms and have a role in tumour stabilisation. Antidiarrhoeal agents may help to control intractable diarrhoea.

Radical surgery may result in complete remission. Resections of hepatic metastases are often carried out during the excision of the primary tumour.

The prognosis for carcinoid tumours is highly variable. Some patients have a very poor prognosis with rapid deterioration and death while others, even with metastatic disease, live more than 20–30 years.

Carcinoid crisis is a severe, life-threatening form of carcinoid syndrome. It is caused by the sudden release of a large amount of vasoactive peptides. This can be triggered by surgery, so prophylactic somatostatin analogues are used.

Insulinomas

Insulinomas are neuroendocrine tumours arising from the beta islet cells of the pancreas that secrete excessive insulin. These tumours are rare, with an annual incidence of fewer than four cases per million in the general population. Most insulinomas are small (<2 cm), solitary and benign; only about 5% of cases are malignant. Up to 10% of insulinomas are familial, some of which occur as part of MEN type 1. Insulinomas associated with MEN type 1 tend to be multiple and are often malignant.

Clinical features

Patients with insulinomas present with symptoms of hypoglycaemia, such as tremor, sweating, palpitations, anxiety and hunger. In the most severe cases, patients may develop profound hypoglycaemia, leading to confusion, seizures and coma. The hypoglycaemic symptoms in insulinoma typically occur in a fasting state, although patients may occasionally present with the symptoms after a meal. Patients with insulinomas tend to eat more frequently to prevent hypoglycaemic symptoms, so weight gain is common.

Diagnostic approach

Insulinoma is considered in patients presenting with Whipple's triad:

- symptoms consistent with hypoglycaemia
- a low blood glucose concentration at the time of the symptoms
- relief of the symptoms once blood glucose concentration is normalised

Diagnosis is made on the basis of the patient developing hypoglycaemia during a 72-h fast; this is associated with increased insulin and C-peptide concentration at the time of the

hypoglycaemia (see page 109). In contrast, hypoglycaemia caused by exogenous insulin is associated with increased insulin and decreased C-peptide (Table 10.6). Hypoglycaemia resulting from the use of sulfonylurea drugs, such as gliclazide, is associated with increased insulin and C-peptide concentrations similar to those in insulinoma; however, sulfonylurea can be detected by screening serum or urine (Table 10.6).

After the biochemical diagnosis of insulinoma, CT, MRI or endoscopic ultrasound is used to localise the tumour.

Management

Definitive treatment of an insulinoma is surgical removal of the tumour. Medical treatment (with diazoxide or somatostatin analogues) is sometimes used:

- while awaiting the surgery
- when the tumour cannot be localised
- in the presence of inoperable metastatic disease
- if the patient is unfit for surgery

Differential diagnosis of spontaneous hypoglycaemia			
Test	Insulinoma	Exogenous insulin	Sulfonylurea
Insulin	↑	↑	↑
C-peptide	↑	↓	↑
Sulfonylurea screen	Not detected	Not detected	Positive

Table 10.6 Differential diagnosis of spontaneous hypoglycaemia

Other neuroendocrine tumours

Other neuroendocrine tumours such as gastrinoma, glucagonoma, vipoma and somatostatinoma are rare, and present with diverse clinical syndromes.

Gastrinomas

Gastrinomas (also known as Zollinger-Ellison syndrome) are rare gastrin-secreting

neuroendocrine tumours arising from the duodenum or the pancreas. About two thirds of gastrinomas are malignant, and one third are associated with MEN type 1.

Clinical features include:

- multiple, severe and recurrent peptic ulceration (caused by excessive production of gastric acid in response to the hypersecretion of gastrin)

- diarrhoea and malabsorption (resulting from inactivation of intestinal enzymes, as well as intestinal mucosal damage caused by excessive gastric acid secretion)

Patients with gastrinomas have increased fasting plasma gastrin. After biochemical diagnosis, various imaging techniques are used to localise the tumour; they include CT, MRI, endoscopic ultrasound, scintigram using radiolabelled somatostatin analogue and selective angiography.

Treatment of gastrinomas includes surgery (if the tumour is operable) and proton pump inhibitors (to reduce gastric acid production).

Glucagonomas

Glucagonomas are very rare neuroendocrine tumours arising from the alpha islet cells of the pancreas and secreting excessive glucagon. Most of these tumours are highly malignant.

Clinical features include:

- a characteristic skin rash called necrolytic migratory erythema
- diabetes or impaired glucose tolerance
- weight loss
- anaemia
- deep vein thrombosis

Diagnosis is made by showing markedly increased plasma glucagon concentration. Treatment of glucagonoma includes surgery (if the tumour is operable), chemotherapy and somatostatin analogues (for symptom control).

Vipoma

Vipomas are very rare neuroendocrine tumours that secrete vasoactive intestinal polypeptide (VIP). Over 90% of these tumours arise in the pancreas.

Clinical features include:

- intractable and profuse watery diarrhoea (typically > 3 L/day, sometimes up to 20 L/day)

- dehydration and occasionally circulatory collapse (resulting from diarrhoea)
- electrolyte disturbance (particularly hypokalaemic alkalosis caused by loss of potassium and bicarbonate through diarrhoea)

The biochemical diagnosis is made by showing increased plasma VIP concentration. After biochemical diagnosis, imaging modalities, including CT, MRI and scintigram using radiolabelled somatostatin analogue, are used to localise the tumour.

> Vipoma crisis is a life-threatening emergency characterised by circulatory shock and electrolyte disturbance as a result of profuse diarrhoea in a patient with vipoma. The patient must be resuscitated with intravenous fluid.

Surgery is the treatment of choice if the tumour is operable. Somatostatin analogues are effective in controlling the diarrhoea.

Somatostatinoma

Somatostatinomas are somatostatin-secreting tumours arising from pancreatic delta islet cells and the small intestine. They can be malignant.

Clinical features include:

- diarrhoea or steatorrhoea
- gallstones
- glucose intolerance
- achlorhydria (little or no production of gastric acid in the stomach)

Biochemical diagnosis is based on increased fasting somatostatin concentration. Imaging modalities CT, MRI and scintigram using radiolabelled somatostatin analogue are used to localise the tumour.

Treatment options include surgery if the tumour is operable, and chemotherapy in cases of metastatic disease.

Answers to starter questions

1. Rarely, autoimmune Addison's disease occurs as a component of type 1 autoimmune polyendocrine syndrome (APS), which is associated with chronic candidiasis, hypoparathyroidism and other autoimmune disorders. The presence of chronic Candida infection in a patient's nails provides a clue to diagnosing this condition.

2. Only about 10% of carcinoid tumours cause carcinoid syndrome, most commonly by midgut carcinoid tumours alongside liver metastasis. Tumours without liver metastasis do not produce the syndrome because vasoactive peptides secreted by the tumour (such as serotonin) are metabolised by the liver before reaching the systemic circulation. Most hindgut carcinoid tumours are nonsecretory and do not cause carcinoid syndrome.

3. Vasoactive intestinal polypeptide secreting tumours (VIPoma) are usually located in the pancreas and cause watery diarrhoea. This can be as profuse and intractable as in patients with cholera and is therefore referred to as pancreatic cholera.

Chapter 11
Endocrine emergencies

Introduction

Diabetes-related emergencies such as severe hypoglycaemia and diabetic ketoacidosis are common causes of admission to hospital. In contrast, some endocrine emergencies, such as thyroid storm and pituitary apoplexy, are very rare, so their recognition and diagnosis are frequently delayed.

Endocrine emergencies have one of two causes:

- excessive hormone secretion, for example oversecretion of catecholamines resulting in a hypertensive crisis

- hormone deficiency, such as insulin deficiency in cases of diabetic ketoacidosis

Rarely the emergency is the first presentation of an endocrine disease. Usually in a patient with a known endocrine condition.

An endocrine emergency may be precipitated or made more severe by coexisting illness, thus revealing the underlying endocrine abnormality. For example, chronic cortisol deficiency progresses to an acute adrenal crisis in the presence of a infection such as pneumonia.

Case 13 Diarrhoea, vomiting and lethargy after a meal out

Presentation

Jane Fletcher, a 44-year-old woman with a 30-year history of type 1 diabetes mellitus presents with a history of diarrhoea, vomiting and lethargy after a meal out the evening before. The monitor shows her capillary blood glucose concentration to be 25 mmol/L, and her blood ketone concentration is 5 mmol/L.

On arrival at hospital, the patient's heart rate is 108 beats/min and her blood pressure is 100/68 mmHg. A venous blood gas test is done (**Table 11.1**).

Initial interpretation

Mrs Fletcher has the three key features necessary for a diagnosis of diabetic ketoacidosis:

- known diabetes mellitus or blood glucose concentration > 11 mmol/L
- serum bicarbonate concentration < 15 mmol/L, venous pH < 7.30, or both
- blood ketone concentration > 3 mmol/L or urinalysis with 2+ ketones or more

The diabetic ketoacidosis is likely to have been precipitated by a gastrointestinal infection, given that the symptoms of diarrhoea and vomiting started shortly after a meal out. Food poisoning was probably responsible for the diarrhoea and vomiting.

> **Diabetic ketoacidosis is the consequence of absolute deficiency of insulin.** The insulin deficit causes intracellular glucose deficiency, increased insulin counter-regulatory hormones [acute cortisol, growth hormone, glucagon and adrenaline (epinephrine)] and production of acidic ketones.

Further history and examination

Mrs Fletcher had tried to control her blood glucose at home with additional doses of subcutaneous insulin, but she was unable to keep food or fluids down. She appears dehydrated and has generalised abdominal tenderness.

Interpretation of findings

Diabetic ketoacidosis precipitated by a gastrointestinal infection remains the most likely cause for the patient's symptoms. Food poisoning causes abdominal tenderness, and dehydration can result from diarrhoea and vomiting.

Hyperosmolar hyperglycaemic state (HHS) (see page 303) also presents with hyperglycaemia but does not tend to occur in patients with type 1 diabetes mellitus, so this condition is less likely. HHS occurs in those with type 2 diabetes mellitus who still have some circulating insulin present (preventing ketoacidosis).

Acute pancreatitis is more common in people with diabetes and can present in a similar manner to diabetic ketoacidosis (with abdominal pain and vomiting). Pancreatitis is ruled out by normal serum amylase.

Women of childbearing age presenting with vomiting must have a pregnancy

Venous blood gas test results		
Measurement	Value	Normal range
pH	7.04	7.35–7.45
Bicarbonate (mmol/L)	12	22–26
Potassium (mmol/L)	6.2	3.5–5.5
Sodium (mmol/L)	135	135–145
Glucose (mmol/L)	27	3.6–6.9

Table 11.1 Venous blood gas test results for a patient with diarrhoea, vomiting and lethargy after a meal out

Case 13 *continued*

test. A negative test excludes morning sickness as a cause of vomiting. The risk of miscarriage in a woman with diabetic ketoacidosis is high, so urgent obstetric review is required if the pregnancy test is positive.

Immediate intervention

Intravenous access must be obtained and intravenous fluid resuscitation with saline started immediately to begin the process of rehydration. An intravenous insulin infusion is required (at a dose of 0.1 units/kg/h) to run simultaneously with the intravenous fluid. The insulin infusion turns off the process of ketone body formation and acts to reduce the elevated blood glucose levels.

Mrs Fletcher requires regular monitoring of her serum electrolytes, especially potassium. Potassium levels can decrease rapidly in cases of diabetic ketoacidosis, leading to life-threatening cardiac arrhythmias due to hypokalaemia.

Regular recording of physical observations (blood pressure, heart rate , respiratory rate, oxygen saturation and urine output) and electrocardiographic monitoring are required to assess response to treatment.

Once blood glucose concentration begins to decrease, an intravenous infusion of dextrose is needed to maintain a blood glucose >4 mmol/L. The insulin infusion rate is reduced only when:

- DKA fully resolves (blood ketone concentration < 1 mmol/L)
- pH increases above 7.3
- bicarbonate is > 18 mmol/L.

Stool and vomit samples are sent for microbiological analysis to identify any infective organisms.

Diabetic ketoacidosis

Diabetic ketoacidosis arises from a state of total insulin deficiency. The condition occurs in:

- patients with newly developed or pre-existing type 1 diabetes mellitus
- patients with long-standing type 2 diabetes and insulin deficiency if they miss insulin doses or if illness increases their insulin requirement

Pathogenesis

Without insulin, glucose from the blood cannot enter the cells. Therefore absolute insulin deficiency results in hyperglycaemia (caused by glycogenolysis and gluconeogenesis) and intracellular glucose deficiency.

To address the energy deficit resulting from the lack of intracellular glucose, lipids are metabolised to generate energy. This process (lipolysis) leads to high circulating levels of free fatty acids. When these free fatty acids are metabolised, abundant acidic ketone bodies (acetoacetate, β-hydroxybutyrate and acetone) are produced as a by-product. Accumulation of ketones causes metabolic acidosis which inhibits normal cell metabolism.

Hyperglycaemia results in osmotic diuresis and dehydration, electrolyte loss and hyperosmolarity. Whole body stores of sodium and potassium are reduced.

Clinical features

DKA is characterised by the following clinical features:

- nausea and vomiting
- hypotension and tachycardia (due to dehydration)
- tachypnoea (rapid respiratory rate as respiratory compensation for metabolic acidosis)

- reduced levels of consciousness
- hyperglycaemia
- acidaemia
- ketonaemia
- hyperkalaemia
- hyponatraemia

Management

Diabetic ketoacidosis requires management in an appropriate setting, such as a high-dependency unit (**Table 11.2**). The steps in the management of diabetic ketoacidosis are as follows.

- Gain intravenous access
- Do blood tests (e.g. venous blood gas analysis, full blood count, liver function tests, urea and electrolytes)
- Start aggressive fluid replacement with 0.9% saline (fluid deficiency in diabetic

ketoacidosis is often 100 mL/kg, so a 70-kg patient may be 7 L fluid-deplete)
- Start fixed rate insulin infusion (0.1 units/kg/h) to reduce ketosis
- Begin potassium replacement after the first litre of saline unless the potassium >5.5 mmol/L (as the potassium will fall rapidly once insulin infusion is commenced due to movement of potassium from the extracellular to intracellular space)
- Monitor blood glucose and ketones hourly, as well as serum electrolytes 1–2 hourly
- Carry out electrocardiographic monitoring (required because of potassium abnormalities)
- If necessary, insert a nasogastric tube to prevent vomiting and aspiration caused by gastric stasis
- Administer low-molecular-weight heparin to prevent deep vein thrombosis

Diabetic ketoacidosis resolves when blood ketone concentration is < 1 mmol/L, pH is > 7.3 and bicarbonate concentration is > 18 mmol/L.

When the patient has recovered and is awaiting discharge, they are visited to discuss 'sick day rules' (guidelines for patients with diabetes on how to control their blood glucose in times of illness), to develop a written management plan and to review injection sites and usual glycaemic control. Provision of home ketone testing (blood or urine) may help the patient to avoid further admissions to hospital with diabetic ketoacidosis.

Diabetic ketoacidosis: criteria for admission to a high-dependency unit	
Indicator	Value
Blood ketone concentration (mmol/L)	>6
Serum bicarbonate (mmol/L)	<5
Venous or arterial pH	<7.1
Hypokalaemia on admission (mmol/L)	<3.5
Glasgow coma score	<12 out of 15
Oxygen saturation (%)	<92
Systolic blood pressure (mmHg)	<90
Heart rate (beats/min)	<60 or >100

*One or more of these criteria may necessitate admission to a high-dependency unit.

Table 11.2 Diabetic ketoacidosis: criteria for admission to high-dependency unit*

> **Most cases of diabetic ketoacidosis occur in patients whose diabetes has already been diagnosed.** The condition is less likely in patients without known diabetes.

Hyperosmolar hyperglycaemic state

Hyperosmolar hyperglycaemic state is characterised by the development of a very high blood glucose concentration. The condition usually develops over days in patients with type 2 diabetes mellitus.

The very high blood glucose causes polyuria and consequent fluid deficiency and dehydration. Hypernatraemia and hyperosmolarity develops as a result of the water deficit.

Clinical features

Hyperosmolar hyperglycaemic state is characterised by:

- hypovolaemia
- severe hyperglycaemia (blood glucose usually > 30 mmol/L)
- increased serum osmolality (> 320 mOsm/kg)

> **Osmolality is calculated when hyperosmolar hyperglycaemic state is suspected.** Serum osmolality > 320 mOsm/kg is one of the diagnostic criteria for this condition. The following equation is used to calculate serum osmolality (all concentrations in mmol/L):
>
> 2 [sodium] + 2 [potassium] + [glucose] + [urea]

Hyperosmolar hyperglycaemic state is distinct from diabetic ketoacidosis, because patients with the former have less ketonaemia (ketone concentration, < 3 mmol/L) and a lesser degree of acidaemia (pH typically > 7.3 and serum bicarbonate > 15 mmol/L).

Patients with hyperosmolar hyperglycaemic state tend to be > 60 years and have type 2 diabetes mellitus. They often present with a coexisting illness, such as myocardial infarction or infection, or have had a gradual onset of hyperglycaemia over a few days and as a result are severely dehydrated (sometimes up to 20 L fluid-deficient).

Management

Treatment depends mainly on fluid resuscitation, which corrects the hyperglycaemia and dehydration. Insulin infusion is sometimes required if blood glucose concentration fails to decrease with rehydration.

Potential complications of hyperosmolar hyperglycaemic state are:

- pulmonary emboli (patients with the condition have higher thrombotic risk)
- myocardial infarction or stroke
- heel ulceration or pressure sores (in neuropathic skin)
- hypoglycaemia (caused by overtreatment with insulin)

Patients with hyperosmolar hyperglycaemic state often have a prolonged hospital stay as these patients are often elderly and take time to recover to their previous mobility and independence. Mortality associated with the condition is high (up to 15%), mainly because of the risk of complications in the older patients who tend to be affected.

Severe hypoglycaemia

Hypoglycaemia is defined by blood glucose concentration < 4 mmol/L. Mild hypoglycaemia can be treated by the patient at home. However, severe hypoglycaemia requires assistance from others, including treatment by health care professionals, but patients rarely require hospital assessment or admission. In addition, the symptoms of severe hypoglycaemia (see page 157), which include falls and confusion, may be non-specific in the elderly. Hypoglycaemia can be caused by:

- an excessive dose of insulin or an oral hypoglycaemic agent
- one or more missed meals
- intercurrent illness (especially if it causes vomiting)
- acute renal failure (causing insulin or sulfonylureas to accumulate)

- development of an autoimmune condition, such as Addison's disease and coeliac disease
- altered absorption of insulin (lipohypertrophy or lipoatrophy) or oral hypoglycaemics (gastroparesis)

If the patient is conscious, their hypoglycaemia can be treated by taking rapid-acting glucose (glucose tablets, a sugary drink or pure fruit juice).

Severe hypoglycaemia (causing reduced consciousness, coma or seizures) can be treated with:

- buccal glucose gel
- intravenous dextrose
- intramuscular glucagon

Case 14 Collapse and agitation

Presentation

Anne Castle, a 76-year-old is found by her son at home, collapsed on the floor. There is evidence of recent vomiting. Mrs Castle is agitated and the attending paramedic reports that she has a Glasgow coma score of 10 out of 15. Her son reports that she has had a dry cough for several weeks and has lost weight.

Initial interpretation

Sepsis causes reduced consciousness and presents without fever in the elderly. Metabolic abnormalities cause reduced consciousness, agitation and vomiting. Alternatively, the vomiting may be a sign of intercranial pathology, such as ischaemic or haemorrhagic stroke.

The recent cough and weight loss raise the possibility of the development of lung cancer or possibly a chest infection.

Further history and examination

Mrs Castle appears euvolaemic, and her blood pressure is 142/90 mmHg. Her temperature is 36.1°C.

Mrs Castle has a history of hypertension, for which she takes amlodipine. She has been a smoker for many years. Last month, she had her annual check, which included blood tests, and was told by her general practitioner (GP) that everything was normal.

The results of the patient's blood and urine tests on admission to hospital are shown in **Table 11.3**. A computerised tomography (CT) scan of her head is unremarkable. However, a chest X-ray shows a mass-lesion in the right upper zone.

Interpretation of findings

Mrs Castle's symptoms (reduced level of consciousness, agitation and vomiting),

Blood and urine test results		
Test	Value	Normal range
Sodium (mmol/L)	107	135–145
Potassium (mmol/L)	4.4	3.5–5.5
Creatinine (µmol/L)	80	50–110
Urea (mmol/L)	3.6	2.5–7.8
Serum osmolarity (mOsm/kg)	265	275–295
Urine sodium (mmol/L)	70	>30
Urine osmolality (mOsm/L)	450	300–900

Table 11.3 Blood and urine test results for an elderly patient found collapsed and agitated

coupled with the low serum sodium concentration (107 mmol/L; normal range, 135–145 mmol/L), mean that she has severe hyponatraemia in the context of euvolaemia. It is uncertain if the hyponatraemia is acute (<24 h duration) as there are no other biochemical results in this time frame. Hyponatraemia causes reduced consciousness.

The low serum sodium in the context of dilute serum (low osmolarity) and concentrated urine (elevated urine sodium and osmolarity) support syndrome of inappropriate antidiuretic hormone (SIADH) (see Figure 2.27), of which lung cancer is a recognised cause. However, it is wise to also consider other causes for hyponatraemia (**Table 11.4**), including hypothyroidism and cortisol insufficiency.

The cause of hyponatraemia is considered in the context of the patient's fluid state and fluid state will also determine the management of hyponatraemia. Certain causes are more likely in patients who are hypovolaemic or euvolaemic, or who have fluid overload therefore assessing the patient's fluid state is an essential first step in classifying the cause of hyponatraemia. (see **Table 11.4**).

Case 14 *continued*

Causes of hyponatraemia		
Hypovolaemic	Euvolaemic	Fluid overload
Gastrointestinal fluid loss	Syndrome of inappropriate antidiuretic hormone	Cardiac failure
Renal fluid loss		Renal failure
Haemorrhage	Hypothyroidism	Liver failure
Skin fluid loss	Cortisol insufficiency	
	Water intoxication	
*The cause is frequently multifactorial.		

Table 11.4 Causes of hyponatraemia*

The diagnosis is severe hyponatraemia due to SIADH secondary to underlying lung malignancy (seen on chest X-ray).

Immediate intervention

The aim of treatment is to rapidly correct the hyponatraemia to resolve the acute neurological symptoms. Correction of hyponatraemia is done using hypertonic saline in an intensive care setting. This requires careful monitoring of serum sodium concentration as overly rapid correction of hyponatraemia (>12mmol/L increase in serum sodium per 24 h) can cause permanent neurological damage from central pontine myelinolysis.

Hyponatraemia

Hyponatraemia (low serum sodium) is associated with increased morbidity and mortality, as well as longer hospital stays for inpatients. The condition is a sign of poor prognosis in cancer and in cardiac and hepatic failure. However, there is currently no evidence that correcting serum sodium improves prognosis in these patients.

Hyponatraemia has various symptoms and signs. Symptoms of hyponatraemia include:

- Nausea and vomiting, headache
- Loss of energy and fatigue,
- Irritability
- Muscle weakness or cramps
- Confusion and reduced conscious level
- Seizures and coma

Its causes are listed in **Table 11.4**.

Syndrome of inappropriate antidiuretic hormone

In this syndrome, the release of antidiuretic hormone is freed from the usual physiological controls. The resulting hypersecretion of antidiuretic hormone causes aquaporin channels to be deployed in the renal collecting ducts when ADH binds to V2 receptors on the cells surface.

The aquaporin channels allow excessive reabsorption of free water in the kidney. The result is excessive free water in the serum and dilutional hyponatraemia in consequence, but the patient appears euvolaemic. In turn, the urine becomes more concentrated.

Clinical features and diagnostic approach

If there is evidence of a euvolaemic state (i.e. no fluid overload and no evidence of dehydration, such as dry tongue, postural hypotension and tachycardia) (See Figure 2.27) in a patient with hyponatraemia, it is helpful to measure:

- serum osmolality
- urine osmolality
- urine sodium concentration

The results may allow SIADH to be diagnosed (**Table 11.5**). SIADH is a state of hypo-osmolar hyponatraemia.

The cause of the SIADH needs to be identified and treated. When the underlying cause is treated, the SIADH will resolve. There are a number of causes of SIADH (**Table 11.6**), but if none is identified the condition is termed idiopathic SIADH.

Management

When managing hyponatraemia, it is vital to establish if the condition is chronic or acute. Acute hyponatraemia can be rapidly corrected, whereas chronic hyponatraemia needs to be corrected more slowly. Often it is impossible to establish the speed of onset, but some

Diagnostic criteria for SIADH	
Essential	Supportive
Serum osmolality < 275 mOsm/kg	Urea < 3.6 mmol/L
Urine osmolality > 300 mOsm/kg	Failure of sodium to correct after 1 L 0.9% saline administration
Urine sodium > 30 mmol/L	Correction of sodium with fluid restriction
No recent use of diuretics	Low serum uric acid concentration
Euvolaemia	
Normal thyroid and adrenal function	

Table 11.5 Diagnostic criteria for syndrome of inappropriate antidiuretic hormone (SIADH)

patients have had a recent normal result and others have a history of hyponatraemia, which can provide clues. The severity of symptoms also needs to be established, as severe symptoms such as vomiting, seizures, drowsiness or coma need to be corrected rapidly until the symptoms improve (even if established to be chronic with sudden deterioration).

Chronic hyponatraemia

Hyponatraemia of > 24 h in duration (chronic hyponatraemia) results in large intracellular proteins being shifted out of the brain to

Causes of SIADH		
Group of causes	Category	Example(s)
Neoplasia	Pulmonary	Small-cell lung cancer and mesothelioma
	Gastrointestinal	Pancreatic cancer and colon cancer
	Genitourinary	Cancer of the cervix, bladder, prostate and ovary
	Other	Brain cancer, nasopharyngeal cancer and lymphoma
Pulmonary disease	Infective	Pneumonia, empyema and tuberculosis
	Inflammatory	Chronic obstructive pulmonary disease, asthma and sarcoid
Central nervous system	Infective	Meningitis, encephalitis and cerebral abscess
	Vascular	Cerebrovascular event, subarachnoid haemorrhage and subdural haematoma
Pharmacological	Prescribed drug	Opiates, tricyclic antidepressants, sodium valproate and selective serotonin reuptake inhibitors
	Recreational drugs	MDMA (ecstasy)

Table 11.6 Causes of syndrome of inappropriate antidiuretic hormone (SIADH)

equalise oncotic pressure between the brain and the dilute extracellular fluid. If serum sodium concentration is corrected too rapidly, large fluid shifts can occur from the extracellular to the intracellular space; this leads to cerebral oedema and central pontine myelinolysis. Central pontine myelinolysis results in irreversible confusion, drowsiness, delirium, ataxia and dysphagia.

Therefore care must be exercised when correcting chronic hyponatraemia. Sodium concentration must not be allowed to increase faster than 10–12 mmol/L in 24 h. Acute treatment of severe hyponatraemia continues until the patient stops having seizures or their Glasgow coma score normalises to minimise the risk of central pontine myelinolysis from over rapid correction.

Acute hyponatraemia

In cases of acute hyponatraemia (< 24 h in duration), no shift of proteins in the brain occurs (as it does in chronic hyponatraemia).

Therefore a patient with acute hyponatraemia and severe symptoms can be safely treated by rapid correction of serum sodium concentration with hypertonic saline.

After the initial resolution of symptoms fluid restriction is started for hypervolaemic or euvolaemic patients. For this treatment to succeed, their fluid intake during recovery needs to be less than their normal fluid intake (which needs to be assessed).

Patients with SIADH whose condition fails to respond to fluid restriction are treated:

- with vasopressin receptor antagonists to block the excessive antidiuretic hormone
- with demeclocycline, which causes renal insensitivity to antidiuretic hormone
- by increasing solute intake with 0.25–0.50 g/kg of urea daily
- low-dose loop diuretics and oral sodium chloride

The key to success in reversing hyponatraemia is successful treatment of the underlying cause of the SIADH.

Case 15 Abdominal pain, vomiting and drowsiness

Presentation

A 32-year-old man, Mr Cowan, attends the acute medical unit. He describes a 2-month history of progressive lethargy, weakness, weight loss and low mood. Over the past 24 h, he has had abdominal pain and has been vomiting.

Mr Cowan is drowsy and has a heart rate of 115 beats/min. He is hypotensive, with a blood pressure of 85/60 mmHg.

Initial interpretation

Mr Cowan's symptoms could be caused by one of a number of conditions.

- An inflammatory disorder such as inflammatory bowel disease is possible but unlikely without a history of

diarrhoea or blood or mucus in the stool
- Acute abdominal pathology, such as appendicitis, is possible, but this condition would not explain the prodrome (symptoms leading up to the presentation)
- Malignancy could be the cause and he may have other symptoms, such as cough in lung malignancy or change in bowel habit in colonic malignancy
- Chronic infection, such as subacute bacterial endocarditis, is also a possibility
- Depression, although this alone will not cause hypotension and tachycardia

However, the chronic and non-specific nature of the progressive symptoms indicates an endocrine cause, such as diabetes mellitus or Addison's disease.

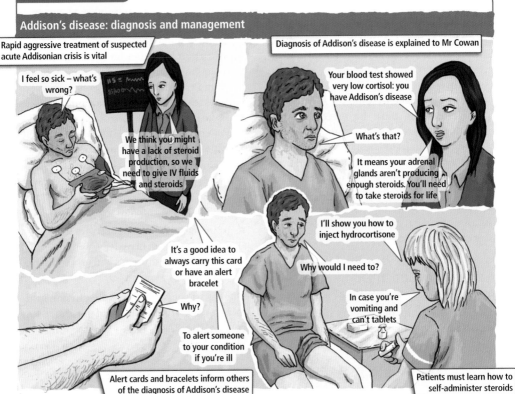

Case 15 *continued*

Addison's disease: diagnosis and management

Rapid aggressive treatment of suspected acute Addisonian crisis is vital

Diagnosis of Addison's disease is explained to Mr Cowan

I feel so sick – what's wrong?

We think you might have a lack of steroid production, so we need to give IV fluids and steroids

Your blood test showed very low cortisol: you have Addison's disease

What's that?

It means your adrenal glands aren't producing enough steroids. You'll need to take steroids for life

It's a good idea to always carry this card or have an alert bracelet

Why?

To alert someone to your condition if you're ill

I'll show you how to inject hydrocortisone

Why would I need to?

In case you're vomiting and can't tablets

Alert cards and bracelets inform others of the diagnosis of Addison's disease

Patients must learn how to self-administer steroids

Further history and examination

Mr Cowan's parents accompany him to the hospital. They are concerned that he has been unwell for some months. They worry that he may be depressed. Mr Cowan's mucous membranes are dry, he is unable to cooperate with the examination and his skin appears surprisingly pigmented for the time of year.

The results of a serum electrolyte test carried out yesterday by Mr Cowan's GP show hyponatraemia (132 mmol/L; normal range, 135–145 mmol/L) and hyperkalaemia (potassium concentration, 5.6 mmol/L; normal range, 3.5–5.5 mmol/L). The results of his blood count and liver profile are normal.

Interpretation of findings

The combination of a chronic deterioration in health, followed by vomiting, dehydration, hyperpigmentation and the biochemical findings of hyponatraemia and hyperkalaemia is in keeping with Addisonian crisis (acute adrenal failure) (**Table 11.7**). In a patient who has been vomiting, the potassium concentration would be expected to be low rather than high, as in this case.

Immediate intervention

Mr Cowan is given immediate saline replacement and intravenous cortisol replacement (in the form of hydrocortisone). The aim is to resolve shock.

Case 15 *continued*

Addisonian crisis: clinical features		
Symptoms	Signs	Investigations
Nausea and vomiting	Shock (often refractory to fluid resuscitation)	Hyponatraemia
Abdominal pain		Hyperkalaemia
		Increased serum urea
Weight loss	Dehydration	Low or undetectable serum cortisol
Fatigue	Hypoglycaemia	
Confusion		

Table 11.7 Clinical features of addisonian crisis

Mr Cowan requires 5 L of intravenous fluid over the first 12 hours of admission in order to treat the shock. His vital signs (BP, heart rate, urine output and GCS) are recorded hourly by the nursing staff to monitor his progress.

Mr Cowan has repeat electrolytes after 4 hours of treatment that demonstrate normalisation of his sodium and potassium. Later that day the laboratory call the ward to inform the doctors that Mr Cowan had a random serum cortisol level of 55 nmol/L. This is extremely low given the physiological stress he is under (expected to be >550 nmol/L in acute stress) and is diagnostic of cortisol deficiency.

Addisonian crisis

Addisonian crisis presents with shock, hyponatraemia and hyperkalaemia resulting from cortisol deficiency. If the condition is suspected, serum cortisol concentration is measured and the following treatment administered without delay:

- 50–100 mg intravenous (or intramuscular) hydrocortisone four times daily
- intravenous 0.9% saline infusion
- intravenous dextrose to treat hypoglycaemia
- antibiotics for coexisting sepsis

The patient also requires electrocardiographic monitoring, especially if hyperkalaemia is present.

If the patient is unwell, treatment is not delayed while a synacthen test is carried out. In such a case, a serum cortisol concentration <100 nmol/L is diagnostic of cortisol deficiency.

The diagnosis can be confirmed by the results of a short synacthen test done when the patient is well. The test is done after withholding the hydrocortisone dose for ≥8 h.

In cases of suspected Addison's disease, adrenocorticotrophic hormone (ACTH) is measured at baseline in the short synacthen test. The baseline ACTH concentration is increased in primary adrenal insufficiency, because of the loss of negative feedback from cortisol to the pituitary gland.

Case 16 Weight loss, sweats and anxiety

Presentation

Deborah Stack, aged 38 years, presents to the emergency department accompanied by her husband. She gives a history of worsening agitation, fevers, sweats, palpitations, vomiting and tremor.

Her symptoms worsened dramatically over the past few days, but she had not been her usual self for a few weeks. Her husband says that she has lost weight and had become increasingly anxious, hot, sweaty and shaky. She had not wanted to see a physician during that time due to the anxiety.

Case 16 *continued*

Initial interpretation

There is a wide differential diagnosis here.

- Sepsis is likely, because of the sweats and fever
- Arrhythmia is possible, but this would not explain the fever and other symptoms
- Anxiety disorder is also possible, but the presence of fever makes this less likely
- Alcohol withdrawal is a possibility in patients with a history of excessive alcohol intake

The history of recent symptoms of thyroid overactivity must be interpreted to make the correct diagnosis. Thyroid storm can be precipitated by infection or stress (such as surgery) in a patient with underlying hyperthyroidism, particularly if they do not adhere to medication.

Further history and examination

Deborah's symptoms worsened after she developed urinary frequency and loin discomfort. On direct questioning, her husband states that his wife has a history of vitiligo and has a sister who has had a thyroid problem.

Deborah looks unwell and has signs of respiratory distress. She has a temperature of 39.5°C, tachycardia (120 beats/min), hypertension (BP 180/128 mmHg) and respiratory rate of 36 breaths/min. More careful examination finds evidence of a smooth goitre and thyroid eye disease in the form of proptosis (forward displacement) of both eyes.

Immediate intervention

The evidence of thyroid disease (goitre and thyroid eye disease), personal and family history of autoimmune disease and clinical features of hyperthyroidism point to a diagnosis of Graves' disease. The fact she is severely unwell with fever, tachycardia, hypertension and respiratory distress indicate the diagnosis of thyroid storm. Deborah is treated in the high-dependency unit. She is given rapid intravenous fluids, as well as beta-blockers to slow her pulse. Intravenous antibiotics are given to treat urinary sepsis.

The results of blood tests done on admission show fully suppressed thyroid-stimulating hormone and markedly increased free thyroxine (T_4) (> 100 pmol/L). These results confirm the diagnosis of hyperthyroidism. Deborah is started on anti-thyroid therapy with carbimazole.

Thyroid storm

Transfer to a high-dependency unit is vital. The mainstays of treatment are managing airway, breathing and circulation. Specific treatments include:

- beta-blockers to control tachycardia
- antithyroid drugs (carbimazole or propylthiouracil) to reduce the release of T_4

- high-dose corticosteroids, which can reduce the effects of excessive T_4
- active cooling by intravenous fluid infusion
- treatment of coexistent infection

Table 11.8 summarises the potential complications of thyroid storm.

Once the patient's condition has stabilised after a thyroid storm, medical management of thyrotoxicosis with oral beta-blocker and antithyroid drugs continues (see page 200).

Complications of thyroid storm	
System	Consequence(s)
Cardiovascular	High-output cardiac failure
	Cardiac arrhythmias
	Myocardial ischaemia and infarction
Respiratory	Respiratory distress
Central nervous	Confusion
	Agitation
	Seizure
	Coma
Metabolic	Hyperpyrexia
	Hypermetabolic state (increased oxygen demand)
Gastrointestinal	Vomiting
	Diarrhoea
	Jaundice

Table 11.8 Complications of thyroid storm

Myxoedema coma

Myxoedema coma is a life-threatening but rare presentation of severe hypothyroidism. Its presenting features are those of extreme hypothyroidism:

- hypothermia
- bradycardia
- slow respiratory rate
- reduced consciousness
- slow relaxing reflexes

The condition is usually diagnosed in patients with a known history of hypothyroidism (and poor medication adherence). However, myxodema coma can be caused by previously undiagnosed hypothyroidism.

Treatment is supportive, with airway support, intravenous fluids, oxygen and slow re-warming, alongside thyroid hormone replacement.

Case 17 Worsening palpitations, headaches and tremor

Presentation

Paula Gough, a 36-year-old woman presents with a history of palpitations, headaches and tremor. These symptoms had been coming and going over the past few weeks. Today, the symptoms became dramatically worse and are associated with chest pain and breathlessness. Her heart rate is 118 beats/min and her blood pressure 235/100 mmHg.

Case 17 *continued*

Initial interpretation

Acute myocardial infarction or aortic dissection with undiagnosed hypertension is possible because of the acute onset chest pain. Thyrotoxicosis can present with palpitations and tremor. The combination of intermittent symptoms and severe hypertension and tachycardia raise the possibility of phaeochromocytoma. Breathlessness indicates a hypertensive crisis.

Further history and examination

The patient has no notable medical history or family history. In addition to the tachycardia and hypertension, Mrs Gough is tachyopnoeic, with an oxygen saturation of 92% on air.

Chest examination detects bibasal crackles.

> Phaeochromocytoma is considered in patients with anxiety, hypertension, tachycardia, tremor or electrocardiographic signs of cardiac ischaemia. Phaeochromocytoma is rare, but it is vital not to miss this life-threatening condition especially as there are a some very specific treatment steps (such as avoiding beta-blocker medication in the early stages of management).

Interpretation of findings

Breathlessness and bibasal lung crackles signify acute left ventricular failure. This can result from myocardial infarction. Myocardial infarction is often associated with acute hypotension rather than hypertension. The patient's young age and absence of significant ischaemic risk factors raise the suspicion of a secondary cause of hypertension such as phaeochromocytoma that could account for the other features of tachycardia, tremor and headaches.

No rapid test is available to confirm the diagnosis. However, all the clinical features point to a phaeochromocytoma with hypertensive crisis.

Immediate intervention

Mrs Gough is transferred on oxygen therapy to a high-dependency unit. Intra-arterial pressure monitoring begins, and shows paroxysms of severe hypertension (**Figure 11.1**). An electrocardiogram shows tachycardia and ischaemic changes with ST-segment depression and T-wave inversion (**Figure 11.2**).

Because phaeochromocytoma is suspected, beta-blockers must be avoided. Intravenous infusion of alpha-blockers are commenced to reduce blood pressure.

> Beta-blockers, a commonly used first-line treatment for acute coronary syndrome, are contraindicated in patients with phaeochromocytoma. In these patients, the use of beta-blockers (without adequate alpha blockade) can lead to massive vasoconstriction and life-threatening intracerebral haemorrhage or pulmonary oedema.

The following results confirm the diagnosis of phaeochromocytoma.

- Chest X-ray confirms pulmonary oedema
- An echocardiogram shows a globally hypokinetic left ventricle with a reduced ejection fraction but no evidence of aortic coarctation or dissection
- Increased 24-h urine metadrenaline (metanephrine) identifies excess catecholamine production confirming the diagnosis of phaeochromocytoma

Case 17 *continued*

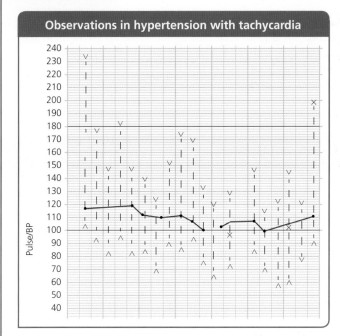

Figure 11.1 Observation chart showing paroxysms of hypertension and tachycardia.

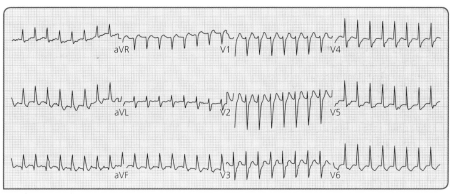

Figure 11.2 Electrocardiogram showing features of tachycardia and ST-segment depression and T-waves inversion in the lateral chest leads (V4-6).

- Computerised tomography of the abdomen is arranged; the scan shows normal-sized kidneys (making a renal cause of severe hypertension less likely) but a 3-cm right adrenal mass

Once Mrs Gough's condition is stabilised, her treatment is converted to an oral alpha-blocker, phenoxybenzamine, allowing more complete alpha blockade. Once alpha blockade is established, if the patient remains tachycardic, a beta-blocker can be safely added at this stage.

Hypertensive crisis

The general principle for managing a hypertensive crisis due to a phaeochromocytoma is to safely reduce the blood pressure with alpha-blockers. Once the patient has been established on alpha-blockers, beta-blockers can be added.

Supportive care, such as titrated oxygen therapy and intravenous fluids, maintains adequate perfusion of vital organs.

Case 18 Severe headache and double vision

Presentation

Stephen Gardiner, a 68-year-old man presents to the emergency department with a 6-h history of a sudden onset severe headache and double vision. He is drowsy, afebrile and tachycardic (106 beats/min), with a blood pressure of 92/58 mmHg.

Initial interpretation

Severe headache and drowsiness suggest a severe intracranial pathology, and the sudden onset of symptoms suggests a vascular event. Other possibilities include intracranial infection, such as meningitis.

Further history and examination

Mr Gardiner had been previously fit and well. Examination finds a visual field defect in both temporal fields (bitemporal hemianopia). He has a gaze palsy; the left eye is unable to abduct, causing diplopia on leftward gaze, consistent with left 6th cranial nerve palsy.

There is no fever, rash or neck stiffness.

Interpretation of findings

Subarachnoid haemorrhage or carotid dissection could cause this presentation with sudden onset headache, reduced level of consciousness and gaze palsy. The combination of headache, reduced consciousness and hypotension could indicate meningitis, but fever would be expected in such a case.

Although uncommon, pituitary apoplexy is the best unifying diagnosis. The clinical features of sudden onset headache, hypotension, gaze palsy and visual field defect support this diagnosis.

Immediate intervention

Once the clinical diagnosis of pituitary apoplexy is recognised, the priority of treatment is to give fluid resuscitation and intravenous corticosteroids to treat the life-threatening cortisol deficiency.

A CT brain shows signs of acute blood in the pituitary fossa. A pituitary MRI confirms haemorrhage in a large mass in the pituitary, compressing the optic chiasm (**Figure 11.3**).

Case 18 *continued*

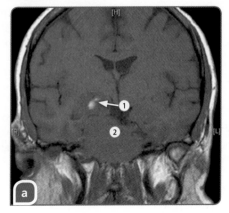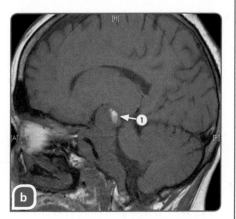

Figure 11.3 Magnetic resonance imaging of the pituitary gland. (a) Coronal section. (b) Sagittal section. Acute haemorrhage ① is present in an enlarged pituitary gland ②; this finding is consistent with pituitary apoplexy in a pituitary macroadenoma.

Blood samples are drawn to test other pituitary hormones. The patient's care is discussed with the local pituitary surgeon and endocrinologist to determine if acute transsphenoidal surgery is indicated.

Pituitary apoplexy

Pituitary apoplexy is an endocrine emergency characterised by haemorrhage or infarction of the pituitary gland which usually contains a macroadenoma (tumour > 1cm diameter). The condition results in sudden onset headache, visual disturbance and cranial nerve palsies. It can cause life-threatening cortisol deficiency. The typical clinical features are described in **Table 11.9**.

■ If the patient's level of consciousness is reduced, intensive care may be required to protect the airway

Pituitary apoplexy: clinical features		
Symptoms	Signs	Investigations
Severe headache	Hypotension	Hypoglycaemia
Nausea and vomiting	Tachycardia	Hypopituitarism (low cortisol, free thyroxine, thyroid-stimulating hormone, luteinising hormone and follicle-stimulating hormone, growth hormone, prolactin and sex hormones)
Reduced vision or double vision	Reduced Glasgow coma score	
Confusion	Ptosis, ophthalmoplegia and visual field defects	Haemorrhage or infarction in the pituitary adenoma on computerised tomography or magnetic resonance imaging

Table 11.9 Clinical features of pituitary apoplexy

- Intravenous hydrocortisone 50–100 mg four times daily is administered without delay; this treatment may be life-saving
- Blood is drawn for measurement of electrolytes, clotting factors and blood count, as well as concentrations of cortisol, prolactin, free T_4, thyroid-stimulating hormone, luteinising hormone, follicle-stimulating hormone, growth hormone and sex hormones
- An urgent CT or preferably contrast magnetic resonance imaging scan of the brain is required to look for a haemorrhage in the pituitary fossa

Haemorrhage extending into the cavernous sinus can result in cranial nerve palsies and compression of the optic chiasm, causing visual field defects. Formal visual field testing and visual acuity are assessed urgently and the results help guide the decision on the need for an immediate operation.

Pituitary surgery is sometimes considered if symptoms fail to resolve rapidly (as blood regresses) or if the nerve palsies progress.

Patients are often left with hypopituitarism requiring full hormone replacement. The residual tumour needs regular radiological assessment.

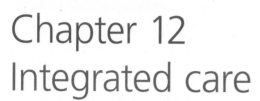

Chapter 12
Integrated care

Starter questions

Answers to the following questions are on page 331.

1. How can self-management of a chronic illness be encouraged?
2. What influence does the government have on diabetes management?
3. Why are thyroid function tests used so commonly?
4. Why are women often diagnosed with diabetes sooner than men?

Introduction

Chronic health conditions are expensive to manage. Patients require regular medical check-ups to ensure the medication is at the appropriate dose, that healthy lifestyle measures are in place and that complications have not developed. For this reason, focus is given to preventing diseases that have a major lifestyle component (such as type 2 diabetes) and educating the public of symptoms, to encourage an early diagnosis and to avoid development of complications.

Coordination between primary (general practice) and secondary (hospital) care allow conditions to be managed locally by doctors who have a good grasp of the patient's family and lifestyle, whilst using the expertise of specialists in secondary care. Rarer conditions often need to be discussed with tertiary centres (hospitals with particular specialist interest in the rare condition).

The majority of countries do not have a unified computer system for their health service which means communicating between centres involves transferring information (often in paper form) when a patient moves. However, most hospitals have developed, or are developing, electronic health records (online medical notes, pathology and X-rays) which help to share information rapidly. The electronic health records will also allow easier access for research and audit, to encourage change that will improve patient care.

Case 19 Poorly controlled diabetes mellitus

Presentation

The practice nurse has been trying to contact Sue, aged 45 years, for a diabetes review, because results from recent blood tests suggest poor glycaemic control. Sue keeps cancelling appointments and rarely answers the phone. The nurse notices that she has not picked up her prescriptions recently.

> **Most general practitioner (GP) services in the UK have computer systems that show when patients last collected their prescription.** This information enables assessment of patients' adherence to treatment.

Initial interpretation

Many GP appointments are missed because of patients' failure to attend. The underlying reason for low attendance needs to be determined and dealt with in order for treatment to be successful. Patients do not engage with treatment for various reasons (**Table 12.1**), including:

- forgetting to attend appointments, or other life events taking priority
- difficulty getting to the clinic
- denial or not wanting to consider certain diagnoses or treatments
- depression and anxiety
- not appreciating the necessity of the appointment
- not wishing to appear a failure if their blood glucose control is poor
- loss of income if missing work
- feeling intimidated by the physician or nurse

Further history

The nurse eventually talks to Sue over the phone. Sue has recently lost her job, and her

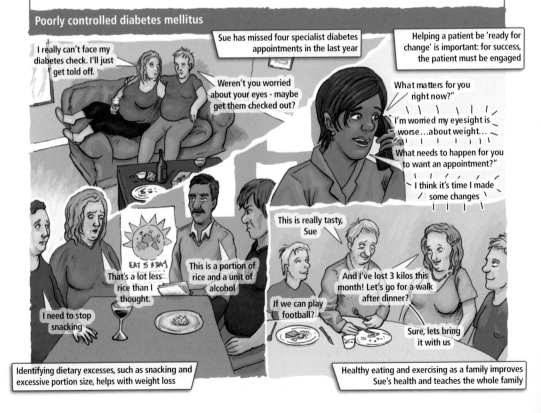

Poorly controlled diabetes mellitus

I really can't face my diabetes check. I'll just get told off.

Sue has missed four specialist diabetes appointments in the last year

Helping a patient be 'ready for change' is important: for success, the patient must be engaged

Weren't you worried about your eyes - maybe get them checked out?

What matters for you right now?"

I'm worried my eyesight is worse...about weight...

What needs to happen for you to want an appointment?"

I think it's time I made some changes

EAT 5 A DAY

That's a lot less rice than I thought.

This is a portion of rice and a unit of alcohol

I need to stop snacking

This is really tasty, Sue

If we can play football?

And I've lost 3 kilos this month! Let's go for a walk after dinner?

Sure, lets bring it with us

Identifying dietary excesses, such as snacking and excessive portion size, helps with weight loss

Healthy eating and exercising as a family improves Sue's health and teaches the whole family

Case 19 *continued*

	Solutions for dealing with non-concordant patients	
Area of non-compliance	Causes of non-concordance	Solutions
Appointments	Difficulty to attend (transport, location, time off work, disability)	Phone and email consultations Home visits Assistance with transport
	Forgot or mistaken time	Text, email or telephone reminder
	Patient's denial of a problem or not ready to discuss it	Psychological support Change personnel (nurse/doctor)
Lifestyle adjustments (diet, exercise, smoking)	Peer pressure	Family education (change as a family)
	Habit/addiction/apathy	Psychological and drug support (e.g. nicotine replacement for smoking cessation)
	Not feeling well due to symptoms associated with chronic disease	Improve control/modify treatment
	Cost saving unhealthy options (e.g. unhealthy food options are cheaper to buy than healthier food choices)	Government support for low cost healthy options and education
Drug treatment	Patient does not read information, hear instructions or forgets them due to physiological factors (hearing, vision or memory impairment)	Family assistance or help from district nurses. Pill (dosette) boxes and blister packs
	Behavioural factors (no symptoms of disease, no immediate consequence to non-concordance, lack of motivation, low priority, denial of a problem)	Education about importance or self-monitoring (e.g. blood pressure) so can see benefit of medication Motivational interviewing Text, email or telephone reminder
	Treatment factors (multiple tablets a day, size and tolerability, and side effects)	Slow release preparations Alternative preparations or combination tablets Liquids/tablets
	Relationship to healthcare provider (motivation and education about efficacy of tablets)	Computer prescription logs to flag non-compliance to allow early intervention Patient-centred care

Table 12.1 Underlying causes of non-concordance in patients and possible solutions to deal with them

son is being bullied for being overweight and she has been feeling low in mood. Last time she saw the GP, he discussed stopping smoking and losing weight and suggested that she needs insulin, and she said that she 'doesn't need another lecture' and feels like she is being 'told off' or criticised. Her husband also has diabetes and has recently had a heart attack. However, she admits having had some blurred vision and is worried about going blind.

> The first stage in making a change towards better health involves understanding the patient's 'readiness to change' and recognising what they consider important. Engaging patients in their care often involves engaging the whole family.

Case 19 *continued*

Examination

From information in the GP's records, it is clear that Sue is obese; she has a body mass index of 36 kg/m². Her last recorded blood pressure was 150/90 mmHg.

Interpretation of findings

Non-compliance, obesity and hypertension result in Sue's poorly controlled diabetes. She also has limited understanding of healthy living. Helping her set three simple, manageable targets can start to integrate her diabetes care into her life:

■ attending appointments
■ taking tablets
■ seeing a dietician with her family

When these targets have been achieved, three new targets can be set. Trying to achieve too much, too quickly is likely to discourage engagement.

Allowing Sue a 'holiday' from capillary blood glucose testing but agreeing targets such as those described here could help her to work with health care professionals to manage her own health.

> **The traditional approach of 'scare tactics' rarely leads to behavioural change.** Allowing patients to set their own agenda is usually more successful.

Helping Sue to look after her health involves engaging and motivating her whole family to practise self-management and to make changes in their lives (**Figure 12.1**). Exploring her fear of going blind, or concerns about her family, may encourage Sue to participate in this process.

If Sue is unprepared to make immediate changes, she may be prepared to set a date to consider change. For example, she may agree to stop smoking in the New Year. This agreement could mark the start of her 'readiness to change'. Low mood and clinical depression are common in people with diabetes and makes change more difficult to contemplate.

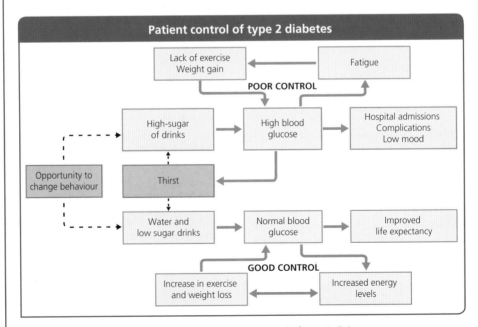

Figure 12.1 Patient habits leading to good and poor control of type 2 diabetes.

Community management of diabetes mellitus

Management of diabetes mellitus is expensive, and patients require lifelong review. Diabetes mellitus accounts for 5% of all healthcare costs in the UK and 12% of health expenditure globally. In 2010 this equated to $376 billion globally and this is predicted to rise to $490 billion by 2030.

Diabetes care requires a multidisciplinary approach, with integration between the patient, their primary care providers (e.g. a GP) and secondary care providers (based at a hospital). Many patients gain extra support from patient organisations (**Figure 12.2**).

The roles of primary care providers are to:

- identify patients at risk of diabetes mellitus (universal screening is not currently considered cost-effective)
- provide education and lifestyle advice after a diagnosis of diabetes mellitus
- coordinate the vital regular monitoring of patients with diabetes mellitus (the annual review)
- provide healthy living advice to prevent diabetes mellitus in patients at risk of developing the condition

Diabetes prevention

The onset of type 2 diabetes mellitus is prevented or delayed by maintaining or achieving a healthy weight (BMI 20–25 kg/m^2) and a healthy level of physical activity.

Each year, about 11% of patients with impaired fasting glucose or impaired glucose tolerance develop diabetes mellitus. Impaired glucose tolerance is associated with an increased risk of premature cardiovascular disease, and early lifestyle changes (especially

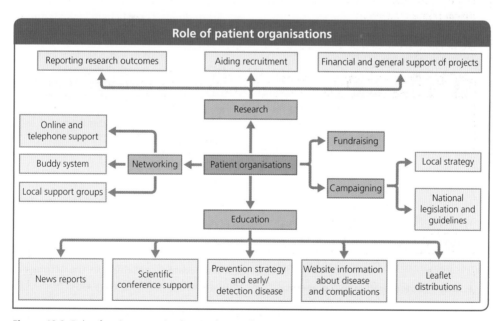

Figure 12.2 Role of patient organisations such as Diabetes UK. These groups are used by patients and professionals.

weight loss) reduces progression to diabetes mellitus. More dramatically, established diabetes mellitus is commonly reversed after significant weight loss. This occurs in more than half of patients with diabetes after bariatric surgery. GPs can help by targeting weight and exercise opportunistically when patients attend for another reason, or through screening of high risk groups. In addition, national campaigns and school education help to ensure people engage in healthy living.

Early diagnosis

About 0.75 million people in the UK have undiagnosed diabetes. Up to half of patients with type 2 diabetes mellitus have early complications of the condition at the time of diagnosis, particularly retinopathy.

There is a long latent asymptomatic period during which diabetes mellitus can be diagnosed. Early diagnosis is being targeted via government strategy, by encouraging testing in high-risk populations and advertising campaigns to make people aware of the symptoms of diabetes mellitus.

Diabetes screening

Aggressive case finding of high-risk patients by GPs, using practice computer databases, is done to identify a significant proportion of patients with asymptomatic diabetes mellitus.

The following high-risk groups are offered regular aggressive case finding for type 2 diabetes mellitus:

- Patients with impaired glucose tolerance or impaired fasting glucose
- White people > 40 years old and black people, Asian people and people in minority ethnic groups > 25 years old with one or more of the following risk factors:
  - a first-degree relative with diabetes
  - overweight (body mass index > 25 kg/m^2) and sedentary lifestyle
  - waist measurement > 94 cm in white and black men, > 90 cm in Asian men or > 80 cm in women

- Patients with a history of hypertension or vascular disease
- Women with a history of gestational diabetes
- Women with polycystic ovary syndrome with obesity (body mass index > 30 kg/m^2)
- Patients with severe mental health problems and receiving antipsychotics such as risperidone

The criteria for universal population screening for diabetes mellitus are not satisfied, because of a lack of cost-effectiveness. However, the incidence of diabetes mellitus continues to increase, so population screening may eventually become appropriate.

The criteria for a successful screening programme are as follows:

- The condition is an important health problem for the population
- The epidemiology and natural history of the condition are understood
- Screening uses a simple, safe, precise and well-validated test that is acceptable to the population
- Treatment is available that improves outcomes
- The findings of cost:benefit analysis are favourable

Pregnant patients with diabetes are often highly motivated to maintain good glycaemic control and to try to improve their blood glucose readings. However, post-pregnancy they sometimes find it harder to maintain this motivation solely for their own long-term benefit, particularly when they do not see the difference on a day-to-day basis.

Organisation of diabetes care

Diabetes care is provided in the settings of both primary and secondary care.

Initial care

Once type 2 diabetes mellitus is diagnosed, the initial care of the patient is usually coordinated in a primary care setting.

Coordination between primary and secondary care

Regular interaction is required between primary and secondary care providers. Clinics run by specialist diabetes consultants in local practices can provide care closer to home and integrate with primary care. Joint clinics or 'virtual' clinics enable individual cases to be discussed by diabetes specialists, practice nurses and GPs in the patient's absence. This allows practice nurses and GPs to be more comfortable with some of the traditionally challenging aspects of diabetes care, such as starting patients on insulin.

> A new diagnosis of diabetes can cause people to experience some of the stages of grief gone through in bereavement: denial, anger, bargaining and depression. Compared with people without diabetes, patients with diabetes mellitus are twice as likely to have depression, and poor well-being is associated with worse glycaemic control. Recovery from depression leads to an improvement in diabetes control.

Lead GPs for diabetes

Many general practices have a lead GP for diabetes who has a specialist interest in the condition, maintains a depth of knowledge and keeps up to date with developments in the field, which is not possible for all GPs who have a multitude of chronic conditions to look after. General practices have a key role in ensuring that all patients have an agreed care plan and appropriate, regular screening for complications.

In the first year after diagnosis, the following are addressed.

- An agreed self-care plan (which includes dietary improvement, an increased level of exercise, and smoking cessation)
- Structured education and written support in appropriate language, with the offer of engagement in patient groups
- Psychological support, if needed
- Discussion of effects on occupation, driving and insurance
- Discussion of annual screening for complications and treatment of other risk factors
- Capillary blood glucose monitoring (if receiving treatment that occasionally causes hypoglycaemia)

This care is usually delivered by the practice nurse and the GP working together, with help from members of other teams, such as dieticians and podiatrists.

Referral to secondary care

Referral to secondary care is usually considered for the following patients with diabetes mellitus.

- Patients with type 1 diabetes mellitus
- Children and adolescents
- Women considering pregnancy and those who are pregnant
- Patients with significant complications, including:
  - foot ulceration or Charcot's joint
  - significant nephropathy
  - retinopathy requiring laser or specialist treatment
  - neuropathy that is difficult to treat
- Patients with recurrent hypoglycaemia
- Patients with resistant hyperlipidaemia
- Patients for whom bariatric surgery is considered

Diabetes mellitus in adolescents

Diabetes mellitus in adolescent patients is challenging, both in cases of a new diagnosis of diabetes and in cases of diabetes persisting from childhood. It is not uncommon for children going through adolescence to:

- experience a deterioration in diabetes control

- require more emergency admissions to hospital
- fail to attend their appointments.

Support services

Diabetes services are adapting to try to engage and support adolescents by using age-appropriate education and communication. These services aim to prevent a feeling of abandonment by paediatric care, which has traditionally been much more intensive and supportive.

Good care of adolescents with diabetes mellitus involves understanding:

- the past (issues associated with diagnosis, hospital admissions, absence from school, etc.)
- issues associated with puberty
- the importance of a safe, independent and planned future

Management

Looking after teenagers involves communicating with them on their terms, such as letting them run the consultation and using email and text to communicate, while keeping them safe. Parents have often tried to 'protect' them from too much information in childhood. Developing independence means:

- attending clinic appointments on their own

- managing their own insulin injections
- learning about managing illness, alcohol, drugs and contraception
- learning about control in the long term
- discussing pregnancy and contraception openly

Complications

Adolescent patients who have had diabetes mellitus since childhood often have reduced independence. They may have been socially isolated or adopted the sick role. They may also be egocentric or feel insecure about their self-worth.

Adolescent patients in whom diabetes mellitus has been newly diagnosed may find the condition particularly difficult to adapt to. They are already coping with the demands of early adulthood, such as increased calorie intake, increased hormone levels and social changes (e.g. more adult relationships and use of alcohol or drugs).

The changes that patients experience at this time of their life often underlie:

- poor adherence to treatment
- risk-taking behaviour (e.g. chaotic eating, smoking, alcohol and drug abuse, and sexual risk taking)
- difficulty imagining the future and a feeling of being 'bulletproof' or invincible
- rejection of parents and health professionals

Monitoring thyroid function

Thyroid disease is common; it affects 0.5% of the population at any one time. However, its prevalence increases to 2% in women over 40 years old, and some studies show that 2-5% of patients on elderly care wards have thyroid disease. Thyroid disease in the elderly is frequently asymptomatic, so there should be a low threshold for checking thyroid function if the patient has atrial fibrillation, non-specific confusion or weight loss. Thyroid function is commonly checked by a

GP when a patient presents with non-specific symptoms such as weight gain and tiredness.

Management

Most patients with hypothyroidism are treated in the primary care setting by GPs. These patients need thyroid function tests annually (more frequently if their levothyroxine dose needs to be adjusted). Discussion with secondary care providers is indicated if:

- the patient's symptoms worsen or do not improve despite levothyroxine therapy
- the results of thyroid function tests are abnormal (e.g. high thyroid-stimulating hormone) despite full-dose levothyroxine therapy
- hypothyroidism coexists with active ischaemic heart disease
- the hypothyroid patient is pregnant
- the hypothyroid patient is a child

Most patients with hyperthyroidism are referred to secondary care for investigations to determine the cause of the condition and to plan its management. Follow-up is then usually shared between primary and secondary care with regular monitoring done in primary care and changes in treatment made in secondary care.

Pregnancy

It is important to consider thyroid disease during preconception counselling and in cases newly diagnosed in pregnancy. Risk factors for thyroid disease in pregnancy include:

- previous thyroid disease
- a strong family history of thyroid disease
- other autoimmune conditions (e.g. type 1 diabetes or coeliac disease)
- the presence of goitre
- symptoms of thyroid disease

New models of care for patients with chronic conditions are being developed in the UK. Conditions such as polycystic ovary syndrome, erectile problems, mild hypercalcaemia and vitamin D deficiency are commonly managed in primary care.

Answers to starter questions

1. There is a variety of resources available to encourage and help patients to manage their chronic conditions. These include websites and information sheets, educational courses in diabetes, blood glucose monitoring meters, sending clinic letters to patients and patient groups.

2. Government policies should encourage the prevention, early detection and appropriate management of diabetes. Prevention includes education programmes in schools, promotion of physical activity (such as funded schemes in the workplace), legislation on food labeling and promoting healthy eating. Early detection includes screening at-risk populations and making people aware of the symptoms. Management strategies include financial targets for the successful control of outcome measures that affect morbidity and mortality, such as blood pressure, HbA1c and urine albumin: creatinine ratio in patients with diabetes.

3. Feeling 'tired all the time' and unexplained weight gain are two common complaints for people attending primary care. Both are associated with hypothyroidism, which requires a thyroid blood test to confirm the diagnosis. Missed cases of severe hypothyroidism do occur but are extremely rare because tests are performed frequently.

4. Around 5% of women develop diabetes while pregnant, so they are already more aware of the risk of developing diabetes later in life. They also tend to present to their doctors earlier with symptoms, which means they receive a diagnosis before their symptoms are too severe. Men develop diabetes at a lower BMI than women and doctors may therefore not consider the diagnosis immediately.

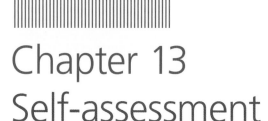

Chapter 13
Self-assessment

SBA questions

Diabetes, obesity and lipid disorders

1. A 19 year-old woman has a 3-week history of polyuria, polydipsia and tiredness. She has been losing weight and vomiting.
What is the single most appropriate test to perform?

A GAD antibodies
B Glucose tolerance test
C IA2 antibodies
D Random blood glucose
E Ultrasound of pancreas

2 A 55 year-old man is admitted to hospital with cellulitis. He has a history of hypertension and hyperlipidaemia, is overweight and smokes. His blood glucose is 30 mmol/L and his BP is 150/86 mmHg.
Apart from antibiotics for his cellulitis, what is the single most immediate problem to tackle?

A Hypercholesterolaemia
B Hyperglycaemia
C Hypertension
D Smoking
E Weight

3. A 40 year-old woman with type 1 diabetes has severe, unrecognised hypoglycaemic episodes. She is on haemodialysis for end-stage renal failure secondary to her diabetes, which is managed with an insulin pump. She has a donor that has been matched for a renal transplant. What is the single best treatment for long-term management of her hypoglycaemia?

A Basal bolus insulin via an insulin pen
B GLP-1 analogue injection
C Islet cell transplant
D Peritoneal dialysis
E Porcine insulin

4. A 38 year-old woman has type 2 diabetes (HbA1c 68 mmol/mol). Her BP is 150/78 mmHg and BMI is 51 kg/m². She takes metformin 500 mg daily as a higher dose had made her feel bloated.
What is the single most effective treatment for her diabetes?

A Bariatric surgery
B GLP-1 analogue
C Increase metformin again
D Insulin
E Sulphonylurea

5. An 86 year-old lady has a fall. Her HbA1c is 49 mmol/mol; she has been on low-dose gliclazide for 20 years. Her daughter has noticed she is intermittently confused and is worried about her managing on her own.
What is the single most appropriate next step?

A Add metformin to gliclazide
B Change to a long-acting sulphonylurea
C Increase gliclazide
D Start basal insulin
E Stop gliclazide

6. A 68 year-old man has an HbA1c of 49 mmol/mol on a routine blood test done after a consultation with his GP for his hypertension.
What is the single most appropriate next step?

A Arrange oral glucose tolerance test
B Give lifestyle advice and inform him of diagnosis of diabetes mellitus
C Repeat HbA1c test
D Repeat HbA1c test and give lifestyle advice
E Start metformin and inform him of diagnosis of diabetes mellitus

7. A 26 year-old woman has a 10-year history of type 1 diabetes. She has recently started exercising more and wants to run a marathon this year. She is worried about the effect of exercise on her blood glucose control.

What is the single most appropriate piece of advice?

A Avoid carbohydrate before the race
B Avoid exercise
C Decrease insulin before the race
D Increase insulin before the race
E Only exercise if starting capillary blood glucose is > 15 mmol/L

8. A 60 year-old woman has an infective exacerbation of chronic obstructive pulmonary disease being treated with a short course of antibiotics and steroids. Her diabetes mellitus is usually controlled with lifestyle measures. Her capillary blood glucose is 7–12 mmol/L.
What is the single most appropriate management for her diabetes?

A No additional treatment necessary
B Treat with metformin
C Treat with short-acting insulin injections at meal-time
D Treat with sulphonyluria
E Stop the antibiotics and steriods

9. A 23 year-old woman with type 1 diabetes has had a cold for 2 days. She has vomited several times since the morning. Her blood glucose is 20 mmol/L, and urine dip shows +++ ketones.
What is the single most appropriate next step?

A Advise withholding blood glucose monitoring temporarily to prevent anxiety
B Antibiotics
C Anti-emetic drugs to stop vomiting
D Hospital admission for IV fluids and insulin
E Withhold insulin injections to prevent hypoglycaemia

10. A 50 year-old man with type 1 diabetes mellitus has had erratic fluctuations in blood glucose readings recently, which he has found difficult to explain through dietary changes. Physical examination is unremarkable apart from subcutaneous lumps at insulin injection sites.
What is the single most appropriate next step in the management?

A Admit to hospital to monitor blood glucose levels
B Change insulin injection site
C Change insulin regime to porcine insulin
D Refer for an insulin pump
E Start metformin in addition to insulin regime

11. A 45 year-old woman has a serum cholesterol level of 7 mmol/L. She cycles 5 miles 3 days a week and drinks about 5 units of alcohol per week. She takes carbimazole for thyrotoxicosis and ramipril for hypertension. Her urine dip shows ++++protein. Her serum creatinine is 76 umol/L.

What is the single most likely cause of her elevated cholesterol?

A Alcohol
B Cycling
C Proteinuria
D Ramipril
E Thyrotoxicosis

Diabetes complications

1. A 53 year-old man has had type 1 diabetes mellitus for 35 years. He has proliferative retinopathy, diabetic nephropathy and diabetic neuropathy. He has a red left foot which has been present for 3 days. There is no ulcer. The foot is warm and swollen but not painful. Full blood count and C-reactive protein are normal. There is no fracture on X-ray.
What is the single most appropriate treatment?

A Intravenous bisphosphonate
B Observe and review
C Oral antibiotics
D Strict bed rest and elevation of the foot
E Total contact cast of the foot

2. A 34 year-old man has type 1 diabetes and background diabetic retinopathy. During annual review, his urine albumin-creatinine ratio (ACR) showed 10.6 mg/mmol. His serum, creatinine is 94 μmol/L. His repeat urine test shows persistently elevated ACR at 11.4 mg/mmol with no evidence of urinary infection. His BP is 144/92 mmHg.
What is the single most appropriate medication?

A ACE inhibitor
B alpha-blocker
C beta-blocker
D Calcium channel blocker
E Thiazide diuretic

3. A 60 year-old man with type 1 diabetes has a sudden painless loss of vision in his left eye for 10 hours. He has not attended his diabetic retinal screening appointments for 3 years. He has diabetic nephropathy and dense peripheral diabetic sensory neuropathy. His BP is 164/91 mmHg.
What is the single most likely cause of the loss of vision?

A Acute close angle glaucoma
B Amaurosis fugax
C Background retinopathy with macular oedema
D Cataract
E Vitreous haemorrhage

4 A 42 year-old man with type 2 diabetes has progressive diabetic renal disease. He complains

of fatigue and breathlessness on exertion. His blood tests show creatinine 304 μmol/L, urea 14.3 mmol/L, sodium 135 mmol/L, potassium 5.0 mmol/L, Hb 78g/dL, ferritin 509 μg/L.
What is the single most appropriate treatment?

A Activated vitamin D
B Erythropoietin
C IV iron infusion
D Haemodialysis
E Peritoneal dialysis

5. A frail 85 year-old man with type 2 diabetes has a necrotic right 5th toe. There is dry gangrene and no surrounding cellulitis. He is symptom-free. No foot pulses are detectable on hand-held Doppler. Femoral and popliteal pulses are palpable.
What is the single most appropriate next step?

A Above-knee amputation
B Below-knee amputation
C Long-term antibiotics
D Observation only without active intervention
E Toe amputation

6. A 45 year-old woman with type 2 diabetes has a new plantar ulcer. She has a history of prolif-erative retinopathy treated with laser photoco-agulation and dense peripheral neuropathy. The ulcer looks infected with purulent discharge and surrounding cellulitis.
What is the single most likely infective organ-ism?

A *Candida albicans*
B *Clostridium perfringens*
C *Escherichia coli*
D *Pseudomonas aeroginosum*
E *Staphylococcus aureus*

Thyroid disease

1. A 22 year-old woman has a 2 cm thyroid nodule which she noticed incidentally. She is otherwise well and has no symptoms. Her serum TSH is 1.3 mIU/L and thyroid peroxidase antibodies are negative.
What is the single most appropriate investiga-tion to perform?

A CT scan
B Flow volume loop
C Positron emission tomography
D Radionuclide uptake scan
E Ultrasound and fine needle aspiration cytol-ogy

2. A 66 year-old woman has breathlessness and stridor due to a large multinodular goitre compressing her trachea. She undergoes total thyroidectomy, and commences daily levothy-roxine 100 μg. Her breathlessness and stridor improve but 2 days after surgery she develops paraesthesia and painful spasms of her hands.
What is the single most likely cause of her symptoms?

A Damage to recurrent laryngeal nerve
B Hypocalcaemia
C Side-effect of anaesthesia
D Side-effect of levothyroxine
E Transient ischaemic attack

3. A 48 year-old man has palpitations, heat intol-erance and tremor following a flu-like illness. He has no goitre but his neck is tender. His thy-roid function tests show TSH <0.01 mIU/L and free T4 38 pmol/L. TSH receptor antibodies are negative and radionuclide scan show no uptake in the thyroid.
What is the single most appropriate treatment?

A Carbimazole
B Propranolol
C Propylthiouracil
D Radioactive iodine
E Thyroidectomy

4. A 36 year-old woman has palpitations, tremor and a small diffuse goitre. Her test results include TSH <0.01 mIU/L, FT4 96 pmol/L and positive TSH receptor antibodies, consistent with the diagnosis of Graves' disease. She starts carbimazole and propranolol, with which her symptoms gradually improve. However, 3 weeks later, she develops severe sore-throat and high fever (38°C).
What is the single most appropriate manage-ment?

A Check full blood count and continue car-bimazole and propranolol
B Check full blood count and stop carbimazole
C Check full blood count and stop propranolol
D Send throat-swab for culture and continue carbimazole and propranolol
E Start antibiotics and continue carbimazole and propranolol

5. A 71 year-old man has tiredness, cold intoler-ance and dry skin. His thyroid function tests include TSH 98 mIU/L and FT4 5 pmol/L. He has a history of hypertension, raised cholesterol and angina, and takes atenolol, aspirin, simvastatin and GTN spray.
What is the single most appropriate manage-ment for this?

A High dose (100–125 μg) of levothyroxine
B Levothyroxine and carbimazole
C Levothyroxine and liothyronine (T3)
D Liothyronine (T3) alone
E Small dose (12.5–25 μg) levothyroxine

6. A 31 year-old woman is 6 weeks pregnant. She has lost 5 kg of body weight in 3 months. She also has palpitations, heat intolerance, tremor and a small diffuse goitre. Her thyroid function tests show TSH <0.01 mIU/L and FT4 35 pmol/L. TSH receptor antibodies are positive.
What is the single most appropriate management?

A Carbimazole alone
B Carbimazole with levothyroxine
C Propylthiouracil alone
D Radioactive iodine
E Total thyroidectomy

7. A 55 year-old woman has a moderately-sized goitre. Her hands are warm and clammy and she has a tremor. Her heart rhythm is irregularly irregular and she has protruding eyes (exophthalmos). Her thyroid function tests reveal TSH <0.01 mIU/L and FT4 45 pmol/L.
Which single clinical sign is most indicative of Graves' disease?

A Atrial fibrillation
B Exophthalmos
C Goitre
D Tremor
E Warm, clammy hands

8. A 40 year-old woman has a lump in her neck. Fine needle aspiration cytology under ultrasound guidance shows malignant cells. She undergoes total thyroidectomy. Histology confirms papillary thyroid carcinoma. She is on long-term levothyroxine replacement.
What is the single most appropriate target when monitoring her levothyroxine dose?

A Keep serum FT4 above the reference range
B Keep serum FT4 below the reference range
C Keep serum TSH above the reference
D Keep serum TSH below the reference range
E Keep serum TSH within the reference range

9. A 38 year-old man undergoes a total thyroidectomy for medullary thyroid carcinoma. His has no evidence of phaeochromocytoma or primary hyperparathyroidism. He has no family history of medullary thyroid carcinoma and his genetic testing shows no evidence of mutation in the RET gene.
Which is the single most appropriate test for regular monitoring to detect recurrence of his carcinoma?

A CT neck
B PET scan
C Radioiodine uptake scan
D Serum calcitonin
E Serum thyroglobulin

Pituitary disease

1. A 65 year-old man has 'pins and needles' and pain in his both hands and fingers, which is worse at night. Nerve conduction study shows features consistent with bilateral carpel tunnel syndrome. He also reports headaches, sweating and increasing shoe size. He has thick skin and a large tongue. His BP is 170/100 mmHg and urine dip shows glycosuria.
Which of the following biochemical investigations is most likely to reveal the unifying diagnosis of his clinical features?

A 24-hour free urinary cortisol
B Glucose tolerance test
C Insulin stress test
D Serum prolactin
E Serum TSH and FT4

2. A 24 year-old woman has gained weight, which she is unable to shift despite rigorous dieting. She has been bruising easily, her menstrual cycles are irregular and her muscles feel weak. She also has a history of epilepsy, diabetes and hypertension. She takes phenytoin for her epilepsy.
What is the single most appropriate investigation?

A 24-hour urinary cortisol
B 9am serum cortisol
C Low-dose dexamethasone suppression test (LDDST)
D MRI pituitary
E Plasma ACTH

3. A 28 year-old woman has a history of headaches and intermittent galactorrhoea. An MRI scan shows a pituitary mass and visual fields that show a bitemporal hemianopia. Fundoscopy shows no evidence of optic atrophy. She is hypopituitary on testing except for a raised prolactin of 600 mU/L.
What single feature would be an indication for an operation?

A Bitemporal hemianopia
B Headaches
C Hypopituitarism
D Galactorrhoea
E Prolactin 600 mU/L

4. A 52 year-old man has weakness of his leg muscles and easy bruising. His BMI is 36 kg/m^2 and BP 160/100 mmHg. Tests show fasting blood glucose 9.2 mmol/L, 24 h urinary cortisol 386 nmol/24h, serum cortisol after overnight dexamethasone suppression test 150nmol/L and plasma ACTH <1 ng/L.
What is the single most appropriate next investigation?

A CT adrenal
B CT chest, abdomen and pelvis
C Inferior petrosal sinus sampling
D MIBG scan
E MRI pituitary

5. A 25 year-old woman has thirst, polyuria and nocturia. Her serum Ca^{2+} is 2.4 mmol/L and fasting glucose is 4.5 mmol/L. She undergoes a water deprivation test. After 6 hours of fluid restriction, her serum osmolality is 300 mOsm/kg and urine osmolality 250 mOsm/kg. At the end of the test, she is given DDAVP spray. After the spray, her serum osmolality is 296 mOsm/kg and urine osmolality 776 mOsm/kg.
What is the single most likely diagnosis?

A Cranial diabetes insipidus
B Diabetes mellitus
C Nephrogenic diabetes insipidus
D Primary polydipsia
E Syndrome of inappropriate ADH secretion

6. A 40 year-old woman has a history of schizo-phrenia, diabetes and hypertension managed with risperidone, metformin, insulin, amlodip-ine and ramipril. She has spontaneous bilateral galactorrhoea but continues to have menstrual cycles. Her serum prolactin is 1900 mU/L.
What is the single most appropriate next step?

A Consult with psychiatrist to change risperi-done
B Mammogram
C MRI pituitary
D Start cabergoline
E Stop metformin

7. A 26 year-old woman has been diagnosed with a prolactinoma and has recently got married. She asks about the impact on her fertility if she decides not to have treatment.
Which of the following is the single most appropriate statement?

A She will have an increased chance of having twin pregnancies
B She will have an increased risk of miscar-riage
C She will have difficulty breastfeeding
D She will have difficulty conceiving
E The baby will have an increased risk of con-genital abnormalities

8. A 35 year-old man has features of acromegaly. His nadir growth hormone on glucose tolerance test is 5.1 ug/L and IGF-1 80 nmol/L. His MRI shows a 1 cm left-sided adenoma in the pituitary.
What is the single most appropriate treatment?

A Cabergoline
B Somatostatin analogues
C Standard beam radiotherapy

D Stereotactic radiotherapy
E Transphenoidal surgery

9. A 40 year-old woman has a pituitary mass. She is otherwise well. Her BP is 110/74 mmHg. Her biochemistry results show normal pituitary function except cortisol 140 nmol/L (rising to 380 nmol/L on short synacthen test, and plasma), ACTH 5 ng/L.
Which one of the following is the single most appropriate hormone replacement for her?

A ACTH
B ACTH and aldosterone
C Aldosterone (fludrocortisone)
D Aldosterone and cortisol
E Cortisol (hydrocortisone)

10. A 70 year-old man has a bitemporal hemiano-pia. MRI pituitary reveals a large mass com-pressing and distorting the optic chiasm and extending into the temporal lobe. He is sched-uled for immediate transphenoidal surgery.
What single test result would alter the decision to perform surgery?

A 9am serum cortisol 67 nmol/L
B IGF-I 4 nmol/L (age related normal range 5 -26 nmol/L)
C Prolactin 26 000 mU/L (NR 86 -324)
D Testosterone 6 nmol/L (NR 6.7 -25.8)
E TSH 5 mU/L (NR 0.35 -4.5)

Adrenal disease

1. A 72 year-old man has chronic obstructive pulmonary disease and a history of fatigue, dizziness, weight loss and lethargy. His blood pressure is 100/60 mmHg. He has had recurrent courses of high-dose prednisolone for exacer-bations of his lung disease. Blood results show Hb 144 g/L, Na^+ 135 mmol/L, K^+ 4.3 mmol/L, corrected Ca^{2+} 2.24 mmol/L and random blood glucose 3.8 mmol/L.
What is the single next best investigation to perform?

A 24-hour urinary cortisol
B Low dose dexamethasone suppression test
C Overnight dexamethasone suppression test
D Plasma ACTH
E Short synacthen test

2. A 50 year-old woman has aldosterone excess. An adrenal CT shows bilateral adrenal hyperplasia. It is recommended that she continue with medical treatment as surgery would not be curative.
What is the single most effective antihyperten-sive drug for her to take?

A Atenolol
B Bendroflumethiazide

C Doxazosin
D Ramipril
E Spironolactone

3. A 52 year-old woman is overweight and has recently been diagnosed with diabetes mellitus. During a recent admission with abdominal pain an abdominal CT showed an incidental 1.5 cm left adrenal mass. Her BP is 170/100 mmHg.
What is the single most appropriate next investigation?

A 9am cortisol
B Adrenal vein sampling for cortisol measurements
C MRI adrenals
D Overnight 1mg dexamethasone suppression test
E Serum testosterone

4. A 32 year-old woman with congenital adrenal hyperplasia (CAH) at birth is due to have laparoscopic cholecystectomy. She takes hydrocortisone and fludrocortisone.
What is the single best action regarding her medication during the perioperative period?

A Increase fludrocortisone dose
B Increase hydrocortisone dose
C Increase hydrocortisone and fludrocortisone doses
D Stop hydrocortisone
E Stop hydrocortisone and fludrocortisone

5 A 27 year-old woman has had type 1 diabetes mellitus since 15 years of age. She has been tired and losing weight for 5 months. Her BP is 100/76 mmHg and drops to 85/60 mmHg on standing. Her heart rate is 70 bpm. Her HbA1c is 60 mmol/mol.
What is the single most likely cause for her symptoms?

A Addison's disease
B Coeliac disease
C Graves' disease
D Poorly controlled diabetes mellitus
E Primary hypothyroidism

6. A 32 year-old man has hypertension that is not controlled by ramipril, doxazosin and amlodipine. His BP is 166/98 mmHg in both arms and there is no radiofemoral delay. His BMI is 26 kg/m^2; other physical examination was unremarkable. His tests show, creatinine 68 umol/L, Na$^+$ 137 mmol/L and K$^+$ 3.2 mmol/L
What is the single most likely cause of his hypertension?

A Conn's syndrome
B Cushing's syndrome
C Medication non-concordance
D Phaeochromocytoma
E Essential hypertension

7. A 31 year-old woman has episodes of palpitations, sweating and tremor. She denies diarrhoea, weight loss or wheeze. She has regular menstrual cycle. Her BP is high at 180/100 mmHg.
What is the single most appropriate next investigation?

A 24 hour urinary 5-hyroxyindoleacetic acid (5-HIAA)
B 24 hour urinary metanephrines
C 24 hour urinary vanillylmandelic acid (VMA)
D CT of adrenal glands
E MIBG scan

Calcium homeostasis and metabolic bone disease

1. A 62 year-old man has a history of thirst, polyuria and vomiting. He has primary hyperparathyroidism and is awaiting surgical removal of a parathyroid adenoma. He is dehydrated. Serum biochemistry reveals corrected Ca^{2+} of 3.12 mmol/L, phosphate 0.64 mmol/L and creatinine 260 umol/L.
What is the single most appropriate next step?

A Aggressive fluid resuscitation
B Cinacalcet
C IV pamidronate infusion
D Systemic steroids
E Urgent haemodialysis

2. A 44 year-old woman has lethargy. She moved to the UK from the Middle East 2 years ago. She is normally fit and well, maintains a strict Halal diet, wears a Hijab (headscarf) and has no significant family history. Her serum Ca^{2+} is 2.0 mmol/L, phosphate 1.1 mmol/L, Mg^{2+} 0.87 mmol/L and eGFR is >90 mls/min/1.72m^2.
What is the single most likely cause of her hypocalcaemia?

A Dietary calcium deficiency
B Hypervitaminosis D
C Primary hyperparathyroidism
D Primary hypoparathyroidism
E Vitamin D deficiency

3. An 82 year-old man has a 20-year history of type 2 diabetes mellitus and stage 4 chronic kidney disease. Recent blood tests show serum calcium 2.04 mmol/L and serum PTH 10 pmol/L. He also has a normocytic anaemia with Hb 102 gm/L.
What is the single most likely cause of his elevated serum PTH level?

A Dietary calcium deficiency
B Familial hypocalciuric hypercalcaemia
C Primary hyperparathyroidism
D Secondary hyperparathyroidism
E Tertiary hyperparathyroidism

4. A 75 year-old woman has a history of poor appetite, weight loss, lethargy and constipation. Blood tests reveal Hb 101 g/L, MCV 75 fL, creatinine 122 mmol/L and corrected Ca^{2+} 2.78 mmol/L.

What is the single most appropriate next test?

A CT chest, abdomen and pelvis
B Neck ultrasound
C Parathyroid hormone
D Serum electrophoresis and urinary Bence Jones protein
E Sestamibi scan

5. A 71-year-old man has a fall. An X-ray shows a fractured neck of femur. Subsequent DEXA scan shows osteoporosis. His serum testosterone is 8 nmol/L. He is non-smoker and drinks about 4 units of alcohol per week and takes over-the-counter multivitamins.

What is the single most appropriate treatment?

A Avoid exercise
B Bisphosphonate
C Prednisolone
D Stop alcohol completely
E Testosterone

6. A 63 year-old man has pain in his legs. There are no obvious clinical signs on examination. Blood tests show serum ALP 312 iU/L, corrected Ca^{2+} 2.2 mmol/L, phosphate 1.1 mmol/L, Hb 134 gm/L, eGFR 90 ml/min/1.73m^2 and serum 25 OH vitamin D 68 nmo/L. His other liver enzymes are normal.

What is the single most likely diagnosis?

A Multiple myeloma
B Osteoarthritis
C Osteomalacia
D Osteoporosis
E Paget's disease

Reproductive system disorders

1. A 40 year-old man has erectile dysfunction. He is divorced but recently met a new partner. Examination is unremarkable with normal secondary sexual characteristics and testicular volume (25 ml bilaterally). A blood test shows serum testosterone 8 nmol/L.

What is the single most appropriate next step?

A Karyotype analysis of chromosomes
B MRI pituitary
C Repeat serum testosterone
D Start testosterone replacement
E Testicular ultrasound

2. A 20 year-old man has general lethargy and loss of libido. He had orchidopexy surgery for unde-scended testes at the age of 2 years. Investigations show serum testosterone 4 nmol/L, serum LH 40 iu/L and serum FSH 48 iu/L , consistent with primary hypogonadism. He starts testosterone replacement with injections.

Which single most important test would you perform annually to monitor side-effects?

A CT prostate
B DEXA scan for bone density
C Full blood count and haematocrit
D Mammogram
E Serum electrolytes

3. A 24 year-old woman has had hirsutism for 3 years and has irregular menstrual cycles. She denies easy bruising, muscle weakness or galactorrhoea. Her BMI is 30 kg/m^2 and BP 130/85 mmHg. Investigations show 24 hour urinary cortisol 86 nmol/24 h, serum prolactin 344 mIU/L, serum 17-hydroxyprogesterone 1.5 nmol/L and serum testosterone 2.8 nmol/L. Ultrasound shows normal ovaries.

What is the single most likely diagnosis?

A Androgen-secreting ovarian tumour
B Congenital adrenal hyperplasia
C Cushing's syndrome
D Polycystic ovary syndrome
E Prolactinoma

4. A 28 year-old woman has been having irregular menstrual periods for 2 years. Her last period was 6 months ago. Physical examination is unremarkable except vitiligo in both her arms. Pregnancy test is negative. Tests show serum prolactin 88 mIU/L, serum oestradiol 38 pmol/L, serum LH 56 iu/L and serum FSH 50 iu/L. Ovarian autoantibodies are positive.

What is the single most appropriate hormone treatment?

A Gonadotrophin releasing hormone (GnRH)
B Gonadotrophins
C Oestrogen
D Oestrogen with progesterone
E Progesterone

5. A 17 year-old girl has not started having menstrual cycles. Her breasts and secondary sexual characteristics are poorly developed. She is short (4ft 8in) and has cubitus valgum. Investigations show serum oestrogen oestradiol 20 pmol/, serum LH 60 iu/L and serum FSH 32 iu/L. Chromosomal karyotype analysis confirms the aetiology.

What is the single most likely result of the chromosomal karyotyping?

A 45X0
B 46XX
C 46XY
D 47XX +21
E 47XXY

6. A 20 year-old woman has had secondary amenorrhea for 10 months. She is otherwise well. She eats healthily and runs at least 6 miles a day. Her BMI is 18 kg/m². Other physical examinations are unremarkable. Tests show serum oestradiol 30 pmol/L, serum LH 0.5 iu/L and serum FSH 0.9 iu/L. Pituitary MRI is normal. What is the single most appropriate next step?

A Advise to reduce exercise and gain weight
B Calcium and vitamin D
C Human recombinant leptin
D Oestrogen replacement
E Progestogen challenge

7. A 35 year-old man has secondary hypogonadism due to Kallmann syndrome. He is on daily testosterone gel but admits that he frequently forgets to apply it. He and his partner have been trying to conceive without success for 2 years. He has a low sperm count. What is the single best treatment to improve his sperm count?

A Androstenedione
B Change to injectable testosterone
C Dehydroepiandrosterone (DHEA)
D Human chorionic gonadotrophin
E Multivitamins

Other endocrine disorders

1. A 56 year-old woman has episodes of dizziness, tremor and feelings of hunger. Her husband takes insulin for type 2 diabetes. When she occasionally checks her blood glucose using her husband's glucose testing machine during the episodes, she gets low readings between 2.5–3.5 mmol/L. She has to eat frequently to relieve her symptoms.
What is the single most appropriate investigation?

A 72 hours fasting for c-peptide and insulin level
B CT pancreas
C Glycosylated haemoglobin
D MRI of the pancreas
E Ultrasonography of the pancreas

2. A 46 year-old man has multiple endocrine neoplasia type 1 (MEN1). He has had parathyroidectomy for primary hyperthyroidism and pituitary surgery for acromegaly. Genetic testing shows a mutation in the MEN1 gene. He has a 20 year-old daughter.
What is the single most appropriate advice for her daughter?

A Annual endocrine tests for serum calcium, PTH, prolactin and IGF1, and plasma gastrin
B Annual MRI of pituitary, ultrasound of parathyroid and CT of pancreas

C Predictive testing of the MEN1 gene mutation
D Prophylactic parathyroidectomy
E Reassure as MEN1 occurs only in men

3. A 60 year-old woman has a 6-month history of intermittent flushing, watery diarrhoea and shortness of breath. She denies heat intolerance and sweating. Her periods stopped 4 years ago. Her BP is 110/80 mmHg. Chest examination shows wheeze bilaterally. She also has hepatomegaly.
What is the single most appropriate investigation to perform?

A Oestrogen, LH and FSH levels
B Serum bilirubin, aspartate transaminase (AST) and alanine transaminase (ALT)
C TSH and free T4
D Urinary metanephrines
E Urinary 5-hydroxy indole acetic acid (5-HIAA)

4. A 38 year-old man has episodes of palpitations, headaches and dizzy spells. His BP is 180/110 mmHg. 3 years ago he underwent successful total thyroidectomy for medullary thyroid carcinoma. He has no neck lump and his recent serum calcitonin level is undetectable. What is the single most likely cause of his symptoms?

A Hypoparathyroidism
B Hypothyroidism
C Phaeochromocytoma
D Primary hyperparathyroidism
E Recurrence of medullary thyroid cancer

5. A 20 year-old woman has an episode of melena. She has been suffering from upper abdominal pain and intermittent diarrhoea for 1 year and takes antacids for her symptoms. She is haemodynamically stable. Her haemoglobin is 12 gm/L. Gastroendoscopy shows several large ulcers in her stomach and duodenum. What is the single most appropriate next investigation?

A Fasting plasma gastrin
B Fasting plasma glucagon
C Fasting plasma insulin and c-peptide
D Fasting plasma somatostatin
E Fasting plasma vasoactive intestinal polypeptide (VIP)

Endocrine emergencies

1. An 89 year-old woman has a history of reduced mobility and failure to cope at home. She is alert but not orientated to time or place. Her BP is 130/75 mmHg with no postural blood pressure drop on standing. She is not thirsty and clinically euvolaemic. Serum Na$^+$ is 120 mmol/L, urea 3.2 mmol/L, serum osmolality 245 mosmol/kg, urine osmolality 405 mosmol/kg and urine Na$^+$44 mmol/L. Her serum TSH is 3.0 U/L and morning serum cortisol 575 nmol/L. Her chest X-Ray shows an upper lobe mass.

What is the single most appropriate initial management?

A Commence demeclocycline
B Infuse 500ml of 0.9% sodium chloride over 12 hours
C Infuse 500ml of 3.0% sodium chloride over 12 hours
D Restrict fluid intake
E Vasopressin-2 receptor antagonist

2. A 25 year-old woman with type 1 diabetes has diabetic ketoacidosis. She is treated with fluid replacement and an IV insulin infusion. She is feeling much better. Her most recent venous blood gas results are pH 7.33, HCO$_3$ 12 mmol/L, blood glucose 5.5 mmol/L. Her blood ketones are 3 mmol/L

What is the single most appropriate next step?

A Administer IV bicarbonate infusion
B Continue the IV fluid and insulin infusion
C Stop the IV fluid and insulin infusion
D Stop the insulin infusion and continue IV fluid replacement
E Stop IV fluid and the insulin infusion

3. A 53 year-old man has type 2 diabetes mellitus. His capillary blood glucose is 2.8 mmol/L. He is day 3 post coronary artery bypass graft surgery. He takes isophane insulin 20 units twice per day. He is confused but alert.

What is the single most appropriate initial management?

A 1 mg glucagon IM
B 50 ml of 50% dextrose IV
C 100 ml 10% dextrose IV
D 150 ml pure orange juice
E A small chocolate bar

4. A 45 year-old man with type 1 diabetes mellitus for 14 years is admitted with decreased consciousness. His blood glucose is 32 mmol/L, serum bicarbonate 9 mmol/L, serum sodium 132 mmol/L, serum potassium 5.5 mmol/L, pH 7.1 and blood ketones 5.7 mmol/L.

Which of the following is the single most appropriate statement regarding management of this man?

A Anticoagulants are contra-indicated
B Restrict fluid to 1 L a day
C Treat with an increased dose of his SC insulin regime

D Treat with IV saline, potassium and insulin
E Treat with IM glucagon

5. A 57 year-old woman has an acute, severe headache. Her Glasgow coma scale (GCS) is 12/15 and she is hypotensive with a BP of 94/72 mmHg. Neurological examination reveals left 3rd cranial nerve palsy. A CT scan shows fresh blood in the pituitary fossa.

What is the single most appropriate investigation to perform?

A Carotid doppler
B Cerebral angiogram
C Formal visual field testing
D Lumber puncture
E Pituitary hormone profile

Integrated care

1. A 55 year-old man has a BMI of 27 kg/m^2. His mother, maternal grandmother and sister have all developed type 2 diabetes in later years. He comes to you for advice about how to avoid it.

What is the single most appropriate advice to give?

A Consider bariatric surgery
B Cut down on meals: eat 2 a day missing breakfast if not hungry
C Diabetes is inevitable
D Regular exercise for 30 minutes every day
E Start metformin immediately

2. A 50 year-old woman with thirst has a new diagnosis of diabetes mellitus with an HbA1c of 72 mmol/mol. She smokes and has a BMI of 27 kg/m^2. She is busy at work and doesn't have time to focus on all aspects of her health. She agrees to make simple changes to her lifestyle.

What is the single most appropriate advice to give?

A Cut out sugar in tea and carbonated drinks
B Start insulin injections
C Rapid weight-loss through restrictive diet
D Start taking metformin
E Stop smoking

3. A 28 year-old woman has just had a positive pregnancy test. She previously had a thyroidectomy 3 years ago for Graves' disease and has been on a stable dose of levothyroxine replacement for several years. Her TSH is 4.5 mIU/L.

What is the single most appropriate advice to give?

A Decrease levothyroxine dose
B Continue her current dose of levothyroxine
C Increase levothyroxine dose
D Stop levothyroxine
E Terminate the pregnancy

SBA answers

Diabetes, obesity and lipid disorders

1. D

High random glucose with symptoms of diabetes will confirm the diagnosis so glucose tolerance test is unnecessary. HbA1c and urinalysis are likely to be abnormal, but HbA1c can be normal in a patient with a very short history of probable type 1 diabetes and therefore is not a preferred test if clinical history is very short. GAD and IA2 antibodies do not diagnose diabetes and can be positive before development of type 1 diabetes. Ultrasound of pancreas is not useful for diagnosis of diabetes.

2. B

Stopping smoking might have the best long-term reduction in morbidity and mortality risk, but his immediate risk is hyperglycaemia which, untreated could impede treatment of cellulitis and lead to hyperosmolar hyperglycaemic state. Reducing weight will help to control his diabetes, hypertension and hypercholesterolaemia in the longer term but will not make an immediate difference. The blood pressure may settle as the infection is controlled.

3. C

As she will be immunosuppressed because of her renal transplant, the additional risks of an islet cell transplant are minimal and should improve the hypoglycaemia as well as potentially resolving the diabetes. A pancreatic transplant would be an alternative. Changing insulin pump to basal bolus insulin regime or porcine insulin may worsen control. GLP-1 analogues are not used in type 1 diabetes and changing method of dialysis will not make a significant difference.

4. A

She has morbid obesity and her BMI must be reduced as a priority to improve her diabetes control and prevent further complications. This alone will improve her diabetes and blood pressure. GLP-1 analogues may help her lose some weight, but is unlikely to achieve a normal BMI. Insulin and sulphonylurea will make weight loss more challenging. She has previously been unable to tolerate higher doses of Metformin, so increasing this may diminish compliance.

5. E

The history together with the relatively low HbA1c result would suggest she is having episodes of hypoglycaemia, which may be a bigger risk than hyperglycaemia for an elderly person. Therefore loosening her control is the best option. All other options would lead to increased risk of hypoglycaemia which, at age 86, would outweigh the potential benefits.

6. D

In the absence of symptoms the HbA1c test should be repeated; incorrect diagnosis of diabetes mellitus can have significant psychological and financial consequences. Even if repeat test shows that HbA1c is just below diagnostic cut-off for diabetes mellitus (48mmol/mol), lifestyle advice is important as diabetes mellitus is likely to develop in the future because intense lifestyle modification has been shown to delay its onset.

7. C

Training for a marathon with type 1 diabetes needs careful monitoring avoiding running with very high or very low blood glucose. Blood glucose falls with exercise so reducing insulin can help avoid hypoglycaemia. However, starting with excessively elevated capillary blood glucose can lead to ketosis. She will also need carbohydrates before or during the race to avoid hypoglycaemia

8. A

Her blood glucose level is only mildly elevated, most likely secondary to the short course of steroids. When the steroids are stopped, blood glucose levels are likely to return to normal, therefore she does not require additional treatment for her diabetes. If the blood sugars were much higher insulin would be the best option for rapid control during short courses of steroid treatment. Further episodes of hyperglycaemia are likely with future treatments with systemic steroids.

9. D

It's most likely this patient is developing diabetic ketoacidosis and this warrants urgent assessment and treatment in the hospital. A venous blood gas with pH <7.3 or low serum bicarbonate would confirm DKA. Despite vomiting, she must not stop insulin. In contrast, she may need increased dose of insulin. She must continue to monitor her blood glucose levels closely. Antibiotics are indicated only if there is evidence of a superimposed bacterial infection. Vomiting is likely to stop with IV insulin and fluid treatment for diabetic ketoacidosis.

10.B

This man's subcutaneous lumps at injection sites are likely to be lipohypertrophy. Lipohypertrophy or lipoatrophy can lead to altered insulin absorption and therefore fluctuations in blood sugar. They can develop at insulin injection sites if the same site is used on multiple occasions. He should avoid injecting insulin at areas of lipohypertrophy to prevent fluctuations in his blood glucose levels.

11.C

She is likely to have nephrotic syndrome with heavy proteinuria, which is associated with hypercholesterolaemia. Some drugs such as diuretics can affect lipids, but not Ramipril. Hypothyroidism rather than thyrotoxicosis is associated with hyperlipidaemia. Excess alcohol can be associated with raised cholesterol and triglycerides but 5 units of alcohol per week is unlikely to significantly affect her cholesterol level; exercise tends to improve the lipid profile.

Diabetes complications

1. E

In the absence of infection or fracture, a swollen, warm, red foot in a patient with diabetic neuropathy is typical of acute Charcot's arthropathy. The foot needs immediate immobilisation with total contact cast or Aircast; bed rest is impractical for long periods. Bisphosphonates are effective at reducing pain and inflammation of Charcot's arthropathy but are not first-line treatment. Antibiotics are not indicated unless infection is suspected.

2. A

Persistently raised urinary albumin creatinine ratio (microalbuminuria) in the absence of urinary infection suggests early diabetic nephropathy, which is further supported by the presence of diabetic retinopathy. ACE-inhibitors are the treatment of choice for early diabetic nephropathy and should be titrated to full dose. However, if a target of 130/80 mmHg is not achieved with a single agent, thiazide diuretics and calcium channel blockers may be used in addition.

3. E

Vitreous haemorrhage can occur in patients with proliferative diabetic retinopathy due to new vessel formations that bleed easily. This presents with sudden painless loss of vision. Amaurosis fugax causes temporary unilateral painless blindness due to microemboli, resolving within minutes. Background retinopathy with macular oedema and cataracts do not cause sudden visual loss. In acute close angle glaucoma visual loss is associated with ocular pain.

4. B

The patient's anaemia could be causing his symptoms and is mostly likely to be due to chronic kidney disease. Erythropoietin is the most effective treatment of his anaemia as his iron stores are adequate. Activated vitamin D will not help his anaemia. At present there is no indication for dialysis.

5. D

The toe is dead and will auto-amputate. In the absence of infection or symptoms, he does not require amputation or antibiotics.

6. E

Staphylococcus and *Streptococcus* are the most common pathogens in diabetic foot infections. Other organisms that rarely cause infection in non-diabetic patients with normal immune systems can sometimes become pathogenic (such as *E. coli* and anaerobic organisms like *Clostridium perfringens* and *Bacteriodes*). Pseudomonas is often a colonising rather than infective organism. Candida infection in diabetic feet may be a port for bacterial infection but is rarely a pathogenic organism in ulcers.

Thyroid disease

1. E

About 5% of thyroid nodules are malignant. Fine needle aspiration cytology under ultrasound guidance is the investigation of choice to exclude malignancy, not CT or positron emission tomography. Radionuclide uptake scan is a useful investigation if the patient is also hyperthyroid to exclude a toxic thyroid nodule but this patient is euthyroid. Flow volume loop can be performed to investigate tracheal compression due to a large goitre.

2. B

The symptoms are typical of tetany, caused by hypocalcaemia which is a recognised complication of thyroidectomy secondary to transient or permanent hypoparathyroidism. Recurrent laryngeal nerve injury is another potential complication of thyroidectomy but causes hoarseness of voice. Tetany is not a side-effect of levothyroxine or anaesthesia. Although transient ischaemic attack can occasionally present with paraesthesia, the combination of paraesthesia and tetany is not a presenting feature.

3. B

This patient's symptoms, recent viral illness, neck tenderness, blood results and absence of uptake in the radionuclide scan are consistent with subacute (de Quervain's) thyroiditis. In this condition, thyrotoxicosis results from release of pre-formed thyroid hormones stored in the thyroid, due to inflammation and resolves spontaneously. Therefore, antithyroid drugs, radioactive iodine or thyroidectomy are inappropriate in this condition. A beta-blocker (for example, Propranolol) is useful for symptom control.

4. B
Agranulocytosis is a rare but serious side-effect of anti-thyroid drugs (carbimazole, methimazole or propylthiouracil), often presenting with sore-throat, mouth ulcers and high fever. This patient must stop carbimazole and have her full blood count checked. If this is normal, she could restart the drug. Patients starting on anti-thyroid drugs must be given verbal and written information regarding this side-effect.

5. E
Levothyroxine alone is the treatment of choice for hypothyroidism. In patients with ischaemic heart disease, Levothyroxine may precipitate angina or myocardial infarction. Patients with known ischaemic heart disease and elderly patients (who may have undiagnosed ischaemic heart disease) must start Levothyroxine in a small dose (25 μg or 12.5 μg daily), and titrate up the dose gradually.

6. C
Propylthiouracil is the treatment of choice for Graves' disease in early pregnancy. Carbimazole is associated with rare birth-defects so should be avoided in the first trimester. 'Block and replace' regime (antithyroid drugs with levothyroxine) should also be avoided as antithyroid drugs cross the placenta causing fetal hypothyroidism. In pregnancy, radioactive iodine is contra-indicated, and thyroidectomy is used only for women who can't take antithyroid drugs due to side-effects.

7. B
Exophthalmos is a sign of thyroid eye disease, associated only with Graves' disease, not other forms of thyrotoxicosis. Warm sweaty palms, tremor and atrial fibrillation are associated with all forms of thyrotoxicosis. Many patients with Graves' disease have goitre but this may also be present in patients with thyrotoxicosis due to other cause, in hypothyroidism, or in normal thyroid function.

8. D
In patients with differentiated (papillary and follicular) thyroid cancer, levothyroxine dose should be adjusted to keep serum TSH suppressed. TSH stimulates growth of both normal and malignant thyroid cells, and the suppression of serum TSH below the reference range in patients with differentiated thyroid cancers is associated with lower recurrence rates.

9. D
Serum calcitonin is a tumour marker for medullary thyroid carcinoma and is a useful screening test for early diagnosis of recurrence or metastasis of the carcinoma. CT and PET scans are performed to localise the recurrence or metastasis but because of the exposure to radiation and the cost, these investigations are not useful for regular surveillance. Serum thyroglobulin and radioiodine uptake scans are not useful in medullary thyroid carcinoma (used in papillary or follicular thyroid carcinoma).

Pituitary disease

1. B
Acromegaly is the most likely diagnosis in this man with bilateral carpel tunnel syndrome, enlarging feet, macroglossia and hypertension. The biochemical diagnosis of acromegaly can be made by measuring growth hormone levels during a glucose tolerance test. In a patient with acromegaly, growth hormone levels fail to be suppressed after a glucose load. The insulin stress test is used for diagnosing growth hormone deficiency (and secondary adrenal insufficiency) rather than acromegaly. Although severe hypothyroidism can rarely cause macroglossia, this patients does not have other clinical features of hypothyroidism. Cushing's syndrome (diagnosed with 24 hour free urinary cortisol) and hyperprolactinaemia (diagnosed with serum prolactin level) are not associated with carpel tunnel syndrome.

2. A
Weight gain, easy bruising, muscle weakness, menstrual irregularity, diabetes and hypertension in this woman raise the suspicion of Cushing's syndrome. Low dose dexamethasone suppression test (LDDST) and 24 hour urinary cortisol measurement are both screening tests for Cushing's syndrome. Phenytoin is an enzyme-inducer which increases dexamethasone metabolism so may lead to false positive results on the LDDST therefore 24 hour urinary cortisol is preferred in this case. Plasma ACTH will help identify the aetiology of Cushing's syndrome but is not useful to make the diagnosis. Radiological investigations may reveal "incidentalomas" so should be done after biochemical investigations.

3. A
This patient has a non-functioning pituitary macroadenoma. Visual loss can be reversible if acted on quickly before optic atrophy occurs and may worsen if the pressure is not relieved on the optic chiasm. Headaches are com-

mon and not always relieved by an operation. Hypopituitarism is unlikely to reverse with an operation, and intermittent galactorrhoea with the mildly elevated prolactin of 600mU/l is likely due to pituitary stalk compression. In macroprolactinomas (which are treated medically with dopamine agonists) prolactin is grossly elevated.

4. A

This patient has Cushing's syndrome based on his clinical presentation, increased 24 hour urinary cortisol and unsuppressed serum cortisol on overnight dexamethasone suppression test. His plasma ACTH is suppressed; therefore, the aetiology of his Cushing's syndrome is adrenal. This can be confirmed by a CT of adrenal glands. In case of Cushing's syndrome, due to pituitary (called Cushing's disease) or ACTH-producing non-pituitary tumour (called ectopic ACTH syndrome), plasma ACTH level will not be suppressed. MIBG scan is done for investigation of phaeochromocytoma, not Cushing's syndrome.

5. A

Patients with diabetes insipidus are unable to appropriately concentrate their urine. After fluid restriction, they will continue to pass a large volume of dilute urine. During fluid restriction she concentrates her serum osmolality. In contrast, in patients with primary polydipsia (psychogenic excessive fluid intake), urinary osmolality increases above 750mOsm/kg after fluid restriction in water deprivation. As the patient's urine osmolality increased to above 750mOsm/kg after DDAVP spray, she has cranial diabetes insipidus. In nephrogenic diabetes insipidus, urine osmolality remains low despite DDAVP after water deprivation. Polydipsia and polyuria are not presenting features of SIADH.

6. A

Antipsychotic drugs, such as risperidone are often associated with hyperprolactinaemia, which lead to galactorrhoea and amenorrhoea. Some newer second generation antipsychotic agents (e.g. aripiprazole and clozapine) are less associated with hyperprolactinaemia. The first step in the management of this patient is to consider, in liaison with her psychiatrist, changing the patient's antipsychotic drug before imaging and treatment of her prolactinaemia. Metformin is not associated with hyperprolactinaemia.

7. B

Raised prolactin leads to suppressed oestrogen, amenorrhoea and difficulty conceiving (which improves with treatment). There are no associated risks of prolactinoma once pregnant. Prolactinomas are associated with galactorrhoea so there is no difficulty breastfeeding.

8. E

The primary treatment for acromegaly is surgery, particularly in young people, as this is likely to be curative especially for small tumours. Somatostatin analogues are used first line in those unsuitable for surgery or with unresectable disease. Cabergoline can also help normalise IGF-1 in patients with mild disease without chance of operative cure. Radiotherapy is slow to work and can leave patients with pituitary hormone deficiencies.

9. E

Her suboptimal cortisol response to synthetic ACTH (synacthen) together with low ACTH level suggests secondary adrenal insufficiency (ACTH level will be elevated in primary adrenal insufficiency). She needs regular glucocorticoid replacement. As she has secondary adrenal insufficiency, aldosterone replacement is unnecessary because aldosterone secretion is primarily regulated by renin-angiotensin system, not by ACTH. This is in contrast to primary adrenal insufficiency where both glucocorticoid and mineralocorticoid need replacement. Although this patient's adrenal insufficiency is secondary to ACTH deficiency, glucocorticoid is a more convenient, effective and cheaper hormone for replacement than ACTH.

10.C

The only tumour that would respond rapidly to medical treatment is a prolactinoma. First line treatment for macroprolactinomas (even those causing compression of the optic chiasm) would be dopamine agonists (such as cabergoline). When the vision is under threat in a patient with pituitary mass, the pressure on the chiasm needs to be rapidly relieved surgically unless it is a prolactinoma.

Adrenal disease

1. E

Patients taking chronic supraphysiological doses of corticosteroids can develop adrenal suppression. This patient's symptoms and low blood glucose level raise the suspicion of adrenal insufficiency. Short synacthen test (SST) is the test of choice for investigation of adrenal insufficiency. Urine free cortisol and overnight and low dose dexamethasone suppression tests are investigations used to diagnose cortisol hypersecretion. ACTH is not helpful screening test to detect adrenal insufficiency.

2. E

Spironolactone is an aldosterone antagonist. The other antihypertensives may need to be used in combination to maintain the blood pressure to within the target range.

3. D

Her hypertension, diabetes and being overweight are all potentially consequences of cortisol hypersecretion (Cushing's syndrome) from an adrenal tumour. Overnight dexamethasone suppression test is a screening test for Cushing's syndrome (unsuppressed morning serum cortisol after 1 mg dexamethasone the night before is suggestive of the diagnosis). It is important to rule out a phaeochromocytoma but urine metadrenaline is not an option here. Adrenal vein sampling, 9am cortisol and MRI adrenals are not useful in diagnosing Cushing's syndrome. Adrenal tumours may secrete androgens but her presentation is not suggestive of testosterone excess.

4. B

This woman has classic "salt-wasting" CAH as it was diagnosed at birth. Consequently she is dependent on her steroid replacement so the dose of hydrocortisone must be increased at times of physical stress, severe infection and severe emotional stress. Major surgical procedures will also require an increase in the hydrocortisone dose. The dose of fludrocortisone does not need increasing during the peri-operative period.

5. A

Addison's disease presents with non-specific symptoms of fatigue, weight loss, vomiting and postural hypotension and is associated with pre-existing autoimmune endocrinopathy (eg type 1 diabetes mellitus). Hypothyroidism causes fatigue with weight gain; hyperthyroidism (Graves' disease) causes tachycardia. Coeliac disease causes weight loss but will not usually present with hypotension. Her diabetes is reasonably controlled (HbA1c 60 mmol/mol) and therefore unlikely to be causing her symptoms.

6. A

A young patient with poorly controlled hypertension on multiple agents and with hypokalaemia suggests Conn's syndrome (primary hyperaldosteronism). Cushing's syndrome would tend to have other phenotypical features. Patients with phaeochromocytoma are often symptomatic with paroxysmal anxiety, sweating and palpitation. Both medication non-concordance and essential hypertension are possible but a secondary cause should be ruled out first in a young patient.

7. B

Her symptoms together with hypertension suggest phaeochromocytoma. Urinary or plasma metanephrines are the most sensitive and specific biochemical tests for diagnosing phaeochromocytoma. Urinary VMA is no longer used for testing phaeochromocytoma because the results are often affected by diet. Imaging (CT of adrenal glands and MIBG scan) must only be performed after the biochemical diagnosis of phaeochromocytoma. Urinary 5-HIAA level is measured to investigate carcinoid syndrome; however, the patient's presentation is not consistent with the syndrome.

Calcium homeostasis and metabolic bone disease

1. A

This man is dehydrated with symptoms of hypercalcaemia secondary to primary hyperparathyroidism. Fluid resuscitation must be given prior to administering bisphosphonates. Although he has acute kidney injury with elevated serum creatinine there is no indication for dialysis because his renal function is likely to improve with fluid resuscitation. Cinacalcet is a calcimimetic agent, which is used in refractory hypercalcaemia due to hyperparathyroidism but after rehydration. Systemic steroids are used in treating hypercalcaemia due to malignancy or sarcoidosis. Parathyroidectomy should be performed when he has recovered from this acute illness.

2. E

Severe vitamin D deficiency can cause hypocalcaemia and is common in Northern European countries especially in dark-skinned individuals or those who cover their skin. Vitamin D deficiency is associated with a compensatory rise in PTH (secondary hyperparathyroidism). Dietary deficiency of calcium is less common cause of hypocalcaemia than vitamin D deficiency. Hypervitaminosis D is associated with high serum calcium.

3. D

This man is developing complications of severe renal failure, which include secondary hyperparathyroidism and anaemia. Secondary hyperparathyroidism occurs when renal failure prevents renal conversion of vitamin D to its active form 1,25 OH vitamin D. Excessive PTH is synthesised to maintain normal serum calcium(high PTH, normal serum calcium). Primary hyperparathyroidism, tertiary hyperparathyroidism and FHH (familial hypcalciuric hypercalcaemia) are all associated with elevated serum calcium.

4. C

The commonest cause of hypercalcaemia is primary hyperparathyroidism, in which case serum PTH will be elevated. In this patient, underlying malignancy is possible because of his weight loss and anaemia; serum PTH will be suppressed in this situation. If serum PTH level is low, secondary tests to determine a site of malignancy might include CT imaging, myeloma screen (option D) or gastrointestinal endoscopy. Neck ultrasound and sestamibi scan would only be indicated after the PTH test suggests in the diagnosis of primary hyperparathyroidism and surgery was being considered.

5. B
Bisphosphonates are commonly used drugs to treat osteoporosis. Excessive alcohol is a significant risk factor for osteoporosis; however, 4 units of alcohol per week is unlikely to have a major impact on his bone density. Regular exercise improves bone density. Although testosterone deficiency is an important cause of osteoporosis in men, testosterone treatment is not indicated if the patient has normal testosterone level. Systemic steroids (e.g. prednisolone) case osteoporosis and are not the treatment for this condition.

6. E
Paget's disease is common in this age group and is associated with elevated isolated alkaline phosphatase. Although it is usually asymptomatic, patients can occasionally present with bone pain. Long bone X-rays or a bone scan would help to confirm the diagnosis. Osteomalacia is unlikely with normal vitamin D levels. Osteoporosis is asymptomatic unless a fracture occurs. Multiple myeloma is often associated with other abnormalities such as anaemia, renal failure and hypercalcaemia. Osteoarthritis does not cause elevated alkaline phosphatase.

Reproductive system disorders

1. C
Testosterone secretion is pulsatile and varies diurnally with levels highest in the early morning and lowest in the late evening. Therefore, a single serum testosterone may be low depending upon the timing of the test. The low testosterone level must be confirmed by repeating the test in the morning (for example, 8am) before further investigations and treatment with testosterone replacement.

2. C
Polycythaemia is a recognised side-effect of testosterone replacement. Therefore, patients on testosterone replacement should be monitored for this side-effect by checking haemoglobin and haematocrit annually. Patients on testosterone replacement need annual monitor-

ing for serum prostate specific antigen (PSA) over the age of 40 years but not CT of prostate, mamogram or DEXA scan.

3. D
Her clinical features (hirsutism, menstrual irregularity, obesity and mildly elevated testosterone level) are consistent with polycystic ovary syndrome (PCOS) which is not excluded by normal ultrasound appearance of ovaries. Androgen-producing ovarian tumour tends to have a short history with rapid progression of symptoms. Normal urinary cortisol, serum prolactin and serum 17-hydroxyprogesterone do not support diagnoses of Cushing's syndrome, hyperprolactinaemia or congenital adrenal hyperplasia, respectively.

4. D
This patient has primary ovarian insufficiency; vitiligo and ovarian autoantibodies suggest an autoimmune aetiology. Oestrogen replacement will relieve menopausal symptoms and prevent long-term consequences of oestrogen deficiency. Unopposed oestrogen replacement in a woman with an intact uterus increases the risk of endometrial carcinoma, and therefore this must be interspersed with progestogen. Gonadotrophins and GnRH are ineffective in primary ovarian failure.

5. A
This patient has primary hypogonadism (low serum oestradiol with high gonadotrophin levels) and the physical phenotype suggest Turner's syndrome. This is typically characterised by the absence of an X-chromosome from the normal female karyotype, resulting in the 45X0. 46XX and 46XY are the normal female and male karyotypes, respectively. 47XXY and 47XX, +21 (an extra chromosome 21) are karyotypes for Klinefelter's syndrome and Down's syndrome (female), respectively.

6. A
The most likely diagnosis in this woman is hypothalamic amenorrhoea related to the intensity of her exercise. If she has persistent amenorrhoea despite moderating exercise and gaining weight, calcium/vitamin D and oestrogen replacement are indicated to prevent osteoporosis. Recombinant human leptin has been tried in some forms of hypothalamic amenorrhoea but is not a first line treatment. Progestin challenge is not appropriate in this setting as adequate serum oestradiol is necessary for withdrawal bleeding with the progestin.

7. D
Human chorionic gonadotrophins act like follicular stimulating hormone, and stimulate spermatogenesis in patients with secondary

hypogonadism. Testosterone does not stimulate spermatogenesis so changing his testosterone replacement to injections is unlikely to improve his sperm count. Multivitamins, DHEA and androstenedione will not improve his sperm count

Other endocrine disorders

1. A

Whipple's triad (symptoms of hypoglycaemia accompanied by low blood glucose level and relief of symptoms after blood glucose level is normalized) suggests a diagnosis of an insulinoma. Biochemical diagnosis of insulinoma is made by demonstrating hypoglycaemia during a 72 hour fast, with raised insulin and C peptide levels. Hypoglycaemia due to exogenous insulin is associated with raised insulin level but suppressed C peptide level. Biochemical diagnosis should precede radiological investigations.

2. C

Multiple endocrine neoplasia type 1 (MEN1) is a genetic disorder associated with mutations in the MEN1 gene. It is inherited in an autosomal dominant pattern. Therefore, there is 50% chance that the patient's daughter has inherited the gene mutation. As the MEN1 mutation has been detected in the patient, the daughter could have predictive testing to show if she carries the mutation. If she has the mutation, she will need regular screening with endocrine biochemical and imaging tests. If she has no mutation, she can be reassured. She does not need prophylactic parathyroidectomy.

3. E

This woman has symptoms of carcinoid syndrome (flushing, diarrhoea and wheeze). Flushing in carcinoid syndrome is 'dry' unlike flushing secondary to menopause, phaeochromocytoma or thyrotoxicosis. Carcinoid syndrome typically occurs with midgut carcinoid tumours metastasising in the liver, therefore the finding of hepatomegaly is significant. Carcinoid syndrome can be diagnosed biochemically by measuring 5-HIAA level in 24 hours urine collection.

4. C

Episodic symptoms of palpitations, sweating, headaches and dizzy spells, together with hypertension, are suspicious of phaeochromocytoma. Medullary thyroid carcinoma and phaeochromocytoma can occur together in a patient as parts of multiple endocrine neoplasia type 2 (MEN2). Recurrence of medullary thyroid carcinoma is usually associated with elevated serum calcitonin level. His symptoms are not typical of primary hyperparathyroidism, hypoparathyroidism or hypothyroidism.

5. A

Large multiple peptic ulcerations suggests a gastrinoma (Zollinger-Ellison syndrome). In this condition, increased secretion of gastrin from a neuroendocrine tumour in the duodenum or pancreas causes excess production of gastric acid and severe peptic ulceration. The excessive gastric acid secretion also inactivates intestinal enzymes and damages intestinal mucosa causing diarrhoea and malabsorption. Biochemical diagnosis is made by demonstrating elevated fasting plasma gastrin levels.

Endocrine emergencies

1. D

This patient has low serum osmolality with inappropriately high urine osmolality and is clinically euvolaemic. This together with high urinary sodium and normal thyroid and adrenal function is consistent with inappropriate ADH (SIADH) secretion. Therefore strict fluid restriction is necessary (for example, < 750 ml/24h). Vasopressin-2 receptor antagonists are effective for SIADH but remain second-line treatment. Treatment with 0.9% sodium chloride is useful in dehydration. Hypertonic saline (3%) is only used in emergency situations where severe hyponatraemia is causing seizures or unconsciousness or is known to have occurred very rapidly. Demeclocycline is occasionally used to treat chronic SIADH.

2. B

Although her blood glucose has normalised she still has significant ketosis and unresolved acidaemia (with low bicarbonate). She should continue on insulin and dextrose infusion. Only once pH>7.3, $HCO_3 > 18$ mmol/L and plasma ketones <1.0 should intravenous infusion of insulin be discontinued as stopping this early risks rapid recurrence of diabetic ketoacidosis.

3. D

Oral treatments for hypoglycaemia are the most appropriate management wherever possible. Rapid-acting sugars in fruit juice increase blood glucose more rapidly than those in chocolate as the fat in chocolate slows absorption. 50% dextrose is no longer used as extravasation causes severe irritation. Intramuscular glucagon is reserved for those without intravenous access to administer dextrose or who are unconscious.

4. D

This patient has diabetes ketoacidosis (DKA) and needs urgent treatment with IV insulin and fluid. Although hyperkalaemia occurs commonly in untreated DKA, hypokalaemia is a frequent complication of the treatment of DKA occurring when insulin infusion causes a shift of potassium from the extracellular compartment into the cell. Therefore he will need potassium replacement. Patients with DKA are at increased risk of thromboembolism and anticoagulant treatment is indicated to prevent this. IM glucagon is used in treatment of severe hypoglycaemia, not DKA.

5. E

Acute severe headache and 3rd nerve palsy with the CT finding is suggestive of pituitary apoplexy. MRI pituitary will help to confirm the diagnosis. Haemodynamically stabilising the patient is a priority. Hypopituitarism (including secondary adrenal insufficiency) is common following pituitary apoplexy. She is hypotensive, raising suspicion of hypocortisolaemia.

Integrated care

1. D

Exercise is independently associated with lowering blood glucose and delaying development of diabetes. Weight loss would be advantageous to prevent development of diabetes but he doesn`t fit criteria for bariatric surgery; missing breakfast is not associated with weight loss. Metformin may delay onset of diabetes but is not cost effective for whole populations and lifestyle changes are preferable.

2. A

Patients are often thirsty and drinking excessive quantities of sugary drinks before the diagnosis of diabetes mellitus. Stopping this can dramatically improve blood sugars, hence guidelines recommend for dietary modification, exercise and life-style changes before pharmacological treatment (e.g. metformin) for patients with newly diagnosed type 2 diabetes. Overly-restrictive diets are difficult to sustain, leading to rebound weight gain and should be avoided. Stopping smoking is beneficial but will not affect blood glucose levels.

3. C

In pregnancy, the dose of levothyroxine often needs increasing because of an increased renal excretion and trans-placental transfer of the drug. Furthermore, the TSH should be kept in the lower part of the reference range to ensure adequate maternal levothyroxine replacement. Therefore, although this woman's TSH is at the upper end of population reference range, she needs to increase the dose of levothyroxine in pregnancy. Inadequate levothyroxine replacement is associated with impaired neuropsychological development in the baby and other adverse pregnancy outcomes, such as miscarriages and premature birth.

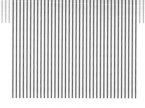
Index

Note: Page numbers in **bold** or *italic* refer to tables or figures, respectively.